AEROBIC NUTRITION

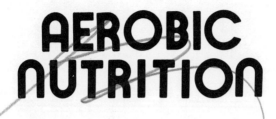

AEROBIC NUTRITION

DON MANNERBERG, M. D., AND JUNE ROTH

Hawthorn/Dutton / New York

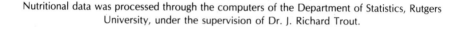

Nutritional data was processed through the computers of the Department of Statistics, Rutgers University, under the supervision of Dr. J. Richard Trout.

Published in the United States by Elsevier-Dutton Publishing Co., Inc.,
2 Park Avenue, New York, N.Y. 10016

Library of Congress Cataloging in Publication Data
Mannerberg, Don.
Aerobic nutrition.

Bibliography: p. 299
Includes indexes.
1. Nutrition. 2. Diet. 3. Triglycerides. 4. Oxygen transport (Physiology).
5. Aerobic exercises.
I. Roth, June Spiewak, joint author. II. Title.
RA784.M34   1981   613.2   80-22284

ISBN: 0-8015-0070-2

Published simultaneously in Canada by
Clarke, Irwin & Company Limited, Toronto and Vancouver

Designed by Barbara Cohen

10 9 8 7 6 5 4 3 2 1

First Edition

With deep appreciation to

Vicky Mannerberg and Fred Roth

for their constant encouragement and

devoted assistance.

And to all those who love life enough

to make the effort to live it

to its fullest and healthiest potential.

CONTENTS

PREFACE

In the spring of 1979, while attending a preventive medicine seminar, I scheduled a breakfast interview for my syndicated newspaper column "Special Diets" with a doctor who was to lecture that afternoon. Dr. Don Mannerberg ordered half a grapefruit (carefully discarded the artificially colored maraschino cherry from the center), hot oatmeal (no sugar), and decaffeinated black coffee. I enjoyed a glass of orange juice, one poached egg on dry whole-wheat toast (no butter, no jelly), and decaffeinated coffee with skim milk (no substitute nondairy chemical-laden food fabrication). We naturally got into a discussion about our mutual concern for what was happening to the quality of the American diet, as we observed the stacks of pancakes dripping with butter and swimming with sugary syrup; three-egg omelets served with butter-drenched white bread toast, to be slathered further with jelly or jam; greasy fried ham slices or fat-striped bacon (loaded with salt, nitrates, and nitrites) along with two fried eggs that had been cooked on a fat-laden griddle. Heavy black coffee was being poured from the time the diner sat down, with constant refills during the meal, sometimes adding up to a three- or four-cup jolt to the nervous system just for starters. It was a typical coffeeshop scene, and it seemed to represent an unstoppable deterioration of cuisine and health.

Remarkably, we were each working on the beginnings of a book that would try to turn around the degenerative disease-causing diet patterns that are becoming common knowledge in the medical community. We were each seriously concerned about the quality of life in the middle years that left too few people with a day-to-day zest and vitality that accompanies good health. Dr. Mannerberg's book was to be from the researched medical viewpoint and from case histories drawn from his private practice in preventive medicine, while mine was planned to deal with the practicality of cooking better food for better health. We both saw the lack of followthrough from the medical community to the home kitchen, where the American diet takes shape. We decided to join our areas of expertise and write a book about nutrition that could affect the nation's deteriorating food habits.

Aerobic Nutrition is the culmination of our joint effort to deliver an informative, youth-prolonging, disease-fighting book, with the sensible application of medical theories to cooking practices. It is for people who value the precious gift of life and who want to prolong the ability to function as a well person. And it is for people who enjoy good food as one of the pleasures of the senses.

Stay healthy,
JUNE ROTH

INTRODUCTION

During the last twenty years we repeatedly have been made aware of risk factors for heart disease and stroke as related to our modern life style, by the continuing release of information concerning the diet/disease connection. We now know that certain living habits begin to produce degenerative disease and loss of life by middle age. Although we read daily about increasing life expectancy, this information is frequently controversial and often contradictory. It is our hope that this book will clarify your knowledge about your role in feeding your body, so that you can enjoy a longer stretch of youthful living and good health.

Of course, no one wishes to become acutely or chronically ill, and everyone would love to have maximum longevity, but the quality of youthful life is often not related to either of these factors. The secret of preserving youth and vitality so that each day can be used to its fullest, both physically and mentally, is to maintain good oxygen delivery to the brain.

Oxygen is the single most important element for survival from minute to minute. A lack of oxygen by the brain for four to six minutes will cause brain damage, and beyond six minutes it will cause biological death. Any interruption of oxygen can cause cell death, tissue damage, and loss of function. If the absence of oxygen for a few moments can produce such dramatic changes in the body, then what do you think happens to the optimal functioning of cell, tissues, and organs of the body when there is a partial interruption of oxygen delivery to all parts of the body during a lifetime? When there is just enough oxygen to permit the body to function and get by, but not enough to enable the body to enjoy its maximum capacity for good health, you can expect trouble. There is a direct relationship of nutrition to the availability of oxygen in the blood. That is what the term *aerobic nutrition* is all about.

Living to your fullest and feeling well until the day you die is positive and productive. It is your birthright. When you feel well throughout the ages and stages of life, you can live with confidence in your ability to cope with current problems and live without fear of the future.

The subject of this book is the relationship of good mental and physical function to the absence of disease and the presence of optimal health. Aerobic exercise and physical fitness often have been written up with the exclusion of the subject of nutrition. The information on these pages establishes a nutrition/oxygen relationship which is just as valid as that now widely known for exercise alone.

A change of daily diet to permit an unblocked flow of oxygen throughout the body, along with a change of attitude that will keep the muscles of the body in frequent motion, could mean a change in your prognosis for a long and vital life. This is not a book about nutrition as related to disease and does not offer a fountain of youth—it is instead a book about nutrition as related to preventive medicine to put the responsibility for your continued good health into your own capable hands.

Youth is a gift to the young, but after that it must be earned.

DON MANNERBERG, M.D.

I
AEROBIC
NUTRITION

1. THE SECRET TO GOOD HEALTH

Aerobic Nutrition is a diet formula that can help you to achieve optimum vitality—to stay as healthy as possible for as long as possible. When combined with the Mannerberg Method of constant physical movement it can help you to feel better now. Today. Tomorrow. Next week. Next month. And then for the rest of your life.

These are not idle promises. Scientific studies prove beyond a doubt that it is true: Aerobic Nutrition can help your body function at its fullest capacity.

You do not have to be a victim of a thoughtless accumulation of habits that can promote the onset of degenerative disease. You can kick those habits. With knowledge comes understanding. With understanding comes change.

How well we perform or how long we live depends on the performance of all the cells which make up the human body. Vitality as well as longevity depends on the performance of these cells and their survival.

What determines cell function and survival? Cells need water, oxygen, calories, and nutrients. When these components are present in less than the required amounts, the cells suffer with improper function or early death.

Our bodies are the sum of all of our cells. The way we feel, our energy and our endurance, depends on how well our cells work. If alcohol can obviously produce altered function in a short period of time, if caffeine in coffee can produce insomnia, then it is easy to understand why all the things we swallow have the potential for affecting our mental and physical abilities.

Aerobic Nutrition is based on medical knowledge of the oxygen delivery system—which in turn is intricately tied into the food you eat and the way you space your meals. The oxygen delivery system is also affected by your personal habits, and depends on regular exercise and sufficient body movement. It plays a major role in maintaining the state of good health. Exercise can increase the body's ability to use oxygen, resulting in increased physical endurance. This is accomplished by increasing the blood flow and function of the lungs. With stronger lungs, better pump (heart), larger blood vessels, and increased oxygen uptake by the muscles being used, there is increased oxygen uptake throughout the body.

Most people assume that as long as they are breathing in air, their bodies will get as much oxygen as they need. But did you know that the air you breathe may never get very far beyond your lungs? It's supposed to be delivered throughout the body by a remarkable system of red blood cell carriers. These cells are free-flowing in the bloodstream, which you can consider to be the superhighway of your body. All the other cells and organs of the body wait for the oxygen delivery to arrive, so they can function well. Partial deliveries leave them gasping for more.

What causes these partial deliveries of oxygen to the cells and organs? When people follow a diet of high fat content, concentrated sugars, and too much alcohol, *triglycerides* reach high levels in the blood and cause the red blood cells to clump together. Clumped red cells are less capable of carrying oxygen, and they clog the capillaries, diminishing the ability to get life-sustaining oxygen to the living cells of the body. This particularly affects such vital organs as the brain, liver, and kidneys, which are not muscular and cannot be exercised as can the muscles of the legs in jogging. When cells of the body do not receive adequate oxygen, they cannot function to their optimum; this can lead to decreased endurance or a sluggish day.

Aerobic Nutrition is based on moderation, common sense, and nutritional wisdom, along with a philosophy of keeping the body in constant movement rather than performing short spurts of drastic exercise. It is a strategy that can bring you optimum health for effective compromises. You will learn delicious ways to limit fats, sugar, salt, and alcohol in the diet, why you should do it, and how to program your body out of a sedentary life. This will result in an aerated bloodstream that has free-flowing red blood cells carrying a full load of oxygen to the other cells and organs of the body. Robust cells and organs produce vital active people.

Partial starvation of oxygen and nutrients eventually produces degenerative diseases: heart disease, diabetes, atherosclerosis, malfunctioning gallbladder, and so on. Instead of blooming, the total body begins to wilt. With poor nutritional habits, deterioration usually begins by age forty and certainly is in evidence by age fifty. This means that several decades of life will be spent talking to doctors about disease control, taking medication, having operations, and sometimes fighting for the right to live.

How many times have you pondered the question with other armchair philosophers, "Which is more important—health or wealth?" After serious discussion, weighing the pros and cons, most people conclude that good health is a form of wealth, but that money wealth without health is a poor way to live. Yet health is a neglected target for many who take it for granted or who feel that fate has already dealt the cards. In reality your health is in your hands every meal of every day.

Many people are now learning to ask questions about healthier guidelines. They are no longer accepting authoritative answers without finding out the *why* behind them. The focus is turning to what produces good health, rather than what to do to turn back the onset of disease. Physicians are taught to recognize disease, make a diagnosis, and then treat the disease with medication. With this background it is understandable that physicians and the public in general can cope with the idea of disease and its consequences, but seldom meet to discuss *preventive* measures. It is important to set *health* as a goal of living. Aerobic Nutrition will help you to achieve it.

Aerobic Nutrition in its very basic form is not a new concept. A version of it is found in the Old Testament. In Daniel 1:8–16, the story is told of a ten-day trial of eating vegetables and drinking water instead of the king's rich food. After this test period, we are told, Daniel and his three friends were judged to be better in appearance than those who had eaten the rich foods. This might be interpreted to be testimony for a vegetarian diet, but in reality it is a contrast of the unhealthful food practices of that day to a simple diet and its obvious benefits.

We too practice unhealthful food choices. The majority of people living in America will eventually suffer the consequences of poor diet. Degenerative disease has become epidemic.

Yet the gamut of good foods is right there in the supermarkets alongside the poor food choices. You just have to learn what the good foods are and where to find them. A rule of thumb is to shop around the perimeter of the store, where the fresh fruits and vegetables, meats, and dairy products are displayed. Then leave, unless you need some staples or cleaning supplies from the center aisles of the store.

Later in this book, these food choices will be discussed in depth. And then a complete recipe section will show you how to cook delicious meals. You'll be cooking with healthier techniques too, and that can mean better-tasting food. You may even develop a more discerning palate. Best of all, you can learn to stretch the middle years of your life into well-nourished healthful and productive living.

HEALTH IS A CHOICE

Aging and degenerative disease have become synonymous in this country. Most people expect that they will lose function and become chronically ill when they grow old. This is a misconception. Recent evidence suggests that how sick or well you are during your later years of life depends a great deal on *how you live* that life in earlier years.

HOW DOES THE WAY WE LIVE AFFECT OUR HEALTH?

The causes of illness and death have changed in the United States since the turn of the century, owing to our modern concepts of health management. When humans live in a more primitive setting, *infectious disease* is rampant, the result of poor sanitary standards. But when infectious diseases are conquered by a modern way of life that includes better sanitary conditions, people live longer. Then the problem of a longer life becomes one of coping with a variety of *degenerative diseases.* So we trade off the acute infectious diseases, which are more likely to kill young people, and now must learn how to prevent the degenerative diseases of an older population. Because we have excellent medical care and improved living standards that eliminate epidemics of infectious disease, we now enjoy a life expectancy of approximately seventy years. In the developing countries of the world, the life expectancy is still at fifty years or less as an average. If you opt for a long life that is free of degenerative disease, improved sanitary conditions are not enough—selected changes in life style should be considered.

WHAT ARE THE DEGENERATIVE DISEASES?

These are the ones that are the most frequent causes of disability, and not always the cause of death. They include arthritis, hypertension, obesity, gallbladder disease, diverticulosis of the colon, and the most common problem of all—dental caries. The three leading causes of death—heart attack, stroke, and cancer—are also included. Degenerative diseases lead to deterioration to a lower level of physical and mental function as we continue to age over the forty- and fifty-year level.

WHAT MAKES US SUBJECT TO DEGENERATIVE DISEASE?

Degenerative diseases are epidemic in the industrialized nations of the Western world but are as rare in the developing countries now as they were in America at the turn of the century. The diet of countries of the modern Western world is a refined, fatty, high-caloric diet. The diet of the developing countries today has more natural complex carbohydrates and a much lower caloric intake. Also, in the lesser-developed countries, where labor-saving devices are not available, physical activity is built into the way of life. We have lost most of our reason to be active, so some people substitute sports and most people sit around and watch them play. Usually they snack on high-fat and high-sugar foods, getting meager activity from raising the hands to the mouth in a steady motion.

IS EMOTIONAL STRESS A FACTOR IN DEGENERATIVE DISEASE?

We differ from the developing countries in the amount of emotional stress we endure. Our complex society creates emotional stress that leads to dramatic physical changes. The amount of emotional stress on a person is directly related to the state of health.

DOES FAMILY STRUCTURE AFFECT DEGENERATIVE DISEASE?

In our modern society moral standards and family structure are challenged by many outside forces which do not exist in less advanced societies. These changes can contribute to emotional stress and can affect the way we eat, the regularity of meals, and who assumes the responsibility for keeping the family in good health. People who live alone tend to have a very narrow variety of foods; they rely more on convenience foods, fast foods, and restaurant fare. Unless conscious of the effect of diet and wholesome food upon health, singles can fall into the trap of catch-as-catch-can eating habits.

WHY IS THE SUBJECT OF NUTRITION CONTROVERSIAL?

At this time, diet is the number one topic on the hit parade of life-style modifications. In the past a lot of attention has been given to exercise and stress modification, and that continues to be productive, but the subject of nutrition leaves many people confused.

There is good reason for this confusion. The subject of nutrition is much like the television panel show *To Tell the Truth,* where three experts claim to be the same person. The final identification comes when the moderator says, "Will the real expert stand up?" In this day and age of so many experts, many of whom are extremely knowledgeable, it is very difficult for the layperson to know whom to believe. Further, because practicing physicians may have little or no education in this area, they usually do not discuss nutrition with patients. Many physicians reject the so-called nonscientific approach to health and disease. Physicians are trained to treat sick people, to deliver excellent crisis care with medication and surgical techniques. Yet the nutrition information needed to maintain a state of well-being may prevent the need for crisis care.

HOW DOES OUR DIET COMPARE WITH THAT OF THE DEVELOPING COUNTRIES?

When we examine the diet of developing countries of the world where degenerative disease is rare, we find that they rely on natural carbohydrates with very little refined food, a limited amount of meat, and a very low-caloric diet of 2,000 calories or less a day along with an active life. On the other hand, our diet is very highly refined, fatty, and of high calories—usually about 3,000 calories a day.

HOW HAS OUR DIET CHANGED?

As we went from a developing country to the present Westernized way of life, we created the roots of our diet problems. A comparison of diet habits from 1910 to 1976 reveals that we have increased our fat intake by 28 percent and decreased the carbohydrate intake from starches by 45 percent. We have also increased our sugar intake by 31 percent. As other developing countries around the world become more modernized, they progressively change to the Western diet. Consequently, where no degenerative disease previously existed, there are now full-time diabetes and hypertension clinics. In Africa and South America this change has occurred only within the last thirty years.

BUT AREN'T WE THE BEST-FED PEOPLE IN THE WORLD?

The average diet for people in the United States now contains 3,100 calories, with 42 percent attributed to so-called empty calories. Empty calories means that there are no nutrient values in the food other than calories. Sugars and syrups account for 17 percent, fats and oils 18 percent, and alcoholic beverages 7 percent of the calories of the average diet. None of these contain any vitamins or minerals. In addition, about 17 percent of the diet is made up of refined and only partially refortified grains in the form of cereals or breads. About two thirds of the sugar consumed in this country has been added to our processed food; the remainder is added to breakfasts, beverages, desserts, baked goods, and routine cooking. Altogether we are consuming over 125 pounds of sugar per person each year.

IF OUR FOOD INGREDIENTS ARE HARMFUL, WHY ARE THEY PERMITTED?

There is a high salt content in processed food, as well as in the fast foods that are becoming a common source of meals for much of the population. Most fast foods have very high sodium content, high sugar, and high-fat ingredients. These particular ingredients in our diet are not necessarily harmful unless they are used in excess of the body's needs for energy or other essential requirements. A diet of processed food and fast food generally adds up to this kind of excessive intake.

WHY IS THERE SO MUCH FUSS RECENTLY ABOUT ADDING HIGH FIBER TO THE DIET?

Our elderly may have the advantage of modern science to prolong life, but many live with the agony of constipation as a result of eating our highly refined diet. Many subsequently suffer from diseased bowels. Dr. Denis Burkitt and Dr. Hugh Trowell of England were the first medical investigators to make us aware of the problems associated with a low-fiber diet. They disclosed that many of the degenerative diseases in Western countries could correlate well with the amount of nutrient fiber in the diet. A change to high-fiber foods can reduce the incidence of colon disease by helping the feces to move quickly through the bowel.

WHAT IS THE USUAL ONSET TIME FOR DEGENERATIVE DISEASE?

Diseases associated with dietary imbalance begin to appear in the middle years of adult life. The medical literature and popular press abound with reports and articles about the excesses of calories, sugar, fats, cholesterol, and the absence of fiber in our diet. Yet most of our population does nothing about it, despite the fact that studies and proofs exist that show why our elderly suffer from degenerative diseases. If you want to ensure a healthier old age, analyze your daily diet and make necessary changes now.

DOES OBESITY AFFECT THE ONSET OF DEGENERATIVE DISEASE?

If we look at only one aspect of the problem of poor health in this country, obesity, we find it is accompanied by a higher incidence of hypertension (high blood pressure), coronary artery disease, gallbladder disease, and diabetes, as well as early mortality. Although obesity is a problem for all age groups, it has a definite correlation with aging; after the age of twenty there is an average increase in weight with each decade. Today, a middle-aged person weighs approximately seven pounds more than did someone of the same height and age a decade ago. The trend is that the statistics will be higher a decade from now.

OTHER PREDICTIVE FACTORS TO CONSIDER

What predictive factors for disease are reflected by our personal makeup or way of life? Some are personal characteristics, such as family history, sex,

THE TEN LEADING CAUSES OF DEATH IN THE UNITED STATES
1900

RANK	DISEASE	PERCENT OF TOTAL DEATHS
1	Influenza	11.8
2	Tuberculosis	11.3
3	Gastroenteritis	8.6
4	Heart	7.9
5	CVA/Stroke	6.4
6	Chronic Nephritis	4.7
7	Accidents	4.2
8	Cancer	3.7
9	Infancy Diseases	3.6
10	Diphtheria	2.3
	ALL CAUSES/100,000	1,719.1

Average Life Span   Male 46.3   Female 48.3

1975

RANK	DISEASE	PERCENT OF TOTAL DEATHS
1	Heart	37.8
2	Cancer	19.5
3	CVA/Stroke	10.2
4	Accidents	5.3
5	Influenza/Pneumonia	3.0
6	Diabetes Mellitus	1.9
7	Cirrhosis of Liver	1.7
8	Arteriosclerosis	1.5
9	Infancy Diseases	1.4
10	Suicide	1.4
	ALL CAUSES/100,000	896.1

Average Life Span   Male 68.7   Female 76.5

*Data from *Vital Statistics of the United States,* 1976.

age, overweight, and level of emotional stress. Add poor habits, such as smoking, overeating, careless nutritional planning, and lack of physical activity. These can cause metabolic disturbances that can lead to an increased incidence of heart disease, stroke, diabetes, high blood pressure, and high blood fats.

HOW IS ATHEROSCLEROSIS AFFECTED BY NUTRITION?

The ideal model to demonstrate the role of nutrition in the development of disease is atherosclerosis, or clogging of the larger arteries with plaques, much like a buildup of rust in the plumbing pipes. This condition eventually leads to loss of blood flow in the circulatory system, followed by damage to organs of the body, such as the heart or brain. This can be in the form of a heart attack, a stroke, or gangrene of the foot. All of these may cause death or, at best, lingering disability.

HOW DO WE KNOW SO MUCH ABOUT ATHEROSCLEROSIS?

As the number one cause of death in this country, atherosclerosis has been studied in both man and animals for over seventy years. We now know that certain elements of our life style, called risk factors, are correlated with the development of atherosclerosis. On the basis of these risk factors, as well as the comparison of populations of the world with varying diets, nutrition emerges as a key factor.

It has been shown that atherosclerosis may be present for many years before its effects are detected. Autopsies performed during the Korean War on men who averaged twenty-two years of age revealed that 77 percent of the American soldiers had various stages of atherosclerosis.

In more primitive areas of the world where extensive epidemiological studies have been done, there is no increase of atherosclerosis with aging. In the primitive areas of the world people die earlier—while in our society there is the ability to prevent early death, which allows more time for the degenerative effects of living to appear.

IS THERE ONE COMMON FACTOR ASSOCIATED WITH DEGENERATIVE DISEASE?

It is difficult to find a relationship among the many apparently unrelated forces that influence our state of well-being. But research shows that there *is one common factor.* It is called a *triglyceride.* This factor plays a key role in health because it has an important relationship to the circulation of blood and utilization of oxygen.

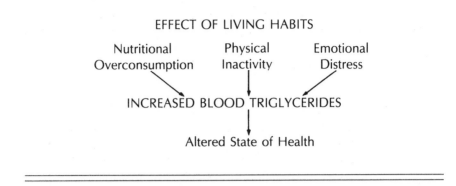

EFFECT OF LIVING HABITS

Nutritional   Physical   Emotional
Overconsumption   Inactivity   Distress

INCREASED BLOOD TRIGLYCERIDES

Altered State of Health

The choice to preserve health involves understanding the triglyceride factor and its function in keeping the cells of our body alive. It is a matter of life or death.

When we examine all the factors that influence triglycerides, and the resulting effects of that triglyceride change in the body, it becomes apparent that triglyceride is indeed the common denominator that is affected by all of the seemingly unrelated aspects of the way we live. These effects are responsible for changes in the way we feel, the loss of ability to function at full capacity, and finally a breakdown that leads to disease.

By the prevention of disease, we erase the need for diagnosis, treatment, and search for a cure. By acknowledging the relationship of the whole lifestyle to triglyceride changes, we can place our need for a healthier way of life into a proper perspective.

The product of a better way of eating and living is enhanced health—*feeling well* with a high level of functioning and a greater resistance to disease.

The relationship of nutrition to the aerobic functioning in the body is established when we look at triglycerides in relation to the oxygen that is required for an energetic way of life. A high triglyceride count means that the blood is sludged with particles that prevent the free flow of oxygen to the brain and vital organs.

Aerobic Nutrition refers to a manner of eating that prevents these particles from forming. When Aerobic Nutrition and the Mannerberg Method of exercise are combined, there is more than a double effect—the benefits of both together exceed the benefits of either one alone.

OPTIMAL HEALTH AND PREVENTIVE MEDICINE

In concept, preventive medicine is the ideal approach to health and resistance to disease. But the term is sometimes used to refer to alternatives to the orthodox medical ways of dealing with disease. Preventive medicine should be geared toward health, rather than toward other ways of treating disease. When we discuss Aerobic Nutrition, we are talking about the way to achieve optimal health and to *increase resistance* to disease.

Optimal health means the best health possible, not merely the absence of disease. It should be a state of extreme social, emotional, and physical *well-being.*

That is not to say that Aerobic Nutrition will not be helpful to those who have health problems and wish to restore themselves to a better level of functioning, even with a disease. Anyone can benefit from the basics of good nutrition. People who suffer chronic poor health can change the situation for themselves—requiring less medication and improving their physical and mental condition.

Certainly there are many people who would not be alive today without the mechanistic or orthodox approach to medicine, so it is unfair and prejudicial to criticize conventional medicine as if it were totally wrong. But if you can prevent the need for crisis medical care, then you are doing a sensible thing for yourself.

Preventive medicine is the preservation of *health* by treating the *root of the problem* rather than the result that shows up as a disease or as symptoms of ill health. The nutrients that get at the root of the problem will provide an absence of disease and an opportunity to live your life in a more satisfying way.

Optimal health is a worthwhile goal. Orthodox medicine has a definite place in the prevention of death or the saving of lives, but after we have saved the life or prevented the death, we must change the system of life that created the problem.

The financial burden of health care and the disability of old age are overwhelming problems for this society. It is important that people learn to take advantage of all we now know so that we can promote good health. It makes good economic sense to diminish disease or to manage it with better results.

One of the ways to achieve this is to have a thorough understanding of the oxygen delivery system of your body, and the role that triglycerides play in your degree of good health.

Think for a moment of what you would do if you bought a brand-new expensive car. You would read the manual to be sure that you didn't use the wrong fuel and to understand the design of that car. You surely wouldn't want to dump anything into the system that was going to clog or gunk up the works. And this is the kind of care you take when you expect the car to last five to ten years. Isn't it strange that most people don't take the time to find out how their bodies work? We'd like to be able to run the physical machinery well throughout a long lifetime, and we can—if we know what fuel the system needs to run well.

The following chapters will help you to learn about triglycerides, the oxygen delivery system, and nutrition, so you can deal more effectively with your fuel system.

2. TRIGLYCERIDES

Triglyceride, to put it simply, is another word for fat. It is the fat and oil we eat, and it also can be the product our livers make from absorbed refined sugars. That is why people with high triglyceride counts are cautioned to cut down on the ingestion of fats and concentrated sweets.

The fat in animals is largely triglyceride, and in humans develops into paunchy bellies and rounded middle-aged torsos. As triglyceride passes from the food we eat to the blubber in our own body, it must also increase the fat particles in the bloodstream. These fat particles, very high-energy components of the fuel transport system, are stored to meet future energy needs.

The problem with the American diet, of which 60 percent to 65 percent is fat and sugars that convert to high-energy particles, is that we don't spend the energy we take in. Unlike having money in the bank for a rainy day, saving triglycerides in your fat cells and in your blood can bankrupt your life. Too much of this necessary substance can cause an imbalance that can be a key factor in triggering degenerative disease.

We gorge ourselves with high-energy foods that are fat and sugar-based yet our life-style needs are for low-energy expenditures. The elevated triglycerides in the blood are a form of internal fatness, much like the external fatness that enlarges the waistline. As the external fatness changes our appearance from willowy to pillowy, high blood triglycerides change our ability to function by slowing down the blood flow and the oxygen delivery to the cells. The sticky triglyceride particles in fatty food, much like glue in the blood, may cause red cells to stick together. With this "sludging," the efficiency of the oxygen delivery system is impeded, and cells do not get life-sustaining oxygen in the amount needed. All the organs and cells in the body must make do with less oxygen because the bloodstream is no longer the free-flowing oxygen delivery system it was designed to be. And that means eventual trouble.

Aerobic nutrition establishes a balance between the fuel transport system and the oxygen delivery system for more effective supply of all the needed ingredients by each cell of our body. When it works efficiently, the cells are not forced to struggle but can thrive to do their best in every tissue and organ in the body. The physical situation under optimum conditions should be that of energy fitness.

DO IRREGULAR MEAL PATTERNS AFFECT TRIGLYCERIDES?

An individual who misses breakfast and has the first intake of calories around noon each day, and then overloads the body with fuel in the evening hours, is taking in most of the calories within an eight- to ten-hour period of a twenty-four-hour day. This evening gorging produces triglycerides within two to nine hours after intake. Blood triglycerides are increased with this sudden influx of fuel that is not needed to produce energy, so the body makes an effort to store them in fatty tissue for when needed. The morning fasting causes a hurry-up call and remobilization of glucose and triglyceride that have been stored during the afternoon and evening gorging sessions. Instead of a regular flow of the small amount of triglycerides needed, giving off just the right amount of energy at the right times, the stored triglycerides travel out of the fatty tissue, sludging up the bloodstream. In any one day when our body is forced to handle gorging and fasting, there are internal consequences that come from the lack of regularity and balance.

Because people vary physically, there are differing degrees of tolerance and adaptability to this type of meal pattern. You can disregard anyone who exclaims, "But I've eaten that way all of my life, and there's nothing wrong with me." Not yet there isn't, but the chance that the imbalance of the triglycerides will not affect your health is slight. Look around you in any shopping center, restaurant, or other place where people are usually grouped together—witness the triglyceride-distorted figures. Every person who appears to have excess weight is a walking bag of triglycerides, or fuel without an energy need. Such people are having an *Energy Crisis* in reverse.

HOW DO WE MANUFACTURE TRIGLYCERIDES?

Triglycerides are made up of three fatty acids attached to a central glycerol molecule. The endogenous triglycerides come from the fats and sugars we eat. High fat intake, mostly in the form of triglyceride, is delivered by the stomach to the intestine, where it is broken down and re-formed after the absorption process, collecting in the lymphatic system which then carries it to the blood. This system bypasses the liver. The resulting clumps of triglycerides, which are fairly large particles, can be removed from the blood by most tissues of the body except the brain.

Triglycerides can also be made in the body by the liver, using fatty acids that have been absorbed from the intestine process, or from the metabolic products of ingested glucose and protein.

WHAT INFLUENCES HIGH TRIGLYCERIDE LEVELS?

The blood triglycerides can be influenced by a number of factors, such as the type of food we eat, the need of calories for energy at the time of absorption, our life habits such as the intake of alcohol, caffeine, and nicotine, the degree and duration of emotional stress, the lack of physical activity, and the use of certain drugs, such as birth control pills, antibiotics, diuretics, and some hormones. Examples of diseases that can cause elevated triglycerides are diabetes, thyroid disorders, gout, and kidney diseases. Those who have a normal triglyceride count are truly fortunate.

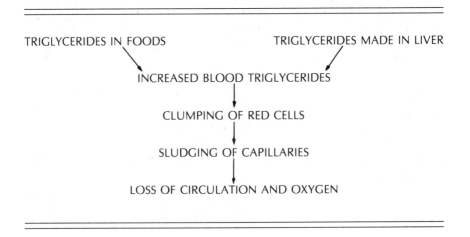

TRIGLYCERIDES IN FOODS   TRIGLYCERIDES MADE IN LIVER

INCREASED BLOOD TRIGLYCERIDES

CLUMPING OF RED CELLS

SLUDGING OF CAPILLARIES

LOSS OF CIRCULATION AND OXYGEN

WHAT IS A NORMAL TRIGLYCERIDE LEVEL?

Most medical tests for triglyceride levels are taken after a twelve- to twenty-four-hour fasting period. The current *normal* value for fasting triglycerides is set at 30–150 mg%. Any value above 200 mg% is considered to be an inborn error of fat metabolism that requires medical treatment. Yet it has been demonstrated repeatedly that this abnormal value of 200 mg% is produced frequently throughout the day in normal subjects who eat the usual American diet that is high in fats and sugars. And there have been very few studies to determine not what the average triglyceride level is, but what it *should be*.

The two doctors in the medical literature who have done the most to help clarify the normal triglyceride question are Meyer Friedman and Peter Kuo.

Dr. Friedman has demonstrated that although the average fasting triglyceride level in a human being might be 100 mg%, it can increase to *as high as 220 mg%* four hours after a meal.

Dr. Kuo also showed that normal subjects on a full diet had rising serum triglyceride curves shortly after their breakfast in the morning. These elevations remained throughout the day and did not return to the base line of a fasting level until late at night. One example was a forty-six-year-old male with fasting triglyceride levels in the range of 90–138 mg% which increased to 225–290 mg% throughout the waking hours after breakfast.

Dr. Friedman's and Dr. Kuo's studies on normal subjects reveal that a significant elevation of triglycerides during the day can be easily attained with the usual American diet.

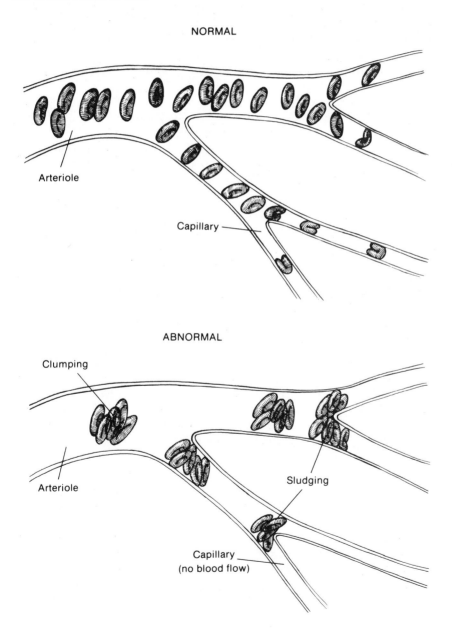

NORMAL

Arteriole

Capillary

ABNORMAL

Clumping

Arteriole

Sludging

Capillary
(no blood flow)

AT WHAT LEVEL DOES CLUMPING BEGIN?

When the studies by Friedman and Kuo are reviewed, we find that there are changes that take place showing that red blood cells begin to clump at approximately the level of 200 mg%. Thereafter, clumping is directly proportional to the elevation of the triglycerides above the level of 200 mg%. With this evidence, we can fully appreciate that high triglyceride levels can be a silent killer of cells in some people, even when the fasting triglyceride level is less than 150 mg%.

Except for rare cases—when a disease, an enzyme deficiency, or a hereditary defect raises triglyceride levels—triglyceride elevations in the bloodstream are directly related to *the way we live and to our diet.*

FASTING TRIGLYCERIDE STUDY IN DR. MANNERBERG'S PRACTICE

From a period of July 1, 1978, through December 1979, a total of 800 patients who had triglyceride tests after a period of fasting were screened to eliminate those who had diseases or were on drugs that influence triglyceride levels.

The resulting 182 males and 247 females were divided into groups and tested to determine variations of fasting triglyceride levels with age and gender.

The males showed a progressive increase in the *mean* triglyceride, especially after the age of forty. The females also showed a progressive increase but not to the same degree as the males, a finding borne out by other reports in scientific literature.

Of the males over the age of forty, 23.6 percent had fasting triglyceride levels over 150 mg%, as compared to 23.4 percent of females. Above the age of fifty, the averages intensify: 43 percent of the males exceeded 150 mg%, while 40 percent of the females tested over 150 mg%.

It was also found that in all people over fifty years of age, the ingestion of a small amount of fat was followed by a twenty-four-hour increase in the triglyceride level, whereas in younger people it returned to normal within five hours. This led to a conclusion that since most people in this country eat fat at least once a day, increased numbers of fat particles circulate in the blood of older people all the time.

When an enzyme was administered with the fat to break down the triglyceride particles, the triglyceride counts of the older people were reduced to the level of the younger subjects. This decrease suggests that older people may not have the enzymes necessary to break down blood triglycerides as they had when they were young. As people age, they are less able to handle fat in the diet, causing blood triglyceride levels to increase progressively. Therefore, the average triglyceride level increases with each decade of increase in aging.

It was also shown that triglyceride levels increase significantly when people consume a high-sugar diet. Increasing the calorie intake by 60 percent above normal had little or no effect on plasma triglycerides or cholesterol, unless there was also an increase in the sugar intake. Patients who had an increase in sugar intake showed serum cholesterol levels that were 50% above normal levels; they returned to a normal level when on a usual diet.

THE EFFECT OF INCREASED BLOOD TRIGLYCERIDES

An extensive study done by Dr. Melvin H. Knisely and reported in 1947 involved more than five thousand animal experiments and evaluation of the circulation in the eyes of fifty healthy medical students and student nurses. Where clumping of red cells and sludging of the capillary circulation was demonstrated, it repeatedly showed the presence of a diseased state. The concluding sentence of his report stated, "The sludges are now ready for study by all the intensive investigative methods our age affords."

Thirty years later Dr. Meyer Friedman conducted studies on patients with type A personalities (impatient, hard-driving, time-conscious individuals) and on those with coronary artery disease. After demonstrating the clumping of red cells and sludging of circulation in these groups, he concluded: "Thus, if these subjects ingest fat in several meals it is probable that they harbor myriad masses of sludge, erythrocytes in the capillary circulation of various organs and tissues for perhaps the greater part of the twenty-four-hour day. At this writing I know of no single phenomenon that has been so consistently neglected in the study of coronary heart disease as this one. Later we may rue this inexcusable oversight."

Dr. Friedman's studies show that a fasting serum triglyceride of above 125 mg% must be considered abnormally high. On review of the studies done to this time it would seem that in some individuals a serum triglyceride above 100 mg% might be abnormally high. From Dr. Knisely's findings and remarks in 1947 through the latest statement by Dr. Friedman, there have been twelve studies that demonstrate clumping of red cells and sludging of the capillary circulation after a fatty meal, along with increases in blood triglycerides.

Dr. Roy Swank, studying the effect of fat and the development of high blood fats following a meal, demonstrated distortion of red blood cells and the tendency to clump together. This slowing of the circulation was demonstrated in the cheek pouch of the hamster. Changes were reversible as the level of blood fats decreased seven to ten hours after the fat meal, and as the blood fat or triglyceride cleared. At this time the clumping was gone and the circulation returned to normal.

Dr. Arthur Williams in 1957 showed that a breakfast consisting of two fried eggs, a large piece of ham, toast with three pats of butter, and coffee with cream produced clumping of red blood cells with plugging of small blood vessels not only in individuals with heart disease but also in normal individuals. Dr. Swank's study in 1959 with rabbits and dogs revealed a reduced surface area of the red blood cells as a possible reason for decreased oxygen-carrying capacity of the red cells.

In a 1960 study Dr. Claude Joyner demonstrated a decrease in the circulation of the skin after a fatty meal, and subsequent research through 1976 revealed that sludging with elevated blood triglycerides affects the circulation and/or the oxygen level of tissues. These studies not only show the relationship of clumping and sludging to high blood triglycerides after a fatty meal, but also to a decrease in oxygen in various tissues.

All these studies show that high blood triglycerides alter the rate of blood flow and decrease the amount of oxygen available to the cells. Since oxygen is not stored in the body, even a slight oxygen deficiency can upset the normal physiology.

It is absolutely necessary that the blood stay unclumped and flow freely, carrying nutrients and oxygen to all the cells of the body, to maintain the highest degree of good health. In order for oxygen and all of the nutrients contained in the blood to sustain life, they must be distributed effectively to the cells. Clumping reduces the surface area of the red cells, which decreases their ability to carry oxygen. When clumps sludge and block the flow of blood through all of the capillaries, there is further decrease of oxygen delivery to the tissues.

WHY ARE THESE STUDIES SIGNIFICANT?

The medical world has focused on cholesterol, cigarette smoking, and hypertension as the major risk factors for heart disease and strokes. Triglyceride is considered a risk factor, but it has been largely overlooked, partly owing to the results of a Framingham, Massachusetts, study which did not prove that triglycerides were of major significance. But the studies of Friedman, Kuo, Swank, and others show that they are of utmost significance.

These studies point up the fact that triglycerides can be a consequence of poor nutritional habits. When we study the whole body rather than the heart alone, it is easy to see that the normal metabolism of an abnormal intake of fats and sugars that exceed the energy requirements of the body over a period of years can indeed have a detrimental effect on our cells.

SLUDGING OF RED BLOOD CELLS

"Sludging" refers to the clumping together of red cells into masses, rather than floating singly in the bloodstream. These clumps may be bunches fifteen to thirty times larger than a single red cell. What causes these red cells to lose their natural coating and change their surface characteristics so that they stick to other cells? Studies show that these changes are related to the high-fat, high-sugar diet.

When sludging occurs, plugging of capillaries is seen on microscopic examination. Clumping not only interferes with the ability of the red cells to enter the capillary to deposit the highly essential oxygen, but also interferes with all the other oxidative processes within the cell which are required to produce energy. Even if there is a very mild degree of this clumping, in which no single vessel is ever completely blocked by sludge, it does upset the precision of the metabolic continuity.

A number of studies in the medical literature demonstrate the effect of sludge on specific tissue or organ functions. Examination of the human eye has revealed the effective plugging of the capillaries and small arterioles by these clumps of red cells, in the presence of a number of different diseases, but also with the intake of certain foods. Sludging can obstruct the blood flow to the liver, kidney, heart, and brain, causing it to take three times longer to circulate than normal. Because brain tissue is extremely sensitive to the need for oxygen, it is easy to understand a possible role obstructed circulation can play in mental disease and aging. An increased loss in brain cells over a lifetime by continuous sludging of the circulation may lead to the most severe problem of later life—the loss of mental functioning so often referred to as senility.

The good news is that sludging is reported not to occur in the healthy person. When blood conditions are ideal, red cells and other cells of the body do not stick together, and there are forces which actually cause them to resist surface contact or adherence. Instead, the red cells bump from side to side through the circulation.

FACTORS THAT INFLUENCE BLOOD TRIGLYCERIDES

Most of the factors that influence triglyceride levels in the blood are directly related to the way we live. Triglycerides do depend to some extent on characteristics we cannot change—for example, levels are often higher in males than in females, and some people inherit a tendency to elevated triglycerides. But for the most part, we can lower triglycerides by changing our nutritional and personal habits.

Excess fats and sugars have a direct effect on the triglycerides and probably are the most common causes of elevated triglycerides from hour to hour through any day.

Single-meal gorging of excess calories—a pattern of skipping breakfast and consuming large evening meals—has a direct effect on the triglyceride storage system, causing warehousing problems for the excess fats and sugars and a traffic jam in the blood vessels when the cells summon oxygen delivery.

Drugs and smoking can also have an effect on blood triglycerides, as both change the chemistry of the body. Smoking is included in this category because it starts as a personal habit but later becomes a true addiction. Drugs and medications mostly increase the blood triglycerides, but a few have an effect on lowering them.

Alcoholic beverages are directly responsible for raising triglyceride levels when taken in excessive amounts along with fatty foods.

Emotional stress plays a role in disrupting fuel transport by causing false alarm signals to summon triglycerides through the blood vessels in unnatural quantities, at an erratic pace that can play havoc with the oxygen delivery system.

Sedentary life styles directly affect triglyceride levels in an adverse way. Constant body movement and exercise, on the other hand, have been proven to lower blood triglyceride levels.

DOES NUTRITION INFLUENCE HEALTH OR DISEASE?

Much of the cited evidence for the influence of nutrition on health and disease has been from epidemiological studies of populations, evaluation of their state of health, analysis of the composition of their diet. Worldwide studies have often divided the populations into two groups: the developing and primitive areas, where life is now similar to the way we lived in this country at the turn of the century; and the Western world, dependent on modern technology that has resulted in a drastic change of life style and the type of foods that are consumed.

Triglyceride levels are lower in people in the developing countries, where they have a natural carbohydrate, high-fiber, low-calorie, low-fat diet, with essentially no processed food. The opposite is true in the Western world, where the diet has become refined with increasing amounts of sugars and fats, with a marked decrease in the amount of fiber and other natural nutrients.

The most significant studies, showing a definite correlation between diet and triglycerides, have been those in which the diet is manipulated within these two groups. One such study, reported in 1961, compared Caucasian and Bantu prisoners in Africa. The Caucasians had had a Western-type diet in which 40 percent of the calories derived from animal fat, whereas the Bantu diet contained less than 15 percent calories from fat and was extremely high in natural carbohydrates. The triglyceride levels of the Bantu were significantly lower than those of the Caucasian prisoners at the beginning of the study. When the Caucasian prisoners followed the Bantu diet over a period of months and the Bantu were given the Western diet, the Caucasians showed a lowering of triglycerides and the Bantu developed higher triglycerides. Diet was the only variable—no other factors, such as weight changes or level of physical activity, were modified—and so the influence of diet upon triglyceride levels was established.

There are other studies that demonstrate the effect of fat on the level of blood triglycerides, showing a decrease when fat intake accounts for 35 percent of consumed calories, which is slightly lower than the usual 40–45 percent in this country. It was shown that triglycerides increased significantly one to three hours after eating and reached another peak four to seven hours after a 35 percent fat meal. These findings show that such a diet could lead to day-long increases in the plasma triglycerides in a majority of humans.

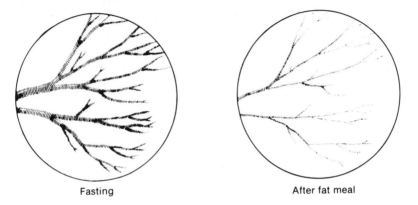

Fasting   After fat meal

WHAT ARE THE EFFECTS OF EATING CARBOHYDRATES?

There is confusion about the role of carbohydrates in the diet, since it has been reported that carbohydrates raise triglyceride levels. But it is important to remember that this increase is caused only by *refined carbohydrates,* such as sugar, honey, and syrups. Sucrose consumption leads to a marked increase in serum triglycerides. Eating unrefined natural carbohydrates, known as *complex carbohydrates,* reduces serum triglyceride levels.

The case for complex carbohydrates was well illustrated by Dr. J. I. Mann, who studied fifty-one healthy office workers between the ages of thirty-six and fifty-five. One third of them were asked to eliminate sucrose and replace it with other foods; another third tried to halve their dietary sugars and substitute starches; and the final third were used as controls who continued their usual diet.

In the low-sugar group, the serum triglycerides showed a significant decrease that persisted until the diets were stopped after a period of five and one-half months. The triglycerides fell more in those whose triglycerides were initially highest. The higher the beginning level, the more drop there was with the dietary change.

On the reduced-sugar diet, the serum triglycerides averaged 22 percent less. In the low-sugar group, serum triglycerides fell in proportion to the loss of weight that resulted from a reduced caloric intake. In other words, triglyceride levels were affected not only by reduction of sugar intake but also by the resulting reduced caloric intake.

Studies have been done in which the caloric intake was maintained in both groups and the only variable was the type of carbohydrate eaten. Again, eating sugar increased the blood triglycerides, which indicates that the dietary habits of an individual and his amount of sugar intake are both important to the production of high blood triglycerides.

A study by Dr. Paul J. Nestel was done with control of the type of sugar, the types of fats, and the variability of caloric intake. The results revealed that glucose and fructose raise triglycerides to the same extent, and that saturated fats invariably led to higher triglycerides. Decreased caloric intake caused a fall in blood triglycerides, whereas overeating led to a marked rise. It has been shown by other studies that triglycerides are raised by fat, whether they be saturated or unsaturated.

So the medical literature does establish that when refined sugars are eaten there is a dramatic increase in the blood triglycerides, even in normal subjects, and that when more calories are consumed than needed for energy throughout any one day, they are converted to triglycerides for storage.

In one study by Dr. Margaret J. Albrink, 215 apparently healthy male factory employees between the ages of thirty and seventy years old were observed for the relationship of triglycerides to certain characteristics. It was concluded that weight gain during adult life was the single most important factor associated with high blood triglycerides in normal men. Those who did not gain weight did not show an increase in triglycerides in the later decades of their lives, as did those who had gained weight.

With decreased sugar intake, increased consumption of unrefined natural complex carbohydrates, fat in the diet that does not exceed our energy requirements, and the *avoidance* of single-meal gorging (which has become habitual in American society), we may avoid the ravages of high serum triglyceride levels.

SHOULD TRIGLYCERIDE TESTS BE DONE IN A NONFASTING STATE?

Examination of people in the nonfasting state is of greater significance than the usual tests done in the fasting state. The measurement of fasting triglycerides helps to uncover those with a possible metabolic disorder, but monitoring the levels of triglycerides throughout a typical, nonfasting day gives a better indication of the effect of our dietary habits. Since we consider that 40–45 percent of the average American diet is fat and 22 percent of our calories comes from sugars, then it's not hard to understand that about 65 percent of the caloric intake of the type which affects the blood triglycerides is being consumed by most of our population. The Western world's habits of cigarette smoking, little physical activity, high emotional distress, and large meal gorging have been proven to increase the level of serum triglycerides. Postprandial testing reveals the effects of our diet.

CAN PHYSICAL ACTIVITY LOWER TRIGLYCERIDES?

It has been shown that exercise has a triglyceride-lowering effect in those with metabolic disorders, as well as normal individuals. Dr. Peter Wood at Stanford University School of Medicine reported that runners have a significantly decreased *mean fasting triglyceride* of 70 mg% versus 146 mg% for those who are not runners. These were men between the ages of thirty-five and fifty-nine years of age. Another study showed that medical students who entered an exercise program significantly lowered their fasting triglyceride levels after seven weeks of activity.

Physical activity or exercise must be habitual in order to have significant benefits. Our sedentary way of living has led to slothful bad habits, and the lack of physical movement is a large contributor to degenerative disease in later years.

HOW DOES EMOTIONAL STRESS AFFECT TRIGLYCERIDES?

It has been shown that acute emotional stress increased the triglyceride fraction of the blood lipids by 50 percent. In a study of race-car drivers, the triglycerides were slightly elevated after a race, but then reached a peak one hour later because the fatty acids mobilized by the body during the race were not expended in physical effort, so were then transformed into triglycerides by the liver. It has also been shown that those individuals with a type A personality, hard-driving people with stress-filled lives, have higher serum triglycerides than those who do not have this characteristic.

HOW DOES SMOKING AFFECT TRIGLYCERIDES?

There have been reports of limited studies that show an association of cigarette smoking and blood triglycerides. Dr. Emanuel Cheraskin reported that heavier smokers have higher serum triglycerides than those who smoke ten or less cigarettes a day. Cigarette smoking has been shown to increase the circulating fatty acids and result in stickiness of platelets of the blood, but red cell aggregation or clumping has not been reported. Smoking cigarettes does have an adverse effect on the body which can be demonstrated in many other ways, but also in relation to triglycerides.

DOES ALCOHOLIC INTAKE HELP TO LOWER SERUM TRIGLYCERIDES?

Alcohol, taken in smaller amounts, has had recent publicity for its possible beneficial effect on blood fats. It has been shown that moderate alcohol intake on a regular basis has definite effect on serum triglycerides. Excess triglycerides in the blood have been shown to increase with the use of alcohol, without the presence of dietary fats or sugars. But the ingestion of *fat and alcohol together* was greater than the effect of either alone. The ingestion of fat alone doubled the fasting level, but the combination of fat and alcohol increased it by three and a half times, beginning at intake and reaching a peak from six to ten hours after ingestion. The effect began to subside after eleven and one-half hours. These findings show that a large fatty meal eaten in the evening, preceded by a few drinks of an alcoholic beverage, can have a profound effect on the body's capillary circulation. This combination is typical at a business lunch or a social evening dining out, and may well affect the oxygen delivery system of the blood.

WHAT KINDS OF MEDICATIONS AFFECT TRIGLYCERIDES?

Many of the medications used to treat conditions such as hypertension, and many commonly prescribed drugs such as estrogens and birth control pills, increase the blood triglycerides. Birth control pill users—even when age, weight, cigarette smoking, and fasting glucose levels were not factors—had fasting blood triglycerides significantly higher than those of women who did not use them. Since past users of birth control pills no longer showed this effect, the change appears to be reversible.

Recent studies show that certain diuretics and a drug called propranolol, used for treating hypertension and other problems, have an adverse effect on the blood triglycerides. Insulin and heparin, an anticoagulant, have the effect of *decreasing* blood triglycerides.

Diseases that may raise the triglyceride level include diabetes, thyroid disease, other endocrine gland disorders, gout, kidney disease, and some pancreatic and liver diseases.

DO PERSONAL CHARACTERISTICS AFFECT TRIGLYCERIDES?

Some personal characteristics that cannot be modified have a definite effect on the level of blood triglycerides. All evaluative studies show an increasing level of blood triglycerides with aging, but this may be related to weight gain. Also, there is a distinct difference between males and females at the same age: males have a significantly higher triglyceride level than females. It may be that higher male triglycerides affect longevity, since females outlive males, but further studies will have to be made to prove this point.

When we examine all of the factors that affect triglycerides, it is easy to understand why the triglyceride is a common denominator among all the aspects of our way of life that have been incriminated in the risk for disease.

WHAT YOU CAN DO ABOUT TRIGLYCERIDES

We assume that our bodies can take anything we put into them and come out with good results. Many people push their bodies to the extent of determining just how much they can get away with before a breakdown occurs. But such practices violate their right to remain healthy. To prevent taking your body for granted, you have to be motivated to strive for better health and to acquire the knowledge that you can use to best advantage.

In our inactive, commercialized culture, all food sources are prepared, stored, and displayed in a fashion that will maximize profits. We have developed food sources that have little or no nutrient value, have unknown effects, or may even be harmful to the body. What takes place in our bodies from hour to hour depends on the fluctuation between desire and need. When we fail to follow basic rules of good nutrition, our bodies must compensate for the errors.

When the advertisements, the food delivery system, and our social eating habits steer us to the opposite of what is good, nutritious food, it is difficult for the average individual to eat properly without being extremely well motivated. In addition, there is confusion about what proper nutrition is. The many authoritative groups hold widely varying opinions about what is good for us. Even in the medical and scientific community, those who seek the right nutrition formula for themselves are finding it a difficult problem to resolve, so it can be even more difficult for those who have less knowledge or experience to evaluate the shifting opinions about nutrition. Yet no one can afford to shrug and say that nutrition doesn't matter. It does matter, and it does affect your body's functioning, especially since abuse can court degenerative diseases. One thing is for sure, the human body does not have the capacity to nourish itself—there is truth to the saying, "You are what you eat."

WHAT HAPPENS AFTER EATING A VERY LARGE MEAL?

The effects of sludging from gorging are often experienced during periods of feasting. The family reunion at Thanksgiving and Christmastime involves a table loaded with all the prime examples of what is good to eat in America, the land of plenty. We witness that after one, two, and very often three helpings of all the best of Mom's cooking, those who fill themselves to the bursting point become sluggish, almost drugged. This sensation occurs because the blood flow is diverted to the stomach and because of sludging and clogging in the small capillaries of the brain, which causes sleepiness due to decreased electrical activity.

When we eat a large meal which is a mixture of fats, protein, and sugars, upon absorption the amino acids derived from the protein go into the amino acid pool for cell replacement and growth. Then unused nutrients are either absorbed and carried to the blood through the lymphatic system as a triglyceride from the diet or as a triglyceride converted from the excess sugars. This flooding of the blood with triglycerides causes stickiness and sludging of the red cells. Overloading of the blood slows oxygen delivery. After a large meal, it is very easy for anyone's triglyceride level to exceed 200 mg%, the critical level at which heavy sludging can begin.

CAN A SLUGGISH OXYGEN DELIVERY SYSTEM BE CORRECTED?

The effect of our diet and of our way of life on triglycerides, and in turn the effect of the blood triglycerides on oxygen delivery, explains why certain nutrition recommendations have a valid scientific basis. If you think of triglycerides as one specific factor in the body and blood that can cause problems, then it is easier to focus on the change in habits that can produce beneficial results. You understand the *why,* rather than follow guidelines of what is good or bad for you; you can adjust your diet to a more beneficial type of nourishment program. The nutrition information and recipes in this book are designed to deal effectively with the triglyceride potential problem to avoid a sluggish oxygen delivery system.

3. YOUR OXYGEN DELIVERY SYSTEM

The five most important elements for survival of man are air, food, water, temperature, and light.

Our relationships with each of these elements is important, but none is as vital as that for air. A candle cannot burn without oxygen, and neither can we survive without it.

The cause of death for each of us in the final moment is the lack of oxygen, which must always be present to preserve the vital functions of the body for living. In other words, oxygen is the cause of our living, and the lack of it is the cause of our death. Not a pleasant thought to be so dependent on an element—but we are. And that simple fact should give us a very healthy respect for the air we breathe and the delivery system through our blood vessels that keeps our cells and organs functioning.

The vital companion to oxygen is the nutrients in the food we eat. While exercise can have a positive effect on our ability to utilize oxygen because of increased physical stress, nutrition can have an effect on the oxygen delivery system as it supplies fuel. The fuel is not just a source of energy, it also helps the metabolic system to work. Fuel influences the availability of oxygen on a minute-to-minute basis.

Who would choose the kind of fuel that would impede the delivery of oxygen to the cells and organs of the body? Would you believe that most of us do?

WHAT IS THE OXYGEN DELIVERY SYSTEM?

It is the uptake of oxygen from the air by the lungs, the delivery of the oxygen by the blood to the capillaries of the body, and the further delivery to and utilization by the cells for production of energy. The following steps are required for the system to work well:

1. Adequate oxygen tension in the air.
2. Lungs to take up the air containing oxygen and pass it into the blood.
3. Red cells and blood to pick up the oxygen delivered by the lungs.
4. Heart to pump the blood and red cells to all parts of the body.
5. Open blood vessels to transport the blood to the tissues.
6. The release of oxygen from the blood and then uptake by the cells.
7. The ability of the cells to utilize oxygen for production of energy.

Since oxygen is not stored in the body, the oxygen supply must be continuous every second of every minute of every day for our survival, whether we are at rest or active. This continuous requirement of oxygen is necessary for all tissues of the body, but especially the brain, which is most sensitive to a deficit in oxygen. Some vital processes can be maintained for a very brief period of time without oxygen, but these are extremely limited.

CAPACITY OF THE LUNGS

Normal breathing at rest is usually at the rate of twelve to sixteen times per minute, and each breath moves a small portion of our total lung volume. The rate of breathing and the depth of each breath determine the respiratory capacity or ability to deliver oxygen.

There are several mechanisms of the body which control respiration, but primarily this is determined by the need of oxygen by the cells. When more oxygen is needed, the message is sent to the lungs to increase respiration and provide the needed air.

The amount of oxygen in the atmosphere depends on the altitude, but man has the ability to adapt to the oxygen tension variability in those areas where we commonly live.

OXYGEN DELIVERY FROM THE LUNGS

Once oxygen is taken in, the lungs deliver air through the air sacs to the blood. This stage is called *diffusion*. Capillaries in the lungs come in contact

OXYGEN DELIVERY SYSTEM

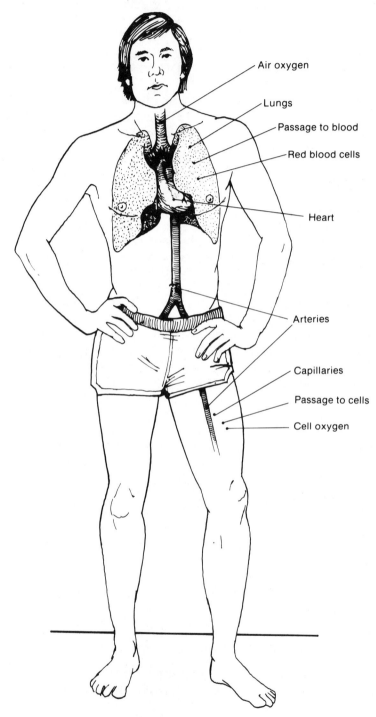

Air oxygen

Lungs

Passage to blood

Red blood cells

Heart

Arteries

Capillaries

Passage to cells

Cell oxygen

OXYGEN DELIVERY SYSTEM

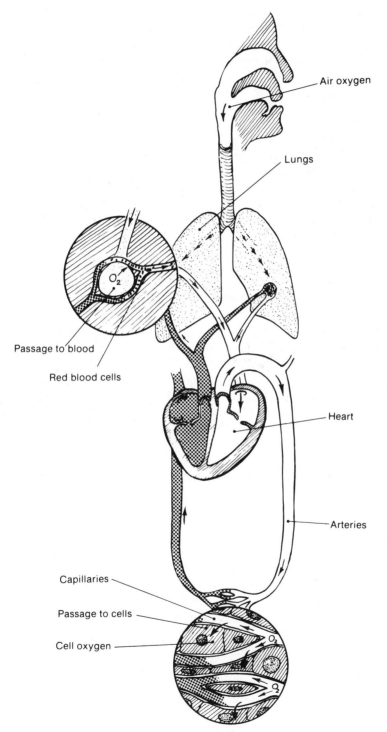

Air oxygen

Lungs

O₂

Passage to blood

Red blood cells

Heart

Arteries

Capillaries

Passage to cells

Cell oxygen

with the air sacs of the lung. As oxygen passes over the red blood cells in these tiny capillaries, it diffuses through their membranes. The red blood cells should be lying side by side to expose the greatest area of surface to the oxygen and permit maximum oxygen pickup. If the surface area is decreased, then so is the oxygen diffusion. After the diffusion takes place, a chemical reaction enables the cells to hold oxygen for delivery to the body.

The red blood cells, which are responsible for the red coloring of the blood, are visible only through a microscope and are a part of the *invisible circulation* (microcirculation). That is the term used to describe what cannot be seen by the naked eye.

The capacity of the red blood cells to carry oxygen depends on the availability of oxygen, the number of red cells, the presence of hemoglobin within the red cells, and several other factors. The percentage of red cells in a given volume of blood is called the *hematocrit*. A red-cell volume of 40 percent to 46 percent of the blood is considered ideal for carrying oxygen. A higher percentage of red cells increases the viscosity or "thickness" of the blood, and slows down the circulation.

ACTIVITY OF THE HEART

The center of the oxygen delivery system, and the most common site of breakdowns in the system or disease, is the heart. Each heartbeat propels the blood containing oxygen through the avenues of blood vessels, called arteries and arterioles.

Physical-fitness training programs produce an increased capacity for pumping larger volumes of blood to accommodate the need for extra energy and extra oxygen. The resting heart rate can increase from a range of 50–80 up to a maximum of 200 with exercise, depending on age and previous training. Developing the ability to propel a large amount of oxygen-containing blood is the so-called aerobic benefit of exercise.

ARTERIES AND ARTERIOLES

The arteries which leave the heart become progressively smaller in diameter and larger in number, until they reach the size called an *arteriole*. An arteriole is the smallest artery leading to the even smaller capillaries.

The ability to circulate and distribute blood depends on the diameter and the number of these vessels. There is a great deal of adaptability and reserve in this system, enabling a distribution of blood and oxygen to where it is needed in the body.

When atherosclerosis (buildup of plaque inside of the arteries) occurs, it reduces the amount of space for the blood to flow through. If the plaque causes complete blockage at any point along the arteries, it means a total interruption of blood flow and lack of oxygen to the cells beyond.

This is the reason for concern about cholesterol and saturated fat in the diet, which is part of the standard approach to preventive medicine. You will be reading further information about the role of cholesterol in the diet in chapter 4, "Biocontamination."

In the so-called normal population, a varying but significant degree of atherosclerosis is present long before symptoms are produced by blockage.

Since most people tend to have some buildup in the arteries after the age of twenty, it is important to keep the red blood cells from clumping together to form a sudden block in the oxygen delivery system, which may be already dangerously narrowed in some vital areas.

CAPILLARIES

The capillary, the smallest blood vessel in which oxygen transfer takes place, operates at the beginning of the system when it collects oxygen in the lung and operates at the end of the system when it delivers oxygen to the cells.

The capillary circulation and the individual red cells are the invisible vital parts of the oxygen delivery system. All of the blood vessels are for transportation of blood, but the capillary is also a place where there is an exchange of water, minerals and other nutrients, and gases such as oxygen. So it is at the level of the capillary that the circulation reaches its goal for delivery and transfer of nutrients to cells of every tissue of the body.

Oxygen-carrying red blood cells travel through the arteries and arterioles until they finally reach the capillaries. But many of the capillaries are so small that only one red cell at a time can pass through them. In these narrow passages, red cells, which are usually round, compress into ellipses to squeeze through, limiting oxygen delivery.

The capillary–red cell relationship is the same in all tissues of the body, but the amount of blood flow or number of capillaries is not under the same control. A muscular tissue of the body, such as a leg muscle, can vary the number of capillaries according to the degree of usage. For example, the average number of capillaries in a muscle in an untrained athlete has been calculated at about 325 per square millimeter of muscle. This can be increased to 460 per square millimeter in a trained athlete. The increased abundance of capillaries is a result of physical stress applied to the muscle on a regular basis.

A working muscle which at rest may receive 15 percent of the total blood supply can increase its allotment to as much as 85 percent of the total blood supply during vigorous muscle contraction. There is a high degree of coordination among the various systems of oxygen uptake from the lungs, transport of the blood, and oxygen supply to the cells in accordance with the body's energy requirements.

In contrast to the leg, where activity of muscles can increase blood flow from 15 percent to 85 percent of total body blood flow, the brain has a fairly fixed blood capacity. It cannot increase blood flow, and its oxygen needs do not vary accordingly. Since the brain's needs are at a constant level, it is even more important that blood flow not be hindered by sludging of red blood cells in the capillaries.

EFFECTS OF HIGH ALTITUDES

It has long been understood that high altitude, where the oxygen pressure is lower than at sea level, interferes with the usual level of activities and performance. The reduced oxygen density of the air at high altitude affects the mechanics of breathing, as well as the amount of oxygen available for uptake by the lungs and blood.

The reduced work capacity at high altitudes was evident in the poorer performances during the 1968 Olympic Games in Mexico City. The effect on the oxygen transport system during maximum work at an altitude such as Mexico City has been found to produce a reduction of available oxygen by 15 percent.

ALCOHOL AND THE OXYGEN DELIVERY SYSTEM

The reason that excess alcoholic intake is condemned, along with excess fats and sugars, is that alcohol interrupts the oxygen delivery system at more than one point. It contributes to the clumping of red blood cells, interfering with the pickup and delivery of oxygen at the capillary level. It also can affect the heart by causing a decreased capacity to pump blood.

Alcohol causes a significant increase in blood triglycerides, which is even more exaggerated when it is combined with the high fat intake of the typical American diet. Whereas the typical American fat intake can double a fasting triglyceride level, when alcohol is added it increases the triglycerides to three and a half times the normal level. The cardiac output has been shown to be decreased by the toxic effect of alcohol on the heart muscle.

There are studies to suggest that moderate ingestion of alcohol in the range of two drinks or less per day may increase the high-density lipoprotein, which then has a favorable effect on the total cholesterol. If you must drink alcoholic beverages, be sure that you do not eat fat at the same time, and do not exceed the two-drink limit. But you don't have to drink for this benefit; the favorable effect can also be obtained with the aerobic nutrition diet plus regular physical activity.

CIGARETTE SMOKING AND THE OXYGEN DELIVERY SYSTEM

The blood triglycerides have been shown to be higher in smokers than non-smokers. This may be related to other health habits that coexist with smoking.

Tars and irritants in tobacco smoke narrow the breathing tubes or bronchi that lead to the air sacs in the lung where oxygen is delivered to the blood. As less oxygen can pass through them, the amount of oxygen that can be delivered is decreased.

Smokers of one or more packs of cigarettes per day have twice the risk of heart attack as nonsmokers. Besides the effect on the small blood vessels, it has been indicated that high-density lipoprotein cholesterol (which is the beneficial type) is decreased in those who smoke. With lowered protective effects of this kind of cholesterol, total blood cholesterol increases and tends to build up in the arteries.

Nicotine also causes the constriction of the small blood vessels, which interferes with blood flow and oxygen delivery to the tissues throughout the body.

It has been shown that smoking two cigarettes can decrease the skin temperature by 4.5 degrees in the toes and 5.8 degrees in the fingers. This produces an increase in the heart rate and blood pressure, which can reflect an increase in the metabolic rate or oxygen need.

Cigarette smoke also contains carbon monoxide. This is the same gas that comes from the exhaust pipe of an automobile, and it is deadly. The reason that exhaust fumes kill is that the hemoglobin in the blood has a greater affinity with carbon monoxide than with oxygen—200 times greater. Red cells chemically bound to carbon monoxide are less able to carry oxygen; the effect lasts for up to a period of twelve hours. Bicycle and treadmill stress tests devised to measure performance relative to the blood level of carbon monoxide have shown that the exercise work time and the maximum oxygen uptake decreased with increased levels of carbon monoxide.

Cigarette smoking increases the free fatty acids in the blood, the precursors of triglycerides. It has been demonstrated that there is a 24.6 percent to 27.2 percent increase in free fatty acids within ten to twenty minutes after smoking, an effect that may persist as long as forty minutes. The increase in free fatty acids of the blood after cigarette smoking was immediate and always present. This effect is demonstrated after smoking two cigarettes, and in any person who smokes continuously at the rate of four cigarettes an hour there is a continuous release of free fatty acids. This is caused by a nicotine effect that stimulates the secretion of adrenal hormone.

So, smoking even a few cigarettes affects the oxygen delivery system in at least six ways:

1. The airways in the lung constrict, which interrupts the flow of oxygen from the air to the lung.

2. The red cells are captured by carbon monoxide and no longer capable of carrying oxygen as long as carbon monoxide is present.
3. There is a possible contribution of triglycerides to sludge and decreased capillary flow at the cellular level which impedes oxygen delivery.
4. In some individuals there is the increase of irregular beats of the heart.
5. There is the effect of decreasing the high-density lipoprotein cholesterol, which then makes the total cholesterol a greater risk in developing blockage of the arteries.
6. The constriction of small arteries decreases blood flow to the skin and other tissues of the body, with the resulting decrease in oxygen.

When all of these effects of cigarette smoking upon the oxygen delivery system are reviewed, it is apparent why early deaths and especially loss of health throughout a lifetime are greatly increased in smokers over nonsmokers, without even considering the data on the potential for development of cancer and chronic lung disease.

The oxygen delivery system of an individual who smokes tobacco is literally smothered by poison. A reduced ability to move air in and out of the lungs will cause a smaller volume of oxygen to reach the blood, causing impaired performance.

STRESS AND THE OXYGEN DELIVERY SYSTEM

The oxygen delivery system can be seriously impeded by reaction to emotional distress. Life is a continuous series of stresses, but the emotional reaction must be stimulated before such stress becomes a problem. As long as stress does not produce an emotional reaction, there is no *fight or flight response.*

The fight or flight response is a very basic reflex in all animals, including man; a perceived threat activates the body mechanism that prepares us to either fight like crazy or run like mad.

In our modern-day society, with its social limitations on our behavior, this basic response has fewer acceptable outlets of the physical type, such as physically striking back or actually running away from the threat. Instead of producing a physical reaction, the response to danger is turned inward and suppressed. When there is no outlet for this very basic emotional arousal, the oxygen delivery system is affected. Actual breakdowns of emotional and physical health can occur.

The oxygen delivery system can be altered by stress in several ways:

1. An increase in triglycerides occurs which can affect the uptake of oxygen by the red cells.
2. The heart can be affected, causing a change in the way the blood is pumped through the system.

3. The arteries can be blocked by new formations of plaque, caused by a rise in the formation of cholesterol as a reaction to stress.
4. The small capillaries can be obstructed by the increase of clumped red cells, resulting in less blood flow to tissue cells.
5. Oxygen requirements of the cells can change.

HOW DO WE KNOW THAT TRIGLYCERIDES INCREASE AS A RESULT OF STRESS?

Scientific tests have proved the point. A 1968 study in Sweden measured free fatty acids and triglycerides in the blood, as well as the byproduct of adrenal hormone secretion, the increased heart rate and blood pressure.

Thirty-three volunteer subjects were divided into three equal groups. The first eleven were subjected to stress and had an elevation reaction in all the areas—fatty acids, triglycerides, heart rate, and blood pressure.

The second eleven subjects were allowed to sit comfortably with no stress and there was no rise in triglycerides or any of the other factors.

The third group of eleven were also given stress, and all of the tests showed elevations. Then they were given three grams of nicotinic acid during a stress test; the results showed a suppression of fatty acids and triglyceride levels while the other factors rose. This clearly demonstrated that without the nicotinic acid, the fatty acids and triglycerides would also have been affected.

HOW DOES STRESS AFFECT THE HEART?

When a stress is interpreted as a threat to the body and becomes a distress, as termed by Dr. Hans Selye, then the result is a higher incidence of irregular heartbeats and high blood pressure, which can contribute to heart disease or damage the pump itself.

During exercise stress testing, anxious patients demonstrated a lower level of oxygen uptake than those with normal anxiety controls. This shows an interference with the oxygen delivery system.

HOW DOES STRESS AFFECT THE ARTERIES?

This effect has been demonstrated in studies of medical students with examination anxiety or patients subjected to stressful interviews. Both groups clearly showed a dramatic rise in blood pressure. The elevation of blood pressure and damage to the arteries that accompany stress also increase the risk of atherosclerosis. Excess cholesterol can form plaques along the walls of the arteries, and may eventually block the vessels. If cholesterol levels are sent soaring by a stress reaction, this danger is increased.

If stress increases cholesterol, then reducing stress should reduce cholesterol. It has been proved medication that promotes relaxation, when used over a period of time, significantly lowers the serum cholesterol.

HOW CAN THE SMALL CAPILLARIES BE AFFECTED BY STRESS?

When stress sends the triglyceride levels up in the blood, clumping and sludging of the red cells occurs. This clogs up the capillaries and interferes with oxygen delivery by the red blood cells.

CAN STRESS ALONE PRODUCE THESE CHANGES?

Stress alone can produce the changes described, but it very seldom acts alone. Stress is often accompanied by detrimental habits, such as cigarette smoking, use of alcohol, obesity, and poor eating habits. These factors affect oxygen delivery system at almost all points, from the extraction of oxygen from the air we breathe to the delivery of oxygen to body cells.

CAN THE NEED FOR OXYGEN BY THE CELLS BE CHANGED?

Yes. Studies on relaxation and its effect on oxygen requirements have shown the cells need less oxygen during physical and mental inactivity, as during a hypnotic sleep. This reduced oxygen need has also been demonstrated during transcendental meditation, which is a change produced without sleep.

The opposite of the fight or flight response has been described in an article by Dr. Herbert Benson, reported in *Psychiatry* in 1974 and also published in 1976 as a book entitled *The Relaxation Response.* These findings reported a 13 percent decrease in requirement for oxygen during relaxation. So it is possible to decrease the oxygen uptake during hypnotic sleep, transcendental meditation, and by the relaxation response. It has also been shown that there is an increase in blood flow to the resting forearm during transcendental meditation.

EXERCISE AND THE OXYGEN DELIVERY SYSTEM

Aerobic exercise has become a part of the widespread physical-fitness movement in the United States. The word *aerobic* pertains to the ability to use oxygen. It is a system that measures the maximum ability to use oxygen to determine the maximum level of physical endurance and the capacity to perform physical work. This involves the oxygen delivery system, whereby oxygen is taken from the air by the lungs, diffused into the blood, and then carried largely by the red blood cells that are pumped to various parts of the body by the heart, using the highways of the arteries to the small capillaries where the oxygen is delivered to the cells.

Exercise improves this oxygen delivery system by increasing the maximum capacity of the lungs. During exercise, the lungs increase their ability to move air from approximately 6 liters per minute at rest to 100–200 liters per minute during maximum effort. Also, the heart can increase its output of blood from 4–6 liters per minute to 20–40 liters per minute at this same maximum effort. Physical stress strengthens the heart (the pump), can help to enlarge the major blood vessels (with high-level endurance training), and can improve the delivery of oxygen to the cells in the muscle group that is being used.

The apparatus for using oxygen in the cells of the exercising muscle are also increased as a result of the training effect. Therefore, with increasing physical fitness with exercise, the ability to utilize oxygen is increased. When you improve the capacity of heart function and blood vessels, there will be continued optimal functioning and survival of all the cells in the body that benefit from a good oxygen delivery system.

Individuals who exercise for endurance-type activities develop enlarged arteries to carry the increased volume from the heart to the capillaries where the exchange of oxygen will take place. This has been shown by autopsies of a marathon runner who was still competing at the time of death and of African tribesmen whose life style requires long-distance walking or running until they die. The capillaries within an exercised muscle group increase in number, owing to the strain, and they can accept increased blood flow with an enhanced ability to exchange oxygen.

The increased ability to deliver and utilize oxygen is not present in muscle groups that have not been exercised. This difference shows in exercise stress testing in this country; it is difficult to do a maximum stress test on a bicycle compared to walking on a treadmill, since the muscles in the legs tend to give out before maximum oxygen uptake can be achieved. Cycling uses a different set of muscles than running. Most Americans have untrained cycling muscles when compared to populations where cycling is a more common method of transportation. This produces a difference in the ability to perform.

Everyone can't participate in extensive aerobic exercises, but there is some level of physical activity that can provide benefits for each person. This must be chosen on an individual basis. If you consider the effects and benefits, including the improvement of oxygen delivery throughout your body, there should be some stimulus to get your body moving. A later chapter on the Mannerberg Method of Movement will show you how to get started on an exercise or movement program of your own.

CHOLESTEROL AND THE OXYGEN DELIVERY SYSTEM

Excess cholesterol contributes to the development of plaques in the arteries. Plaques are accumulations inside artery walls that cause the tubes to narrow, leading to the most common cause of death today—the heart attack.

Although cholesterol gets a lot of medical attention because of this effect, it plays only one role in the entire oxygen delivery system. That is in the arteries. It is part of the visible circulation system and can be easily examined by current medical techniques.

When there is a combination of cholesterol-caused plaques and red cell sludging caused by triglycerides, the oxygen delivery system is drastically impeded. A further explanation of the blood cholesterol can be found in the following chapter.

4. BIOCONTAMINATION

Adaptability has been the key to human survival since the beginning of our history on earth. Behavior—instinctual and learned—is one means of adaptation in response to environmental demands, but not all behavioral adaptations are biologically favorable. Early human behavior was more instinctive; as civilization developed, it became more learned, gaining control of instinctive impulses.

Learning ability and intelligence are centered in the brain. This center of all thought and learned behavior is a prisoner in a bony cage and at the mercy of limited supply lines for all of the essentials for life, including oxygen delivery and fuel utilization. There are limited means for variation or adaptability to change to help protect optimal functioning throughout a lifetime.

Preservation of function of the brain and of all other vital organs throughout a lifetime is related to the rate at which our reserves are lost. During youth there is approximately a 70 percent reserve in these vital organs with a great potential for high levels of function. After the age of twenty or twenty-five years, we spend the remainder of our lives losing that reserve by the process called aging. This wear and tear consists of the degree that living subtracts from the genetic potential of each individual. *The ability to cope with the wear and tear of daily life—adaptability—by using metabolic essentials to produce energy is different in each of us and makes us susceptible to different variables.*

Every thought, heartbeat, and breath require *energy* for survival, and for this we must rely on our environment. How well we function depends on our ability to extract from our environment those essentials needed for each biochemical process of the body. The degree to which these vital factors are used by the brain ultimately determines our ability to survive.

Although we are all exposed to a somewhat similar environment, each of us reacts in an individual way. Nature has provided a great deal of the ingredients in a form which the body, over a period of many hundreds of generations, has used to survive. At this stage in the history of man, the natural ingredients for existence are becoming less and less available. There is now the question of how well our future generations will evolve as a result of an environment which has so dramatically changed within the last seventy-five years. The future changes will be even more rapid, and adaptability will be even more uncertain.

During the early part of this century, Dr. Winston Price traveled 150,000 miles in nine years, studying the health of human populations. His writings describe the nutritional changes that had taken place within one generation. Dr. Price recorded his views of the basic natural food diet requirements for optimal human physical and mental health. During this same period of time, his associate, Dr. Frances M. Pottinger, Jr., studied 900 cats and showed that changes in diet required three generations to produce a point where life of the young could not survive, and also three generations of proper nutrition to reverse these changes. These studies of cats give some clues as to the result of the changes from a natural diet of man in future generations.

For this reason, Aerobic Nutrition promotes the balancing of the fuel and oxygen systems within the human body by using natural foods for improved function and resistance to disease. By modifying the potential implications of the rapidly developing artificial chemical diets of our modern world, we are not only protecting our own good function but that of our children and grandchildren as well.

It is for science to determine what types of diseases may result in the years to come from the nutritional mistakes of today. Each person can opt to improve his or her own diet, to reject most of that which is not natural food, and to be responsible for a body that functions well and healthily for a lifetime.

INDIVIDUAL ADAPTABILITY

The way we eat and live affects triglycerides, with all of the ramifications outlined in the previous chapters. Any intake into the body that produces poor functioning is a part of that ecology of body contamination, just as much as the sludging of our rivers with industrial wastes or our air with oppressive smog.

If you are maladapted to some aspect of your present environment, you should consider making some changes. If you are chronically or symptomatically ill and have never learned why, or if you are just not functioning ideally with a true zest and energy for life, then it is possible that you are suffering from some form of biocontamination. Not all depression, chronic fatigue, undiagnosed headaches, spastic colons, or other illnesses are necessarily the result of the various means of body contamination, but it is surprising to note how many spontaneous remissions occur when offending agents are discovered and removed.

Chemical contamination of our environment includes contamination of our body by the chemicals of our food supply. Chemicals have become part of our way of life, beginning with fertilizers and pesticides in the fields and extending to additives in processed foods for preservation, coloring, or other commercially beneficial effects. Many of these chemicals that are added to the various stages of food production and preparation have been tested and determined to be safe for human consumption, but there are still areas of controversy and disagreement. Perhaps many of these chemicals can be used safely for the general population, but there are individuals who are more sensitive and would do well to avoid them whenever possible.

Most physicians who prescribe medicines are aware of the side effects or potential hazards of these drugs, whether given alone or in combination with other medicines. Yet the medical world seems to have a lack of recognition of allergic or chemical reactions from effects of food technology. That's why it is important for us all to be aware that side effects may occur.

We all want to feel well, but some of us have been more successful than others because we are better adapted to the way we live in the modern world. It is the poor adapters who should not be condemned to a lifetime of illness without a disease. Every effort should be made to discover what part of your own personal environment is causing problems and to alter these for a more compatible existence.

HOW DOES AEROBIC NUTRITION ADDRESS ITSELF TO THE PROBLEM OF BIOCONTAMINATION?

It meets the problem head-on by offering a way of eating that will decrease the overflooding by the fuel transport system and the consequence of sludging the oxygen delivery system.

It is based on foods that are less chemically contaminated than the average American diet, and it shows how to cook better in less time than ever before. It is a fallacy to believe that only fabricated fast food can save time in the kitchen—many recipes in this book can be prepared in fifteen minutes or less with start-from-scratch raw ingredients. It's the best way to decontaminate every mouthful of food you eat.

Aerobic Nutrition suggests that you avoid the use of caffeine products (coffee, strong tea, chocolate, and cola drinks), excess alcoholic beverages, and tobacco.

The concept recognizes that apparent and silent food allergies do exist and are responsible for a wide variety of symptoms of ill health. It also takes into consideration the fact that a large proportion of our population is overweight to the point of being obese, and that this is a self-inflicted biocontamination that can be overcome. You will find a well-balanced Aerobic Nutrition

Weight-Loss Diet just before the recipe section to use as a guide for sensible weight loss of about two pounds a week. You did not put that extra weight on in a week, and it is foolhardy to try to starve it off too fast. Just as the body has adjusted to carrying an extra load of weight and built up extra cell support systems to maintain the unnecessary poundage, so it must slowly adjust itself as the body sheds itself of unhealthy weight excess. Good health and physical vitality are the optimum goals of Aerobic Nutrition.

Many of these biocontaminants are under our direct control and many are not. As Dr. Emanuel Cheraskin says, when lecturing to medical groups, "Your life is affected by the air you breathe, the water you drink, and the food you eat." You may not have control over the air, you could have some control over the water, and you definitely should have full control over your food.

OBESITY

Obesity is self-imposed biocontamination. Obesity is caused by an imbalance of the available fuel that comes from the food you eat and your body's actual needs for energy spent. The unspent fuel is stored as fat.

Just as we have discussed the oxygen delivery system to give a thorough layman's understanding of how the air we breathe reaches every cell that needs it, so we should learn how the fuel delivery system affects the oxygen delivery system. The joining of fuel and energy systems produces continuous life—fuel and oxygen create the energy vital to our capacity for work and play.

The imbalance between fuel and energy requirements has an adverse effect on the oxygen delivery system. The concept of Aerobic Nutrition is to keep a good balance between the fuel taken into the body and the energy that is spent, so that the fuel is burned up as needed and nothing is left for storage as fat. Excess body fat, or obesity, is a product of the way of life in a large percentage of the American population.

DO YOU CALL ALL KINDS OF FOOD THE FUEL FOR ENERGY?

The food we eat provides the building blocks for different cells and tissues of the body, plus vitamins and minerals which participate in metabolism of cells, and the fuel to combine with oxygen for the production of energy which makes possible our existence and accomplishments.

Protein, the most important building block, is used for new cells and tissues during growth and development. It also replaces old cells, which are constantly changing throughout our lives, but is a poor source of fuel for production of energy.

Metabolic processes of the body depend on minerals and vitamins that make possible the use of fuel when combined with oxygen to produce energy. When proteins, fats, and natural carbohydrates are broken down in the process of digestion, they yield amino acids, fatty acids, and simple sugars, in that order. These products are then absorbed into the blood, either directly into the intestinal capillaries or indirectly by the lymphatic system, as in the case of fats and triglycerides. The mechanism of digestion and absorption of food you eat is complicated, and this very simple description offers a general understanding.

WHAT HAPPENS AFTER THE FUEL IS ABSORBED?

Upon absorption of the fuel, whatever its origin, it must be handled in one of two ways. The first priority is to satisfy energy requirements of the moment. Fuel not required immediately is placed in storage for later use. There is a limited space to store the absorbed sugars and an unlimited capacity to store fats. Once the sugar storage capacity is reached, the sugars not needed to produce energy must be converted to triglycerides to be stored as fat. Therefore, *an excess sugar intake ends up as having the same effect as a fatty meal.* Oxygen cannot be stored for later use, so our survival depends on a steady supply from breath to breath, whereas fuel needs tend to vary from activity to activity.

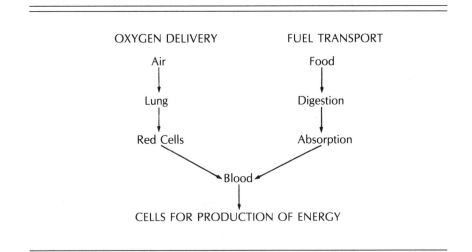

The cells of our body are energy factories, so to speak. In our cells, through the process of oxidation, fuels coming from the food that has been eaten or from stored fat is turned into energy. One byproduct of this process is heat, which maintains our body temperature. Again, it is important to realize that the oxygen delivery system is a continuous dynamic process which must continue from breath to breath, whereas the fuel transport system can rely on storage for satisfying our needs from minute to minute. This explains why a person can fast for long periods of time but can't hold a breath more than about one minute.

WHAT PROVIDES THE GREATEST AMOUNT OF FUEL FOR ENERGY?

It has been known for a long time which types of foods provide the greatest fuel for energy. Carbohydrates are the most efficient source. Although one gram of fat provides more than twice as much energy as one gram of carbohydrate, it requires almost three times as much oxygen to oxidize fat to carbon dioxide and water.

When a muscle group is at rest, most of its energy comes from fat, with its uptake of glucose being less than 10 percent. Within the first ten minutes of exercise, carbohydrate oxidation, rather than fat oxidation, becomes the major energy-producing process. Then, as exercise continues, the triglyceride stored in the fat tissue becomes the major source of energy. After the first few minutes of exercise, the fatty acids in the body are used progressively to a greater extent, so that by thirty minutes they become the major blood-borne fuel for muscle contraction. This is the reason why one period of exercise lowers blood triglycerides to some degree for as long as seventy-two hours.

As work intensity increases, the release of free fatty acids from adipose tissue is greater in the muscles of trained athletes (who have a greater ability to utilize fat at high workloads) than it is in those with untrained muscles. This is one of the benefits in fat metabolism promoting weight loss.

In one study obese women were found to be far less active than nonobese women. The obese women walked an average of 2.0 miles per day for all physical needs, as compared to 4.9 miles per day for nonobese women. Among men, there were comparable figures of 3.7 miles per day for the obese, and 6.0 miles per day for the nonobese. It was also found that the difference in physical activity was parallel to the difference in attitude toward being active in general.

HOW DOES AEROBIC NUTRITION FIT INTO THE PROBLEMS OF OBESITY?

It is not only the content of the diet that affects metabolism and body weight, but also the pattern of meals. *There is more to being fat than just the total caloric content of the diet.*

The meal patterns suggested for good Aerobic Nutrition—calorie consumption spaced evenly throughout the day, with no single-meal gorging—balance metabolism and protect the oxygen delivery system, as well as promote a more normal body weight.

CALORIES FROM FOODS IN THE TYPICAL AMERICAN DIET*		
	% CALORIES	CALORIES PER DAY
Sugars, syrups	17	525
Fats and oils	18	550
Alcohol	7	210
Refined cereals and breads	17	525
Total "empty calories or refined calories"	59	1810

*Average consumption 3,100 calories per day

WHY CAN SOME PEOPLE SEEM TO EAT ALL THEY WANT AND NEVER PUT ON WEIGHT?

Studies indicate that within the human population there is a great deal of individual variability in maintaining weight at either extremely low or high food intake. Overeaters who do not gain weight often show elevated basal metabolic rate and a higher energy need for daily activities. The small eaters who do not gain weight show a much lower activity rate and lower energy need. The main implication of this difference is that those who seem to thrive on low intakes are known to have increased longevity, whereas the high intakers often do not demonstrate this possible benefit.

Most people who have a keen appetite and who have to fight the overweight battle have to learn to increase their activities to match the amount of food they eat. In other words, you must burn off what you take in each day to maintain normal weight. There are 3,500 calories in each pound of stored fat in the body. Overeating and not burning off just 500 calories a day can become one pound of excess weight in a week. That habit can lead to 52 pounds of excess weight in just one year. That is why calorie counts per serving are included in the nutritional information at the end of each recipe in this book.

DOES THAT MEAN THAT EVERYONE MUST BE ON A DIET ALL THE TIME?

No. It just means that everyone should have the facts and then determine a way of eating that satisfies the appetite and also satisfies the desire to live a total healthful life.

Appetite, hunger, and energy are no longer balanced in our present social and economic structure. Most middle-age obesity is the result of a stimulated appetite and the increased availability of foods. The appetite is stimulated—by the senses, sight, smell, taste, touch, and even hearing—without hunger being present. Commercial food advertisements are used with good results for business. But what is good for big business is not always good for you.

Weight gain from an overstimulated appetite, or from routine eating habits that include coffee breaks with doughnuts and sweet rolls several times a day, has its effect on the oxygen delivery system. An average person may not be overweight by the age of twenty-five or when married. But from then on, due to the change in the level of activity and family eating styles there is a progressive increase in weight. This may be initially within the range of 10–15 pounds, reaching 20–50 pounds by middle age. This gradually accumulated weight is affected most by Aerobic Nutrition, since it reverses the very problem that produced the obesity in the first place.

It is amazing how weight tends to normalize when the appetite is controlled and the type of foods that are eaten are modified, without having to struggle with hunger. Knowledge of what really happens when you start wielding that fork toward your mouth is the key to making a change. Aerobic Nutrition is not a short-term approach but rather a way-of-life habit that can promote better health.

In summary, Aerobic Nutrition balances the fuel-energy needs to protect the oxygen delivery system by:

1. Reducing fat and sugar intake.
2. Increasing level of activity.
3. Improving meal patterns.
4. Regulating appetite and energy needs.
5. Accounting for individual variabilities.

CHOLESTEROL

Cholesterol is not necessarily a bad egg! But it is regarded to be one of the three major risk factors for atherosclerosis, a condition that frequently leads to heart attack or stroke. For some unexplained reason, some people seem to manufacture excess cholesterol that lines the artery walls with ever-thickening plaques. This situation is analogous to rust building up in a plumbing pipe. At first, the small amount of buildup doesn't stop the flow of liquid through the pipe, but later as the rust adds many layers, the liquid can only trickle through. Eventually, it may even close at one point and stop the flow entirely. In the human body, the loss of blood flow immediately stops the oxygen delivery system that is vital to life.

WHAT CAUSES CHOLESTEROL TO LINE THE ARTERIES?

After seventy years of research in animals and humans, the answer is still unknown as to why some people develop plaques and other people don't.

Cholesterol is a necessary element, and every tissue in the body has the capacity to make it. Some people manufacture an excess of this substance, and it is this excess that finds a storage place along the arterial walls. Therefore, additional cholesterol in the diet is not an essential requirement, as vitamins and minerals are. When excess cholesterol is consumed in foods that are otherwise good nutritionally, this unneeded cholesterol must be stored in our bodies.

HOW DO WE KNOW IF A FOOD HAS CHOLESTEROL IN IT?

A good rule of thumb is to remember that animal fat is saturated fat (high in cholesterol content) and vegetable fat is unsaturated fat (with no cholesterol content). Animal fat includes the actual fat that marbelizes meat or that is suspended in layers between the meat. It can't be avoided completely. But it can be reduced in your diet if you use only lean cuts of beef and trim them well before and after cooking; pull all excess fat from poultry before cooking; chill soups and stews to let the excess fat solidify into a block at the top that can easily be removed; and completely avoid all fatty cuts of meat, including ham and bacon products, frankfurters, and molded cold cuts. Substitute poultry and fish meals, and use cuts of veal whenever possible because of the lower fat content. Animal fat also includes egg yolks, the butterfat content of whole milk, whole-milk products (cheese, sour cream, regular yogurt), and butter. Choose foods in this category that are lower in saturated fat—skim-milk products or those with less than 2 percent butterfat. Reduce the use of egg yolks to two or three per week. Use vegetable oils to fulfill the body's need for fat.

IS ANY KIND OF VEGETABLE OIL ALL RIGHT TO USE?

Yes, except for olive oil and coconut oil, which are slightly more saturated in content. Corn oil is a good choice and is used in the recipes in this book. But you may interchange any other type of unsaturated vegetable oil that you prefer, such as safflower oil, soybean oil, or cottonseed oil. Instead of butter, use soft margarine and soft vegetable shortening.

WHY SPECIFY *SOFT* MARGARINE AND SHORTENING?

There are studies that indicate that the hydrogenation process has an effect on vegetable oil. The harder in form the product gets, the more saturated the fat content becomes, because of the chemical interaction with the added hydrogen. This has become a highly debated and ongoing conflict in the food and science communities.

WHY WORRY ABOUT ANIMAL FAT IF SCIENCE ISN'T SURE?

These recommendations are primarily based on the fact that, throughout the world, where there is a high intake of saturated fats, there is also a high incidence of atherosclerosis. In those populations with an extremely low intake of saturated fats, there is virtually no atherosclerosis or blockage of arteries. These factors suggest that unsaturated fat actually has a favorable effect in lowering cholesterol blood levels.

WHAT IS CONSIDERED TO BE A NORMAL BLOOD CHOLESTEROL?

"Normal" blood cholesterol is a very misleading concept because the so-called normal range of 150 mg% to 330 mg% (in people over age forty) gives a fivefold change in incidence of atherosclerosis from a low normal to a high normal. It does have some predictive value and is related to risk. For example: If you are an American male playing Russian roulette with a five-chamber pistol and using the heart as the target, a blood cholesterol of greater than 260 (normal) would be playing with four out of five chambers loaded. A blood cholesterol of less than 200 would be playing with one out of five chambers loaded. This is the difference in the risk of the "normal range" of cholesterol in males under fifty years of age, if the trigger is pulled before age sixty-eight.

It has been shown by Dr. Robert W. Wissler of the University of Chicago that in parts of the world where there is virtually no evidence of atherosclerosis, 90 percent of the population has a normal cholesterol range of 100–150 mg%. In our country and in other Westernized countries of the world, where there is a high incidence of atherosclerosis (specifically in our country, where it is related to two of the leading causes of death), the normal value is cited to be 130–330 mg% depending on age. Again, this normal value as determined by an average of our population is not very desirable, as indicated by the health and death statistics.

WHAT DO STUDIES SHOW ABOUT CHOLESTEROL COUNTS IN THE BLOOD?

There is a message of the Masai—a tribe in Africa—that illustrates the pitfalls and dilemma when discussing the relationship between dietary intake of cholesterol, the level of blood cholesterol, and the presence of atherosclerosis.

These African tribesmen survive with and upon the cattle they herd. In the process of herding their animals to grass and water, they average more than twenty miles of walking per day. Their food consists of all parts of the animal, including the blood, soured milk, and meat, which are the main proteins of the diet. By our standards, these foods would be considered to be atherogenic or at least very likely to produce atherosclerosis.

Yet, in these people, there is no *clinical evidence* of coronary disease from atherosclerosis, on the basis of physical evaluation and testing. The average cholesterol in this group is 150–160 mg%. So here is an active group, eating a diet which should lead to high blood cholesterol and evidence of atherosclerosis, that does not fit the simplified conclusion that dietary cholesterol equals increased blood cholesterol and then evidence of disease.

In 1964, this group was first evaluated on a clinical basis by physical examination and electrocardiogram, and at the time it was felt to be quite remarkable that the tribesmen exhibited no evidence of disease on the basis of examination, despite their way of life and food intake. It was felt, on the basis of this initial examination, that physical fitness and exercise was the key to their lack of disease.

In 1972, eight years later, autopsy studies were performed on fifty tribesmen. It was found that there was extensive atherosclerosis present, far in advance of that seen in Western cultures. The arteries were of larger caliber, developed by exercise in the presence of disease, which prevented detection clinically. But then, why did a blood cholesterol testing show levels of only 150–160 mg% when there was actually extensive atherosclerosis present, and a high intake of cholesterol and fat?

In 1974, a further study showed that a large intake of milk led to a decrease in the blood cholesterol. This was proved by feeding fermented milk to these same subjects for a period of twenty-one days. So, a low blood cholesterol does not mean the absence of disease, if the blood cholesterol is decreased by other means than dietary restriction. Decreasing the level in the blood in this case was achieved by increased deposits in the blood vessel walls. The fat was "banked" for the time being, and did not show up in the blood level tests.

There is more to the effect of dietary cholesterol than just the cholesterol content of the diet alone, and a serum cholesterol count does not always indicate the degree of atherosclerosis. Nor does clinical evaluation help to discover these abnormal arteries before symptomatic disease emerges. As is usually the case, there is truth to all sides of the story. We should be limiting the dietary intake of cholesterol in some individuals. The problem is in recognizing those who are susceptible to the effects of cholesterol intake.

WHAT FACTORS INFLUENCE THE DECISION TO CUT DOWN ON CHOLESTEROL-RICH FOODS?

Many factors influence the fate of cholesterol intake in our diet. *It is often only as bad as the company it keeps.* The amount of cholesterol consumed on a vegetarian diet is much less absorbed than that consumed on the usual American high-fat diet. Certain fibers in the diet, such as pectin, can lower total body cholesterol by preventing absorption, whereas wheat bran does not have this effect.

When the blood cholesterol is lowered by other factors in the diet, taking effect after the cholesterol is absorbed, it may not be of any benefit *if the cholesterol is not excreted.* If the lowering of the blood cholesterol is by deposition in the body tissues—which include the arteries—then lowering the blood cholesterol by eating polyunsaturated fatty acids may lead to a false impression about the degree of atherosclerosis. In other words, the cholesterol may be "banked" in the form of plaques on the arterial walls and not show up in the blood level tests.

Again, there is a great deal of *individual variability,* a term that may be overused *but cannot be overemphasized.* The balance of our genetic traits or adaptability to intake of cholesterol, the other nutrients which effect the absorption, utilization, and excretion of cholesterol—all are important when we discuss the fate or destiny of the molecule of cholesterol which, with all of its brother and sister molecules, can end up in the artery wall. This is a gradual process through a lifetime which can be shortened by this buildup.

Cholesterol is not a Lone Ranger but is a member of the Atherosclerosis Gang that works to take away our health by damaging arteries and robbing blood flow. This results in lack of oxygen to the tissue, causing a heart attack or stroke to the victim. The Atherosclerosis Gang is made up of a variety of nutritional variables and metabolic participants. When all of these are considered, it is possible to understand why the *cause of atherosclerosis* is still wearing a mask and is unknown.

The amount of cholesterol in the diet is affected by a variety of other nutritional companions in the food, and also by the metabolic products of the intestinal wall, the liver, and the artery lining and wall.

In populations with a blood cholesterol of 150 mg% or less, owing to restricted intake of cholesterol, all of these influences are evidently working less to produce atherosclerosis. When the blood cholesterol exceeds 150 mg% then all of the variables participate more effectively, in direct proportion to the degree of elevation of the blood cholesterol above 150 mg%. Certainly, when a blood level is above 200 mg%, metabolism in the body is dependent on the composition of the diet.

If all of these nutritional and metabolic factors are in favorable balance, then the dietary cholesterol may not produce atherosclerosis. Our understanding of these factors is becoming more clear as we learn more about the way cholesterol is carried in the blood and about the changes that must take place in the wall of the artery to produce a plaque. These changes are related to:

1. The absorption of cholesterol through the intestinal wall.
2. The effectiveness of excretion of cholesterol in bile.
3. The inhibition of cholesterol production by tissues in the body.
4. Changes in lipoprotein metabolism by the liver.

Cholesterol is carried in the blood in three forms:

1. Low-density lipoprotein (LDL).
2. High-density lipoprotein (HDL).
3. Very low-density lipoprotein (VLDL).

LDL and HDL are the current bad and good guys (in that order) for cholesterol. The LDL is the damaging type of cholesterol, whereas that carried in the form of good HDL is not deposited in blood vessel walls and supposedly is carried to the liver, where cholesterol is excreted. The VLDL is largely triglyceride. As VLDL (triglyceride) increases, the good HDL decreases (so does protection), so that bad LDL can do more damage.

At this time, when predicting the susceptibility to atherosclerosis, the LDL and HDL are in the spotlight. Since the VLDL form is largely triglyceride, less attention is given to this form of lipoprotein. Again, this corresponds with the oversight previously mentioned about the importance of triglycerides. There is some suggestion that the product of the VLDL breakdown may be a stimulant for the entrance of bad LDL into the artery wall. Also, it is known that when the triglycerides are increased, the good HDL is decreased. So the triglyceride perhaps should have some of the spotlight now focused on cholesterol.

We may find that the fractions of blood lipids containing triglyceride have been the silent partner in this whole scheme of atherosclerosis, when the final cause is understood. Certainly, more attention to the nonfasting level of triglyceride and a reevaluation of a true normal fasting triglyceride would seem very much in order. It might be that the relationship of cholesterol and triglyceride to development of disease can be well illustrated by sleight of hand, as in magic. The cholesterol of the right hand has created a diversion so that the triglyceride of the left hand has produced its effects *without being observed.*

WHY DO SOME NUTRITIONISTS SAY TO LIMIT EGG CONSUMPTION AND OTHERS SAY THAT YOU CAN EAT ALL THE EGGS YOU WANT?

It's true that great confusion surrounds the subject of cholesterol. A report on diet by the Food and Nutrition Board of the National Academy of Sciences in May 1980 stated that they found no reason for the average healthy American to reduce the intake of cholesterol and fat. This raised an outcry in the medical and scientific community, who claimed that such a report would be misleading and would undo the excellent progress Americans have recently made in reducing fats (including the saturated fats) in the diet. Take your choice of the expert opinions—but hope that it is the right one, for your life is at risk!

The cholesterol in eggs would seem to be different from crystalline or pure cholesterol, since other nutrients contained in eggs might offset the effects of cholesterol. But in experiments where individuals have attained extremely low cholesterol levels after complete restriction of cholesterol for a period of time, they have returned to the previous level of high cholesterol when given unlimited eggs.

The stand of Aerobic Nutrition is to restrict the use of eggs to several a week, but not to eliminate them entirely. It is the egg yolk that has the saturated fat content, and egg whites may be used in unlimited quantities.

When you plan to have eggs for breakfast or lunch, it would be wise to plan to have fish, veal, or poultry for dinner, thereby cutting down on the high saturated fat content of the day by skipping beef.

HOW CAN A PERSON KNOW HOW MUCH SATURATED FAT AND UNSATURATED FAT IS IN THE DAILY INTAKE?

It's easiest to figure out if you count calories. Aerobic Nutrition permits 10 percent of the calories you eat to contain saturated fat, and 10 percent unsaturated fat. If you eat 1,500 calories during the entire day, 150 may be in the total of all saturated fat and 150 in the total of all unsaturated fat. That adds up to a total of 20 percent of fat in the Aerobic Nutrition way of eating, as compared to the national average of 45 percent.

IF SATURATED FAT IS SO BAD FOR YOUR ARTERIES, WHY DO YOU PERMIT ANY AT ALL?

Interestingly, the United States Department of Agriculture also published a statement in May 1980 that stated: "Eating equal amounts of polyunsaturated fats and saturated fats, as well as fewer total fats, lowered high blood pressure in the U.S. Department of Agriculture experiments."

James Iacono of the USDA's Science and Education Administration reported that in three separate studies of seventy healthy human subjects, both men and women between forty and sixty years old, blood pressure was reduced to the normal range from the moderately hypertensive state by equalizing the amounts of polyunsaturated fats and saturated fats in the diets.

Researchers are now pointing to dietary fats as one of the factors which may increase the occurrence of high blood pressure, a silent killer which claims hundreds of thousands of American lives each year.

Iacono confirmed that pills that reduce blood pressure suppress the symptoms while the disease process continues. While the mechanism of blood pressure reduction still is not fully understood, Iacono suggested that a class of compounds called "prostaglandins" might be involved. These prostaglandins, which arise in the body from polyunsaturated fatty acids, may serve as hormonal type regulators, increasing the salt and water excretion as well as the blood pressure in peripheral blood vessels.

During the course of these experiments, the subjects' weights remained constant, eliminating the known effect of weight loss in reducing blood pressure. These research findings suggest that the types of fats eaten, in equal proportions, are an important factor in lowering both systolic and diastolic pressure.

As part of the experiment, Iacono and his colleagues were able to reverse the process and elevate blood pressure by increasing the proportion of saturated fats relative to polyunsatured fats in the diets.

These findings confirm epidemiological studies done by Iacono and his colleagues in Finland, southern Italy, and the United States.

WHAT OTHER FACTORS MAY AFFECT CHOLESTEROL?

Besides the link to hereditary factors and the balance of saturated and unsaturated fats in the diet, the amount of sugar intake, fiber intake, excess body weight, and frequency of meals can have an effect. Also involved are alcohol intake, the amount of milk and yogurt in the diet, and the level of emotional distress at the time of cholesterol testing.

Good habits that can prevent high cholesterol levels are lowered sugar intake, increased fiber intake, normal body weight, and evenly distributed calories in three fat- and sugar-controlled meals spaced evenly throughout the day. Minimum alcoholic intake and a "cool composure" are your best allies in keeping cholesterol levels on the low side of the normal range.

Lowering the blood cholesterol by any means other than dietary restriction of cholesterol-rich foods may not have a favorable effect on the development of plugging material in the large arteries. It has been shown that when sucrose or sugar is replaced by complex carbohydrates, such as fruits, leafy vegetables, and legumes (beans), there is a decrease in serum cholesterol. Most recently, it has also been shown that protein from plants has a lowering effect on cholesterol as compared to protein of animal origin. The combination of legumes and grains can provide a complete protein meal from plant origin, without any saturated fat (automatically part of animal protein intake).

The distribution of meals is very important, with three equal meals per day having a lowering effect on cholesterol as compared to one large meal or gorging on a daily basis.

Obesity or excess calories also produce higher levels of cholesterol than do normal weight and controlled caloric intake.

The relationship of milk and yogurt to blood cholesterol levels is also significant. The study of the Masais of Africa showed that although they have a diet that promotes atherosclerosis particularly in the males, who eat mostly beef, blood, and milk, the milk in the diet had a cholesterol-lowering effect on the blood. But remember too, that it did not prevent the development of advanced atherosclerosis. The Masai gained some protection by exercise, which enlarged the blood vessels—the only problem is that the Masai had activity at the level required to train for a marathon, which is a level beyond the reach of many of us.

Several good studies have demonstrated that stress has a definite adverse effect on blood cholesterol. Stress significantly increases the blood cholesterol, as has been shown in metabolic ward studies as well as in healthy medical students under stress of examination.

SO, MEASURES TO PREVENT THE FORMATION OF PLAQUES ON THE ARTERIAL WALLS SHOULD HELP A PERSON TO LIVE LONGER?

Possibly. But the prime focus of Aerobic Nutrition is to help a person to live a lifetime that is free of degenerative disease—to live it usefully, with an agile body and an alert mind.

The subject of cholesterol was presented because it affects the oxygen delivery system. Obstruction of blood flow by damage or buildup in the arteries prevents the red blood cells from doing their job of delivering oxygen to the tissues and cells of the entire body. Get those arteries opened up wide all of your life, and then prevent the blood cells from sludging up the oxygen delivery system, so you can enjoy good health every day of your life!

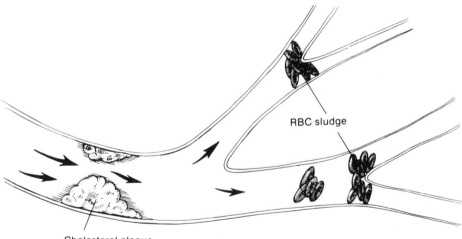

RBC sludge

Cholesterol plaque

FOOD ALLERGIES

Everyone knows that a medical doctor who specializes in the field of allergy can administer scratch tests to determine food or environmental factors to which you may be sensitive. Perhaps you react to these substances with hives, sneezes, or itchy eyes.

What everyone doesn't know is that you might have a silent food allergy that doesn't show up on the scratch tests. It could be responsible for erratic mood swings, headaches, chronic depression, hyperactivity, and a multitude of other strange reactions. Not all doctors acknowledge that this is true, and there is plenty of medication available to mask the symptoms that continue to plague a large group of people.

As many as thirty years ago, Dr. Theron Randolph of Chicago was claiming that food and environmental allergies were causing behavioral disorders. Many doctors all over the country have followed his lead and have developed techniques to uncover these sensitivities. They include intradermal testing, sublingual testing, and the elimination diet. Some sophisticated methods have been developed lately using cytotoxic testing and a blood test known as the RAST test (radioallergosorbent test) that is the most painless of all.

The Huxley Institute in New York City has been set up as an information center for orthomolecular and preventive medicine, keeping rosters of medical practitioners who have specialities in this area of medicine. At this date, the word is out, and doctors who have trouble diagnosing the source of unexplainable headaches and earaches are resorting to these tests to find out whether the cause could be a food biocontamination.

Once the food sensitivity has been established by testing, the usual procedure is to eliminate that food and all of its relatives from your diet. Sometimes that is easier said than done—especially when the allergen is a common food staple such as milk, wheat, eggs, or corn. You must become a master food detective to be able to ferret out such hidden ingredients in your everyday foods. These days, food labels may help you, but it also is important to know the ingredients of fabricated foods so you will be able to avoid a substance to which you may be sensitive.

DAIRY PRODUCTS

If you are sensitive to milk, you are probably also sensitive to buttermilk, chocolate milk, skim milk, cream, dairy sour cream, yogurt, and butter. Watch out for nondairy products that may have milk solids added. Avoid all bakery products that may be made with any of these items, and avoid creamed soups, creamed sauces, and all cheeses. Some people who have a lactose intolerance find that they can tolerate a cultured product that has had some bacterial action, such as yogurt or cottage cheese. Also, there are some special products on the market that can be added to regular milk to make it possible for those people with a lactose intolerance to have it. But generally speaking, those people who have an actual allergy to milk and its byproducts will not be able to use them. Some soy milk products are rather palatable, but they are not much of a substitute for the real thing. Children with this allergy should be guided by a nutritionist to be sure that they get adequate amounts of calcium in the diet from dark green leafy vegetables. When dining out, don't hesitate to ask whether any of these dairy products have been used in the preparation of the dish you are considering. Particularly avoid pancakes, waffles, omelets, puddings, and any creamed dishes.

EGGS

Naturally you will eliminate eggs completely if you are allergic to them. Also, avoid mayonnaise and other creamy salad dressings, meatloaf, pancakes, waffles, malted cocoa drinks, cake mixes, breads, breaded foods, ice cream, pasta, and marshmallows. Read all labels to be sure that dried egg is not listed as an ingredient.

WHEAT

If you are sensitive to wheat, you will have to omit all bran products, pancakes, waffles, breads, cookies, crackers, cakes, breaded foods, pasta, and even some candies. Generally a gluten allergy extends to the gluten relatives of wheat—rye, barley, and oats. The grains that may be used in place of wheat are corn, millet, and a number of others that you may find in a health food store. However, since these grains lack gluten, they will not have the fine texture of wheat when baked and will probably need extra baking powder to leaven them.

When ordering at a restaurant, avoid fried foods as much for the possibility of wheat in the batter as the fact that other wheat products may have been cooked in the deep-fat fryer. Fried foods at home may be dipped into a batter made of seasoned beaten egg whites, or into beaten egg and then cornstarch or crushed corn flakes.

CORN

You may feel relieved when you hear that the allergen is corn, thinking that you don't ever eat much corn anyway. That may not be true, if you consider the fact that cornstarch, popcorn, corn oil, corn syrup, dextrose, hominy, grits, and corn bread can not be used either. Also, do not lick envelopes or stamps, since they often have corn-based glue. Talcum powder, vitamin pills, and many other products rely on the versatility of corn, so it is a tricky substance to avoid. Read all labels with great care.

SUGAR

This is often a culprit in the allergic person's sensitivity profile. Avoid all white sugar, brown sugar, honey, corn syrup, fructose, syrups, baked goods, ice cream, puddings, gelatins, and sweetened desserts. Use only natural fruit juice concentrates for sweetening power, and opt for desserts of fresh fruit and cheese.

5. THE MANNERBERG METHOD OF MOVEMENT

How much you move during each day can affect your health. Notice that the word used is *move* rather than *exercise.*

Think of your body as an object that should be in constant motion. Remember how much a baby moves its legs and arms, wriggles its midsection, turns its head from side to side, creeps and crawls, pulls itself up to climb, walks and falls down only to get up and walk some more, and seems to have more energy than a barrel of monkeys? Spending energy seems to beget more energy as the baby moves to satisfy its curiosity about this wonderful state of being called life.

What happens to that baby when it grows up? If it is like the typical person of this century, that baby learned how to be moved rather than to move itself. It rides on escalators and elevators rather than climbing stairs. It rides in a car rather than on a bicycle. It walks as little as possible, rather than as much as possible. It uses modern machinery to prevent as much bending and stretching, tilling and hoeing, scrubbing and sweeping, as can be avoided.

Instead of yesteryear's sandlot baseball game, our modern grown man is cheering a few fellows who play games on the television set. The body is supine for hours. It is permitted to rest so much that the muscles get weakened, the heart pump is on constant idle, the lungs are not forced to expand, and the sedentary life begins to affect the entire body.

Our kicks are coming from situation comedies instead of participating in a fast-paced country barn dance. By the time age forty or fifty rolls around, the typical American is moving less and less and is sliding into a serious state of degenerative disease onset. Hardly a laughing matter, but we take it as a natural evolution of our human condition. We expect that old age means having sickness and becoming disabled. But it doesn't have to be that way!

THE ALTERNATIVES TO DOING NOTHING

Approximately 60 million people or about 27 percent of the population of this country is exercising regularly, with about 3 percent of those being joggers. Over 40 percent of the Americans have changed their diet in some fashion for health reasons, and 88 percent would like to know more about nutrition as related to health.

Anyone who has been in the practice of preventive medicine or physical fitness for very many years realizes that the major problem facing these programs is *motivation*. Exercise fads come and go, as is demonstrated by the number of pieces of athletic equipment that are gathering dust in garages and attics. If every piece of athletic equipment that has been purchased were used regularly, very few in this country would not be engaging in regular physical activity.

There are many people who, because of their psychological makeup, cannot program themselves to adhere to a long-standing disciplined physical activity under any circumstances. Are these people then to be denied the benefits of feeling well and being resistant to disease?

The evidence available on exercise, nutrition, and stress with regard to the oxygen delivery system, as well as the utilization of oxygen at the cellular level, shows that there are more ways than one to preserve good health. You are not condemned to a lesser state of health because you cannot make yourself exercise with regularity. Those who exercise should be encouraged to continue to do so throughout life to enjoy all the obvious health benefits. But the 73 percent of the population not exercising on a regular basis can also obtain health benefits from a different approach that may work better for them.

Some people may not be inclined to be physically active. The middle-aged person who has developed a pattern of behavior with regard to exercise may not be able to modify it with any degree of enthusiasm. For such a person, a concept of keeping the body in motion (rather than performing regular athletic rituals) is in order.

The key word is *motion*. Keep the body moving. Stop sitting and lying down for long periods of time. Stretch little-used muscles. Walk, hop, skip, bend, reach, sweep the walk, rake the lawn, dance, get on a bike, swim a lap, scrub the floor, wash a window—get yourself moving. Try to keep your body in motion as much as possible during each day.

HOW CAN A NONATHLETIC PERSON BEGIN TO GET ACTIVE AGAIN?

If you want to increase activity in your life style, program motion into your day:

1. Walk the stairs in your office building. If there are too many floors, walk the corridors briskly during your coffee break and skip the doughnut wagon. Use your car less for short trips in the neighborhood and walk instead.
2. Use lunch hours for physical activity that does not require time lost in changing clothes or having to shower. Try a brisk walk around the neighborhood for fifteen minutes before having an Aerobic Nutrition lunch.

3. Arrange your desk and environs so that you will have to move to reach things, especially if you have a sedentary job. Stand up frequently to move your muscles around.
4. Take back some of the jobs you have designated to someone else, like gardening or house-cleaning chores. Use them to bend, stretch, and use as many muscles as you can.
5. Don't sit in front of the television set for long periods of time. You may be entertaining your mind, but you are deteriorating your body.

CAN WALKING AND DOING SIMPLE CHORES BE AS GOOD AS OCCASIONAL SPORTS EXERCISE?

It can be better! Lower levels of physical activity that are done throughout a lifetime are more beneficial than higher levels of exertion that are sporadic or inconsistent. Too often a person who attempts to jog will be successful only a part of the year when the weather is good. The occasional athlete, with his cycle of training and untraining, can be compared to the fad dieter who loses and regains weight within any one year. Extraordinary activity for physical fitness can be a fad too. It's better to program constant movement into your waking hours if you can't have a regular sports exercise regime.

WHY SOME PEOPLE ARE MORE ACTIVE THAN OTHERS

There is an overwhelming natural human instinct that attracts us to the pleasures of gluttony and laziness. This is further promoted by an environment that stimulates this weakness for profit.

Are you nonathletic because of the way you live or because of your personality type? Personality is a major factor in the selection of a type of activity and in the ability to withstand the discomforts of training and to persist throughout a lifetime.

Motivation is the emotional commitment to take a positive action to obtain certain goals. This is undoubtedly the most important psychological determinant in maintaining fitness training in the initial stages of participation. This is the selection factor that separates athletes from nonathletes, a trait apparent even in childhood.

In a study done at the U.S. Military Academy, two distinct groups were found. The athletes were the ones who had been previous letter award winners in school participation. They were more dominant, enthusiastic, adventurous, tough, group-dependent, sophisticated, and conservative than those cadets with little or no previous participation in sports. After four years of compulsive exercise participation as part of the cadet training, the testing was repeated. The personality structure of the nonathletic group did not change. They did not develop the personality traits of the athletes.

This same type of study has been done with students of various categories, comparing low-fitness groups to a high-fitness group and the effect of a training program on the low-fitness groups. Again, a compulsory training period did not produce personality changes. Therefore, we must accept that certain individuals do not have a natural attraction to physical activity or sports. It is this group that should be aware of those effects of exercise beyond its cardiovascular effects.

There is no reason for nonathletic people to be condemned to a lesser level of health fitness because of their intrinsic lack of need for such outlets. Relaxation techniques and yoga may be better suited for them. But people in this personality group need all the benefits of Aerobic Nutrition, since there is no compensation by vigorous regular exercise.

The most important factor necessary for compulsory long-term participation in endurance training is the ability to endure the discomfort of physical stress and fatigue. Perhaps we are measuring the compulsive drives that motivate people to endurance activities when we are evaluating physical fitness. There are truly different strokes for different folks, and it is productive to use this information to individualize your choice of physical activity.

THE DIFFERENCE BETWEEN BED REST AND MARATHON RUNNING

Bed rest and marathon running are obviously two extremes of what you can do with your body. Perhaps by examining these extremes, it will be possible to demonstrate what the problems are in motivation and adherence to a program of exercise.

Continuous bed rest produces many adverse effects on metabolism and endurance. The bones demineralize and become softer through lack of use, causing a loss of calcium even though calcium has been included in the diet. When there is no change in the calorie intake, there is an increase in body fat in the person who has had too much bed rest. Muscle weakness develops, and it is often accompanied by atrophy or loss of muscle mass. These effects can be seen when an arm is placed in a cast for a few weeks; when the cast is removed, comparison of the arms is surprising.

Studies comparing bed rest to physical training show that physical endurance after a three-week period of bed rest is greatly reduced. These are the negative aspects of complete bed rest, which is the extreme example of inactivity.

The opposite extreme of bed rest is the physical endurance required for a marathon runner. The requirements of time, motivation, pain, and persistence are beyond the possible commitment of more than 99 percent of our population. Only an estimated 75,000 people out of the 220,000,000 population in the United States participated in marathons during 1979.

Lack of time is frequently used as a reason for avoiding physical activity.

Thirty minutes a day for three to five days a week is no small matter, and of course much more time must be committed for the extreme of marathon training. But even in the area of lesser achievement for the sake of aerobic physical fitness, there still is a minimal time requirement.

The difficulty of adhering to any physical training program is a major obstacle to large-scale participation. Such training requires a system of deprogramming or unlearning a lifetime of addiction to physical inactivity that results from a society that depends on labor-saving devices and spectator activities. Motivation is needed to counteract the effects of such entrenched behavior.

Pain is very much a part of endurance activities, since there are not only the aches and pains of tired, sore muscles, but also the discomfort of fatigue which is required to improve the physical performance. During the early stages of a conditioning or training program, this is perhaps a major obstacle, since it is our natural instinct to avoid discomfort and pain.

The strain on lower extremities in running or jumping may cause considerable injuries in beginning exercisers. It has been demonstrated that beginning joggers have increased foot, leg, and knee injuries when training is performed more than three days a week and more than thirty minutes per exercise.

A survey has shown that 60 percent of those who run regularly to an endurance level suffer chronic injuries to the lower extremities. It is these resulting adversities of physical training that limit acceptance by the population in general.

Therefore, it is important to engage in these physical stress activities with a degree of caution, especially when they are undertaken in the middle years of life. There are many physical activities that do not involve stress and strain on joints but can produce beneficial physical effect. You don't have to run marathons to get some movement back into your modus operandi!

Many people can be highly motivated for short periods before time pressures and low tolerance for pain destroy the motivation. For every jogger in this country, there are many former joggers. Aerobic exercise, particularly marathon training, requires a commitment of time, motivation, and tolerance of pain with persistence over a lifetime to be effective!

Somewhere between these two extremes is a practical, beneficial, and possible program for everyone. Life itself is a physical activity, and when there is a breakdown in health it is often measured by the limitation in activity. The inability to move or the restriction of the capacity for physical activity can drastically limit participation in work and play. It is a life-spoiler.

After all, in order to survive, we must struggle against gravity throughout our lives. We adapt to this stress for survival. When the body is used in increased levels of activity, there is a stress or strain required that makes this increased level of performance possible.

This chapter on body movement is dedicated to the millions of people who are not receiving the benefits of regular physical activity. On a physical scale of 1 to 10, with bed rest being 1 and a marathon being 10, there should be some area of activity between 4 and 6 that is adaptable to every life style. The problem is finding it and incorporating it into a lifetime habit—a choice we can all make.

LEVEL OF ACTIVITY

The simple statement "Different strokes for different folks" is much more complicated than it seems, when it comes to choosing a form of physical activity that suits you. That's why the more you know about why you need some form of body movement, the more you will analyze what you can do on a continuous basis to meet that need.

There is something for everyone relating to use of the body, from the broad spectrum of relaxation techniques to the extremes of endurance training for marathons. Some relaxation techniques that involve muscle manipulation are body massage and acupressure.

When deciding on an activity for participation for the rest of your life, the key thing to consider is the goal you have in mind. These goals can be any or all of the following:

1. Relaxation or stress reduction.
2. Endurance.
3. Strength.
4. Flexibility.
5. Weight control.
6. Improved figure or appearance.

These can be further modified by:

1. Personality and aptitudes.
2. Age and sex.
3. Life style or financial considerations.

The combination of all of the goals, plus the modifying factors, shows the wide range of the choices to be made—no one need be eliminated from engaging in some form of activity.

It is possible to choose an exercise that helps to improve flexibility, enhance appearance, and aid relaxation or reduce stress without the strain and pain of producing strength or endurance. Combining a conditioning program with a competitive or skilled activity can accomplish several goals at once. Many people who are tennis or racquetball players also engage in jogging and other conditioning programs to improve their skills or their ability to perform on the court. Dancers who develop the body control to create an art form must have strengthening and stretching exercises in order to be able to perform with grace.

Of course it is better to develop physical activity habits early in life to ensure continued participation later on. Often physical decline and loss of health begins with the marriage ceremony, as commitments to the home and marriage reduce the time available for an exercise program. Maybe couples should take an additional vow—that because they love and cherish each other, they will continue a physical fitness program that will allow them a lifetime of health instead of sickness.

Again, be reminded that sporadic impulsive attempts at exercise are more of a hazard than a help. These fall into the same category as fad dieting, which also produces a short-term effect that is not good because it results in a long-term series of failures. Any level of physical activity that is continued throughout a lifetime at some level is bound to produce some long-range benefits. Moving your body more and walking more each day is an easy step in the right direction to good health.

WHY BE PHYSICALLY ACTIVE?

Perhaps you are one of those who finds it difficult to believe such statements as one the philosopher Maimonides made in 1199: "Anyone that leads a sedentary life and does not exercise, even if he eats good foods and takes care of himself according to good medical principles, all his days will be painful ones and his strength shall wane."

While science toils to conquer disease and condemn the ethics of alternative therapies, we must avoid the complete dependence on either of these approaches by changing the real cause of functional decline and loss of health—the way we live. Diagnosis and cures are not needed where disease doesn't exist. When the internal structure of our bodies is kept strong by providing optimal amounts of essentials such as oxygen, we enjoy better health and less loss of physical and mental ability with the process of aging.

Loving rich food and hating exercise, while living at a hectic pace, are health hazards that must be dealt with in a total program. Physical activity plays a major role in health, but it cannot do the job alone.

Better health is the true benefit of being physically active, rather than the prevention of disease (which has yet to be proven). A zestful and productive life that is being lived to the optimal capability is the real goal, and it can be achieved. It is entirely possible that activity makes us more resistant to the breakdown of health. The best insurance of a healthy future is living well today by including some level of physical activity to prevent physical decline.

HOW ACTIVITIES BURN UP CALORIES

If you don't want to store excess calories in fatty sacs all over your body, you have to burn them off. Excess calories are those not used up in your usual daily activities. There are 3,500 calories in each pound of stored fat on your body. They represent 500 excess calories a day for one week.

The calorie expenditures for walking, jogging, and cycling depend not only on speed but on the size of the person. Here is a chart that will help you to determine how much you can burn up if you are moving at the rate of 6 miles per hour:

120 pounds	76 calories per mile
140 pounds	88 calories per mile
160 pounds	100 calories per mile
180 pounds	112 calories per mile
200 pounds	120 calories per mile
220 pounds	136 calories per mile

You can see that a 160-pound person uses 600 calories per hour in comparison to a 200-pound person using 720 calories per hour. The oxygen required and energy used depend on the size of the person as well as the pace and distance traveled. In Aerobic Nutrition, the amount of oxygen used is directly related to the energy expenditure or calories used.

As the Activity Equivalents table shows, you can burn as many calories in

ACTIVITY EQUIVALENTS

ENERGY USED (CALORIES/HOUR)	WALK OR JOG (LEVEL)	CYCLING (LEVEL)	OTHER ACTIVITIES
90–240	2 mile/hour	5 mile/hour	doing light housework, typing, playing musical instrument, mowing lawn, playing golf with power cart, bowling, continuous auto driving, sewing, bartending, climbing up 24 steps, 5 inches
240–300	3 mile/hour	6 mile/hour	high
300–360	3.5 mile/hour	8 mile/hour	dancing Fox trot, roller skating, performing most calisthenics, playing ping pong, playing tennis doubles, hoeing, cross-country hiking, trotting on horseback, climbing up 24 steps, 7 inches
360–420	4 mile/hour	10 mile/hour	high
420–480	5 mile/hour walk	11 mile/hour	playing tennis singles, square dancing, walking upstairs, skiing
480–540	5½ mile/hour jog	12 mile/hour	down hill, water skiing, climbing up 24 steps, 12 inches high
540–600	5.5 mile/hour	13 mile/hour	playing racketball, vigorous shoveling, playing advanced
660 or more	6.0 mile/hour or faster	14 mile/hour or faster	competitive sports, cross-country skiing

daily activities as in heavy exercise. The energy expenditures are based on averages for a 150-pound person, but they can vary widely depending on the intensity of the activity and the degree of individual skill.

AEROBIC EXERCISE

Oxygen is the single most important element for survival of the human body from minute to minute. Oxygen delivery is a dynamic survival process which cannot be interrupted without cell death, tissue damage, and finally death. The word *aerobic* pertains to the ability to *use oxygen.*

Aerobic exercise has become very popular in the physical fitness movement in the United States. It is a system which measures the maximum level of physical endurance and the capacity for performing physical work. It involves the oxygen delivery system whereby air is taken in by the lungs, where it is diffused into the blood, which is carried largely by the red blood cells. The cells are pumped to the various parts of the body by the heart, carried by the blood vessels to the small capillaries, and the oxygen is delivered to other body cells, to keep them in optimum working order.

HOW DOES EXERCISE HELP TO DELIVER OXYGEN TO BODY CELLS?

Exercise improves this oxygen delivery system by increasing the maximum capacity of the lungs, strengthening the heart, enlarging the major blood vessels, and ensuring that oxygen will be delivered to the cells in the muscle group that is being used. As you increase the level of physical fitness with exercise, the ability to utilize oxygen is increased. You also increase the ability to deliver nutrients throughout the body via the same circulatory system.

CAN VIGOROUS EXERCISE CAUSE MUSCULOSKELETAL PROBLEMS?

Striving for an aerobic effect from exercise is shown to be desirable, since cardiovascular benefits are certainly protective against developing the complications of atherosclerosis—mainly heart attack and stroke. When this level of activity is the goal of exercise, then certain complications must be dealt with. One study of a group of sixty-eight middle-aged sedentary men who participated for two months in hard physical training suffered a high frequency of orthopedic problems. The training program consisted of running, muscle strength exercises, and playing ball two to three times a week for eight to ten weeks. During this period of time there were six cases of Achilles tendonitis, eight cases of sprained ankle, eleven cases with symptoms of calf and knee problems, one case of a fracture, and four cases of headache. Muscle pains of the type commonly produced by physical exertion were not regarded as a complication. In the whole group, 19 percent had difficulties to the extent that they quit the training program, but fifty-four of the original sixty-eight were able to complete the two months of training.

DOES ALL AEROBIC EXERCISE HAVE TO BE AS VIGOROUS AS RUNNING AND JOGGING?

Not necessarily. Dr. Michael Pollock reported in 1971 that a significant aerobic training effect could be achieved with vigorous walking. He tested sixteen untrained men who averaged 48.9 years of age. They trained for forty minutes daily, by walking between 2.5 and 3.25 miles. After twenty weeks of this vigorous walking, they showed an increase in the maximum oxygen intake capacity of 28 percent and in pulmonary ventilation of 15 percent. Their resting blood pressure was significantly decreased as well the percentage of body fat. This study concluded that vigorous walking training had a significant effect on cardiovascular function and body composition in adult men. Other studies and measurements of the effects of walking have also indicated that fitness can be achieved with continuous vigorous walking for regular periods of time each day, no matter what age or level of activity you have participated in before you start.

THE MANNERBERG SUPERSTRIDE

When you recognize at last the need to be physically active and decide that a regular vigorous walking program is the best course of action for you, it's time to consider the *Superstride.*

Jogging speed falls in the range of seven to twelve minutes per mile. When you cover a mile in less than than seven to eight minutes, then you can call yourself a runner. The Superstride is to walking what running is to jogging.

The mechanics of walking depend on shifting of the center of gravity and the force exerted by the back leg while in contact with the ground. As demonstrated in the illustration, the walk, the stride, and the run differ in the degree of force applied from the back foot and the length of stride that is achieved by the forward placement of the front foot.

Walking is primarily an up-and-down motion, with a lift from the back foot producing an upward motion and propelling the body forward. In running, there is more of a thrust with the back foot and a lengthening of the stride, with a compensating wider swing of the arms. This increased thrust of the back foot and the increased movement of the upper extremities require increased energy. In running or jogging, the speed or pace depends on the degree of thrust from the back leg as well as the length of the stride, rather than a lift as in walking. In running or jogging both feet leave the ground and the forward foot actually creates an impact on contact with the running surface.

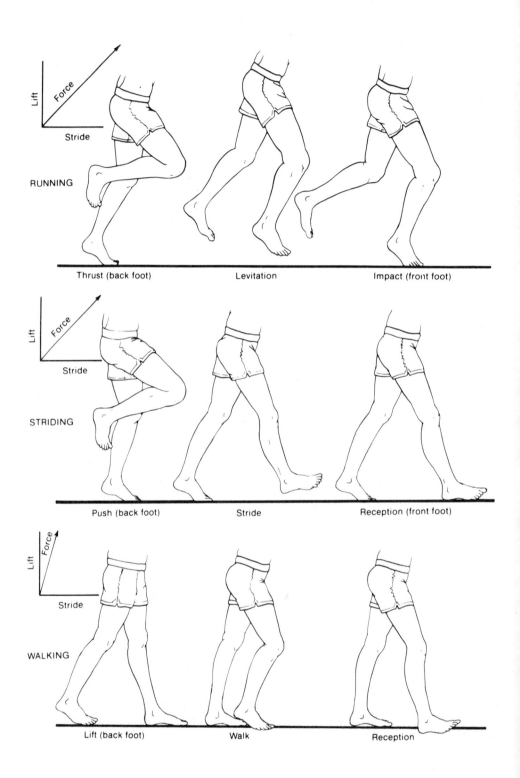

RUNNING

Thrust (back foot)   Levitation   Impact (front foot)

STRIDING

Push (back foot)   Stride   Reception (front foot)

WALKING

Lift (back foot)   Walk   Reception

The difference among these three levels of locomotion is that a stride is an intermediate activity between walking and jogging. Striding has a higher energy requirement than walking but it produces *much less impact* on the joints, since the forward foot touches the ground before the back foot pushes forward.

The forward foot connects with the ground in a rocking motion; as the toe of the back foot is pushing forward, the heel of the forward foot is in contact with the walking surface. As the weight on the forward foot transfers from the heel to the toe, the forward foot becomes the back foot and begins the push for the next step.

The Superstride is designed to increase the pace of walking and emphasize the push of the back foot to lengthen the stride. To create a greater energy need in the upper part of the body as well, your arms should be freely swinging up and down, rather than simply back and forth. This exaggerated stride length and upward movement of the arms will swing most of the body muscles into action, without the jarring impact that can cause the skeletal problems associated with jogging and running. Try to practice the Superstride for thirty minutes a day, at least five times a week.

WILL YOU LOOK RIDICULOUS AS YOU STRIDE AND WAVE YOUR ARMS UP AND DOWN?

Americans have grown accustomed to the sight of joggers and runners sweating and panting in all stages of dress. Striding can be done in your street clothes, with normal walking shoes, and is readily identified as a form of exercise. Degenerative disease onset from lack of body movement is ridiculous, so why should people look askance at a positive effort toward physical fitness? We predict that the Superstride will meet the exercise needs of many who cannot undertake a more vigorous endeavor. We hope that it will spread like an infectious disease to boost the physical fitness of more of the great unmoving population.

6. VITAMINS AND MINERALS

The body depends on vitamins and minerals for continued normal function. If you are interested in prolonging well-being, rather than waiting to do something after your body is in trouble and in need of crisis medical attention, it is important to understand the role of vitamins and minerals in maintaining good health.

Too many people are self-medicating on extreme amounts of vitamins with very little knowledge of what they are doing to themselves. True, there is an area of medical practice in which megadoses of supplements are used as therapy (this branch of medicine is currently called orthomolecular medicine), but such doses are generally used to treat disease and should be established by a specialist who knows what the side effects of overdosing can be.

Aerobic Nutrition is a stay-well system, not a promotion of the use of nutrients as disease therapy. You will find a formula of vitamins and minerals at the end of this chapter to show you what a normal range for each vitamin should be. It would be wise to discuss vitamin and mineral supplementation with a knowledgeable medical doctor before deciding what is best for you.

WHY TAKE VITAMINS IF YOU EAT A WELL-BALANCED DIET?

Often you hear conflicting statements: "If you eat a balanced diet there is no need for vitamins or other supplements." Or, "Vitamins probably won't hurt you, so go ahead and use them if you want to."

Contrast these with statements from those of opposite philosophies that are found in many of the best-selling books on nutrition. Very often our decision on which philosophy to believe depends on our experience with the present health care system, or on the charisma of some high-powered people.

Medical literature leaves many nutritional questions unanswered. Some medical investigators, such as Dr. Roger Williams, have made us aware of individual variability in the area of nutrition. Dr. Emanuel Cheraskin and Dr. William Ringsdorf and their associates of the University of Alabama have given us some insight into possible ideal amounts of specific nutrients that promote *wellness* rather than treat *illness*.

Dr. Cheraskin, using a health survey, correlated the presence or absence of symptoms of disease with the different levels of vitamin intake. The findings of this survey suggested a requirement of five to ten times the RDA (recommended daily allowances) of essential vitamins. Studies on mineral requirements are still in progress, but for magnesium one correlation has been established—those without signs or symptoms of disease had magnesium intakes 15 percent to 34 percent higher than the RDA.

In *Modern Medicine* of April 30–May 15, 1979, a study from Russia showed that supplementation of the diet with vitamins and minerals resulted in improved physical work capacity, rate of muscle work, and movement coordination. Significantly less time was required to make decisions, choose arithmetic problems, and solve logic problems when taking nutritional supplementations.

It seems reasonable, therefore, to give ranges of probable ideal requirements within safe limits and then allow each individual to be an experiment to determine the result or benefit. Certainly, in Aerobic Nutrition, which has the goal of *maintaining good health,* it is necessary to have adequate amounts of all vitamins and minerals to function properly. The ingredients in the recipes of this book also are designed to provide a better variety and amount of nutritive substances than normally found in a routine average American diet. This is all part of a plan to help you to do your best to be your best for the rest of your healthy lifetime.

HOW DO WE KNOW WHETHER VITAMIN SUPPLEMENTS SHOULD BE PART OF OUR DAILY NUTRIENT REGIME?

The needs of an individual can best be evaluated by the way the person feels. This is very subjective and will not satisfy the needs of scientists, but what about you as an individual? Are you feeling well most of the time? Do you have enough vitality and a feeling of well-being to perform all the functions in life that are important to you? Or do you require pills for daily or frequent complaints? Are you tired and listless halfway through the day? Have you been charging all those negative feelings up to older age? Vitamin supplementation within safe limits may solve the problems where conventional drugs have failed.

CAN'T WE JUST TAKE A BLOOD TEST TO FIND OUT WHETHER WE ARE DEFICIENT IN ANY NUTRIENTS?

Such tests are currently expensive and many are not as accurate as would be desired. Many cells and tissues of the body can have deficiencies that exist without detection.

Results of animal experiments cannot reliably be applied to man, since different species metabolize vitamins differently. For instance, the niacin requirement depends on how tryptophan is converted to niacin in the living animal. Chickens and rats can carry out the conversion fairly easily, dogs less easily, while monkeys and humans are relatively ineffective in this process.

Apart from individual metabolic variations, individual living habits affect nutrient requirements. The use of tobacco, alcohol, and medications such as birth control pills, steroids, diuretics, antacids, and laxatives all affect the nutrient needs. These same life habits adversely affect triglycerides and the oxygen delivery system.

All of the controversy concerning nutrition is related to either deficiency or excess. Most commonly, the cited excesses in nutrition are calories, fats, sugars, and cholesterol. Deficiency states are presumed not to exist in the supposedly healthy individual—the person without symptoms of known vitamin-deficiency diseases such as scurvy, beriberi, pellagra, and rickets.

Deficiencies or excesses of nutrients may result from unbalanced intake, but also from the inability to use and excrete them. Deficiency states are largely dependent on decreased intake in the normal person, whereas excess states in the body derive from the inability to use or excrete the amounts above the required quantities. Why make this distinction? Because of the wide variability within the range of the so-called normal. One person's deficiency can be another person's excess, or the reverse. For example, not all people on a vitamin C–deficient diet develop scurvy at the same time. Each person has an ideal amount somewhere between the two extremes.

Many of the degenerative diseases of this country would be prevented if excess calories and cholesterol could be excreted from the body. Without excretion, excess nutrients can have a toxic effect.

IF VITAMINS ARE SO IMPORTANT WOULDN'T IT BE WISE TO TAKE A LOT OF EXTRA PILLS JUST IN CASE?

No, that's how people get in trouble or have the most expensive urine in town. Some vitamins are water-soluble and will be easily disposed of by the body if taken in excess. Other vitamins, such as vitamin A, D, E, and K, tend to be accumulated because of their fat-soluble nature, and can cause effects of toxicity if taken in amounts beyond the body's need.

Excess is a good word to keep in mind when reflecting on those in our society who are gorging themselves with all of the goodies that affect the loss of health and function from degenerative disease! These are the diseases of overconsumption, of excesses that are not excreted.

Here is a diagram that illustrates the effects of deficiency and excess:

Deficiency	OPTIMAL AMOUNT IN THIS WIDE RANGE OF VARIABILITY	Excess
↓		↓
Disease		Potential Toxicity

ARE RECOMMENDED DAILY ALLOWANCES JUST WHAT ALL OF US NEED EACH DAY?

The recommended daily allowances, as established by the National Academy of Sciences, are defined by that organization as not necessarily meeting all nutritional requirements. In their words, "Differences in nutritional requirements of individuals that derive from differences in their genetic makeup are ordinarily unknown. Therefore, as there is no way of predicting whose needs are high and whose are low, RDA (recommended daily allowances) are estimated to exceed the requirements of most individuals, and thereby ensure that the needs are nearly all met."

This definition and explanation does not attempt to define *ideal require-ments,* which is impossible to do on the basis of the scientific evidence on nutrition at this time. Not only does the ideal requirement vary for each person, but we do not know whether the average American diet is adequate in all nutrients without supplementation.

DO MOST PEOPLE EAT A HEALTHFUL DIET?

No. In 1972, Dr. Emanuel Cheraskin and his group at the University of Alabama performed a study on 364 doctors and 296 of their wives from different sections of the country. A dietary analysis revealed that 12 percent of the doctors received less than the RDA of niacin, 10 percent were deficient in vitamin C, 32 percent were low in calcium intake, and 50 percent were less than the RDA for vitamin E. The doctors' wives showed even greater deficiencies than their husbands. Clearly, nutritional deficiencies do not have to result from deprivation or problems of the poor.

A larger survey by the Department of Agriculture, involving 7,500 families, revealed that only 50 percent had diets that met all the recommended daily allowances for essential nutrients. The half who were deficient had diets that failed to meet the minimum requirements in one or more of the essential nutrients. Nutrients most frequently found to be deficient were calcium, vitamin A, vitamin C, iron, thiamine, and riboflavin.

A nutritional assessment of persons over fifty-nine years of age was done in the 1973 Missouri Nutritional Survey. Of the men studied, 20 percent did not meet requirements in iron, 2 percent in vitamin A, 1 percent in vitamin C; of the women 10 percent were low in iron, 10 percent in vitamin A, 1 percent in vitamin C—all judged on the basis of blood analysis. Half of the men and 20 percent of the women had diets with one or more nutrients below 67 percent of the 1974 RDA's.

These statistics are not surprising, since a look at the food that is available from the grocery store reveals the nutritional pillage of natural foods through processing that occurs between the farmer's fields and the marketplace. Much of this processing is economically necessary to preserve food or pro-duce a competitive product. Nature in its own way has provided things required by man to exist on earth since the beginning, but now an artificial diet is becoming more and more the way of life. At this time there are simulated or artificial cheeses, eggs, potatoes, and tomato paste, to list just a few examples. The optimal diet for humans cannot be decided by all the experts in the world, but when we replace nature's own provision for these nutrients, how can we know what is missing in the menu?

The prevalence of refined foods in our diet leaves many of the essential nutrients at just below the recommended values. Too much of the energy intake is obtained from sweet drinks, candy, and alcohol. This type of dietary intake is even more devastating when physical activity or need for all of these calories is diminishing, leaving problems like obesity and high triglyceride blood levels with which to deal.

HOW DOES FOOD PREPARATION AFFECT VITAMIN CONTENT?

There is some loss of vitamins whenever food is cooked. Naturally there will be a greater loss if the food has been through a long processing rather than a fast blanching process.

Vitamins can be lost through your own cooking techniques if you tend to overcook food in large quantities of water or soak raw vegetables in water for a long period of time before cooking.

It is nutritionally better to use fresh food than canned or frozen food. Cook it in as small amount of liquid as possible, and choose a cooking technique that will rapidly prepare the food. Expect a loss of vitamins from fresh food, no matter how you cook it. Vitamin loss begins to occur the moment the fruit or vegetable is picked. If several days pass before the food appears in the marketplace, there will be a greater loss. If you neglect to refrigerate food immediately after purchase (don't drive around with bundles of fruits and vegetables in your car trunk!), there will be additional loss.

In winter, many of our "fresh" vegetables are actually storage foods, particularly the root vegetables such as potatoes, turnips, winter squash, carrots, and beets. Storage vegetables do not have as high a vitamin content as those freshly picked and marketed at farm stands.

Food quality varies, then, no matter what the menu says, and it is very difficult to know whether you are getting adequate daily nutrition.

HOW IS THE OXYGEN DELIVERY SYSTEM AFFECTED BY VITAMINS AND MINERALS?

The quality of the nutrition you choose to provide affects six aspects of oxygen delivery:

1. The integrity or health of the oxygen-carrying red blood cells.
2. The prevention of red cell clumping.
3. The maintenance of proper oxygen delivery for optimal heart function.
4. The effects on the progression of atherosclerosis (blocking of the artery walls).
5. The uptake and release of oxygen by the red blood cells.
6. The utilization of oxygen by the tissue cells.

WHICH VITAMINS AND MINERALS AFFECT THE OXYGEN DELIVERY SYSTEM?

Just as fat, carbohydrate, and protein have their effects, as described in previous chapters, so do these additional nutrients in their separate ways.

Vitamin C, or ascorbic acid, has the most general effect on oxygen delivery. For example, it has been demonstrated that vitamin C improves the release of oxygen from red cells, promotes the excretion of cholesterol as bile acids (therefore lowering blood cholesterol), and favorably decreases the clumping of red cells, thereby increasing the ability of tissue cells to consume oxygen. A prolonged vitamin C deficiency has been shown to decrease the ability to perform aerobic work.

WHAT IS THE IDEAL AMOUNT OF VITAMIN C FOR AN ADULT?

The recommended daily allowance (RDA) has been raised to 60 mg per day for the adult by the United States Food and Nutrition Board. Those who have surveyed the medical literature for animal requirements have given equivalent optimal doses for man in the range of 250 mg per day to 4,000 mg per day for the adult.

It is interesting to note that this vitamin differs from all other vitamins in that it is a requirement in the diet of only a few animal species, and we are one of them. Guinea pigs, the primates or monkeys, and humans are the only species that cannot manufacture their own vitamin C.

Vitamin C has a very low degree of toxicity even in fairly large doses. The problem most often cited is the possible formation of oxalates that may lead to urinary tract stones. There appears to be an insignificant increase in oxalate formation with the ingestion of less than 4,000 mgs of vitamin C per day. Therefore, less than 4,000 mg per day would appear to be safe for almost all individuals. When oxalate formation is suspected, it can be determined by simple medical testing. Lingual (tongue) testing is a simple measure of vitamin C tissue saturation, and urinary losses of vitamin C are easily determined.

Extreme vitamin C deficiency can lead to scurvy, a disease of multiple hemorrhages. In less extreme cases, vitamin C deficiency can cause weakness, irritability, muscle and joint pains, bleeding gums, and loosening of teeth. Clearly we should keep vitamin C intake up to optimum levels to meet our goal of optimum well-being.

SHOULD HIGH DOSES OF VITAMIN E BE TAKEN ALONG WITH VITAMIN C, ACCORDING TO A POPULAR THEORY?

Along with vitamin C, vitamin E has been a nutritional football. Both have been subjects of the pass, kick, and punt contest in nutrition. There seems to be a great deal of variability and individual tolerance to vitamin E. Although some people tolerate extremely high doses without ill effects, there are others who develop side effects at smaller doses. Fatigue is a very frequently reported side effect, especially at a vitamin E intake greater than 400 units per day, and the use of 600 units per day significantly decreases blood thyroid levels and may also cause elevation of the blood triglycerides. In view of this effect on triglycerides, large doses of vitamin E are not recommended as part of Aerobic Nutrition.

Vitamin E should be *used with caution* in any case. Problems associated with high doses include: thrombophlebitis, breast tenderness, elevation of blood pressure, myopathy, intestinal cramps, uticaria (rash), and possible aggravation of diabetes. Those who feel that large doses of vitamin E are required for some health reasons should be aware of the rather common, troublesome side effects.

Adequate vitamin C supplementation may diminish the likelihood of vitamin E deficiency. It has been suggested that vitamins C and E work together, with vitamin E acting primarily as an antioxidant in a reaction with vitamin C to regenerate vitamin E. This recycling of vitamin E at the expense of vitamin C may account in part for the fact that clinically overt vitamin E deficiency has not been demonstrated in humans. The optimal dosage of vitamin E is somewhere between 45 and 75 units per day, which would be three to five times greater than the RDA. This is the safe estimate in the presence of adequate vitamin C. Although many people feel comfortable with vitamin E supplements up to 400 I.U. daily, any amount over that should be taken with medical supervision.

DO THE B VITAMINS PLAY A ROLE IN THE OXYGEN DELIVERY SYSTEM?

All of the B vitamins participate in oxygen metabolism within the red blood cell. It has been shown that thiamine (B_1), riboflavin (B_2), niacin (B_3), pyridoxine (B_6), and cyanocobalamin (B_{12}) affect the oxygen uptake by the red blood cells, as well as the oxygen release from the red cells for uptake by the tissue cells. When thiamine is removed from the diets of rats, studies have demonstrated that there is a decrease in the ability to use oxygen by the red blood cell. Other research has shown that with reduced intake of niacin and a cholesterol-rich diet, there is a hampered aerobic oxidative pathway.

It is in the utilization of fuel for production of energy that all of the B vitamins participate in these enzyme systems within the red cells. Niacin decreases the amount of substrate available for production of triglycerides, which then reduces the conversion of the cholesterol lipoproteins. As a result, there is a decrease in the blood cholesterol and triglyceride with adequate amounts of niacin or nicotinic acid. A decrease in triglycerides lessens the likelihood of clumping of the red cells, and a decrease in cholesterol lessens the likelihood of plaque buildup in the walls of the arteries.

The integrity or health of the red blood cells depends on adequate amounts of vitamin B_{12} and folic acid, and the minerals copper, iron, and potassium. Not only do these nutrients affect the release of oxygen from the red cells, but even optimal oxygen would be of no value without them, since the ability to use oxygen depends on healthy cells.

The heart is affected by a large number of nutrients, and of course is an important part of the oxygen delivery system. The heart provides the force that propels the oxygen-carrying red blood cells throughout the body. Obviously, if the pump fails, then there is no more circulation. It has long been known that thiamine plays an important part in the function of the heart, since a deficiency of this vitamin causes a very specific heart disease, beriberi.

The minerals calcium, potassium, and magnesium work in conjunction with the B vitamins to preserve the integrity of the heart muscle and reduce susceptibility to changes in oxygen consumption. Subjects dying suddenly from ischemic heart disease have lower levels of magnesium and potassium in the heart tissue than individuals dying for other reasons. Possibly a deficiency of one or both of these elements contributes to sudden death in individuals in whom blood flow, and therefore the oxygen supply to the heart muscle, is limited in some way. So the health of the pump and the health of the oxygen-carrying red blood cells are very much affected by B vitamins.

Genetic disposition plays a huge role in determining the vitamin needs for each person, and this is especially true of the B vitamins, which are required for every enzyme system within the body. All the B vitamins have specific functions, but they are also required in combination.

Apart from genetically determined individual requirements, the ability to absorb and excrete vitamins varies from person to person. The need for intake of B vitamins can be markedly changed by the intestinal bacteria content, which may be altered by antibiotics or diarrhea. Diagnosis of a deficiency of a nutrient, as judged by our present criteria—signs or symptoms of disease or a blood test—can be grossly inaccurate. A well-balanced diet with a multiple vitamin supplement that includes all the B vitamins is recommended for those who are concerned about achieving a state of well-being.

IS B_{15} AN IMPORTANT B VITAMIN?

One big question mark in nutrition today is a substance that has been called vitamin B_{15}, or pangamic acid. It is thought to promote oxygen utilization by cells. Most of the literature cited in support of this theory comes from Russia, with other reports from Japan and Canada.

It is proposed that B_{15} produces increased brain oxygen utilization without an increase in the actual blood flow. Because of the inadequate scientific investigation in this country, pangamic acid cannot be recommended with any scientific validity at this time.

The Russian literature suggests that pangamic acid stimulates oxidative metabolism and tissue oxygen consumption. Should this effect on the utilization of oxygen by tissue be confirmed, the substance could very significantly affect the oxygen delivery system. But the use of pangamic acid has never been approved by any federal or state agency in the United States, and is not recognized by the Food and Drug Administration as essential for human nutrition.

The statement by the Food and Drug Administration on pangamic acid as of August 1978 includes, "FDA considers B_{15} to be a food additive for which no evidence of safety has been offered. It is therefore illegal for the substance to be sold as a dietary supplement. No new drug application for pangamic acid has been submitted or approved by the FDA and the substance legally cannot be marketed as a drug."

So, pangamic acid needs further scientific investigation and cannot be designated as a vitamin at this time. The safe limits for the use of this substance have yet to be determined, and therefore the use does carry a risk. If speculation becomes truth about this substance, then there is an extremely valuable future use for B_{15} with regards to the oxygen delivery system.

THEN IS IT REASONABLE TO ASSUME THAT THERE IS ENOUGH SUPPORTING EVIDENCE FOR USING SUPPLEMENTS WITH THE USUAL AMERICAN DIET?

Yes. First, because of the individual variability for optimal requirements and the lack of our ability to measure needs *before* disease develops. Second, there is the question of whether a balanced diet provides adequate intake of all nutrients for everyone. Third, not only the change in the natural composition in our diet, but also our living habits, which add to the individual variability in nutrient requirements, seem to indicate that it is unwise to risk your healthy tomorrow on the risks of uncertainty today. It doesn't make sense to do nothing and hope for the best.

Following is a list of vitamins and minerals to use as a guideline when determining your own individual needs. These suggested ranges are not intended for treatment of disease or abnormal states, but to give ranges for the maintenance of health in normal persons. Need should be determined by the quality of your food and the care you take to retain natural vitamins and minerals during cooking.

BEST SOURCES OF VITAMINS

VITAMIN A.   Found in: fish-liver oils, liver, whole milk, butter, cream, whole-milk cheeses, egg yolk, dark-green leafy vegetables, yellow vegetables, yellow fruits, fortified products.

VITAMIN D.   Found in: fish-liver oils, fortified milk.

VITAMIN E.   Found in: plant tissues—wheat germ oil, vegetable oils (such as soybean, corn, and cottonseed), nuts, legumes

VITAMIN K.   Found in: green leaves such as spinach, cabbage, cauliflower, and liver.

THE AEROBIC NUTRITION STAY-WELL FORMULA		
Vitamin A	5,000 to 25,000	I.U.
Vitamin D	0 to 400	I.U.
Vitamin E	45 to 75	I.U.
Vitamin B_1	5 to 25	mg
Vitamin B_2	5 to 25	mg
Vitamin B_3	10 to 50	mg
Vitamin B_6	10 to 50	mg
Vitamin B_{12}	5 to 25	μg
Folic Acid	400 to 800	μg
Vitamin C	250 to 4,000	mg
Calcium	800 to 1,600	mg
Magnesium	400 to 800	mg
Zinc	15 to 30	mg
Potassium	1,000 to 2,000	mg
Iron	15 to 30	mg
Selenium	25 to 50	μg
Copper	2 to 4	mg
Manganese	2 to 20	mg

VITAMIN C.   Found in: citrus fruits, tomatoes, strawberries, cantaloupe, cabbage, broccoli, kale, potatoes.

FOLIC ACID.   Found in: liver, kidney, yeast, deep-green leafy vegetables.

THIAMINE (B_1).   Found in: pork, liver and other organs, brewers' yeast, wheat germ, whole-grain cereals and breads, soybeans, peanuts and other legumes, milk.

RIBOFLAVIN (B_2).   Found in: milk, powdered whey, liver, kidney, heart, meats, eggs, green leafy vegetables, dried yeast, enriched foods.

NIACIN (B_3).   Found in: lean meat, fish, poultry, liver, kidney, whole-grain and enriched cereals and breads, green vegetables, peanuts, brewers' yeast.

VITAMIN B_6.   Found in: wheat germ, meat, liver, kidney, whole-grain cereals, soybeans, peanuts, corn.

VITAMIN B_{12}.   Amply provided by small daily intakes of animal protein.

BEST SOURCES OF MINERALS

CALCIUM.   Found in: milk and milk products, green leafy vegetables, shellfish, molasses, bone meal.

CHLORINE.   Found in: table salt, seafood, meats, ripe olives, rye flour.

CHROMIUM.   Found in: corn oil, clams, whole-grain cereals, brewers' yeast.

COBALT.   Found in: organ meats, oysters, clams, poultry, milk, green leafy vegetables, fruits.

COPPER.   Found in: organ meats, seafood, nuts, legumes, molasses, raisins, bone meal.

FLUORIDE.   Found in: tea, seafood, fluoridated water.

IRON.   Found in: organ meats, meats, eggs, fish, poultry, molasses, green leafy vegetables, dried fruits.

MAGNESIUM.   Found in: seafood, whole grains, dark-green vegetables, molasses, nuts, bone meal.

MANGANESE.   Found in: whole grains, green leafy vegetables, legumes, nuts, pineapples, egg yolks.

MOLYBDENUM.   Found in: legumes, whole-grain cereals, milk, liver, dark-green vegetables.

PHOSPHORUS.   Found in: fish, meat, poultry, eggs, legumes, milk, milk products, nuts, whole-grain cereals, bone meal.

POTASSIUM.   Found in: lean meat, whole grains, vegetables, dried fruits, legumes, sunflower seeds.

SELENIUM.   Found in: tuna, herring, brewers' yeast, wheat germ, bran, broccoli, whole grains.

SODIUM.   Found in: seafood, table salt, baking powder, baking soda, celery, milk, milk products, kelp, sea salt.

SULFUR.   Found in: fish, eggs, meat, cabbage, Brussels sprouts.

VANADIUM.   Found in: fish.

ZINC.   Found in: seafood, organ meats, mushrooms, brewers' yeast, soybeans, sunflower seeds.

II
THE AEROBIC
NUTRITION
COOKBOOK

Aerobic Nutrition is an easy regimen to follow. It is not extreme, but it does have limitations. Most of the limitations can be met by not bringing the banned food into the house. Health starts at the food market.

Picture your kitchen as it stands today with all of the self-help appliances, self-cleaning or regular oven, cooking range, microwave oven, refrigerator, freezer, dishwasher, and the like. Now into that picture, place the kind of food that was available about one hundred years ago. It was natural. It was unadulterated. It was real food.

That's the kind of food to choose from now on. Whole-grain cereals, such as oatmeal, whole-wheat cooked cereals, and bran-based cold cereals without added sugar are preferred to refined white flour products. Rice should be brown, rather than polished white, but the latter is better than no rice at all. Pasta should be made from unbleached flour or from whole-wheat flour if possible. Breads should be made of whole wheat or other whole grains rather than refined white cottony-soft manufactured loaves. There are recipes for easy-bake breads and muffins later in this book, and you can bake when you have some free time and freeze them for later use.

It's wise to experiment with some grain products that are new to you. For instance, coarse corn meal can be used in the form of tacos or in place of refined white flour when making pancakes.

The average American diet now includes 46 percent carbohydrates, with 22 percent from complex carbohydrates (grains and vegetables) and 24 percent from sugar. The Aerobic Nutrition formula will increase your intake of complex carbohydrates to 63 percent and lower your intake of sugar to a mere 5 percent. The broad term *sugar* includes brown sugar, honey, syrups, and molasses. Fructose is absorbed more slowly than sucrose, as is honey, but all simple sugars should be limited in favor of increased intake of complex carbohydrates. You may find small amounts of sugar in some baked goods recipes in this book—these have been calculated to provide only one teaspoon of sugar per serving, or 18 calories, and are included for special treats rather than everyday indulgences. Desserts should be mostly fruit—either fresh in season or frozen or canned without added sugar. Concentrated fruit juices (frozen) can be used for sweetening power in some desserts and to enhance some main-dish meals.

Don't forget that a baked potato is a good health food. Wash it, bake it, and eat it, skin and all, to get all the vitamins and minerals that you can. What you shouldn't do with it is to cover it with butter, margarine, or sour cream, or mash it with any other high-fat product. Skim-milk yogurt mixed with chopped chives makes an excellent topping for baked potatoes, adding the protein of the yogurt without adding fat. Fried potatoes and creamed potatoes do not fit into the Aerobic Nutrition concept.

Other vegetables should be added to the diet to make it interesting and to add excellent nutrients and fiber. Some of these might be baked acorn squash, baked butternut squash, and all members of the cabbage family including such exotica as kohlrabi and broccoli rabe. Artichokes, eggplant, all leafy vegetables that are high in calcium (including spinach, Swiss chard, turnip greens, and collard greens), peppers of every color and flavor, and carrots in both raw and cooked form are recommended. If you have been eating only a few of the same vegetables every day, you are not only bound to be bored with the fare, you are not rotating enough vitamins and minerals into your meals.

The average American diet includes 42 percent fat every day, with 16 percent in saturated (animal) fat and 26 percent in unsaturated (vegetable) fat. The Aerobic Nutrition plan reduces fat intake to only 20 percent altogether, with 10 percent in saturated fat and 10 percent in unsaturated fat.

This means that all fats should be limited in the diet. Fats include butter, oleomargarine, vegetable shortening, cooking oil, and the fats in whole-milk products and on cuts of meat, poultry, and fish. The recipes in this book are designed to use vegetable oils. There is doubt in the medical world as to whether the hydrogenating process to harden oleomargarine and vegetable shortening will reduce cholesterol counts or actually raise them. But we know that butter is an animal-based fat that contributes to cholesterol production. So it is best to use vegetable-based oil to lower the intake of cholesterol, or soft margarine or soft shortening to avoid the hydrogenated products.

Some people have the mistaken notion that oleomargarine has less fat than butter. They even sometimes think that it has fewer calories. Right here and now, let's state that fat is fat—whether it is butter, oleo, oil, shortening, or lard. And fat has roughly 100 calories per tablespoon. To control the fat intake of your diet, don't spread butter on your bread, and don't pour cream into your coffee. You can certainly use a little oil in your salad, but drop it from a teaspoon so you can limit what you use. In order to meet the 20 percent limit, only 200 calories of a 1,000-calorie day may be in fat, and all animal fat should be included in the count.

Leaner cuts of meat should be the order of the day. All fat should be trimmed before eating. Processed meats, frankfurters, cold cuts, ham, bacon, and other high-fat, high-sodium meats should be avoided. Don't consume huge portions of meat—limit it to 4- or 5-ounce portions.

Poultry meals should be increased, but remember to remove all excess fat from the poultry before cooking—especially the two large pads of fat that are just inside the rear cavity of the bird. Since all poultry skin has a layer of fat under it, cut it all away and just eat the meat.

Eat more fish. Many people don't know how to cook fish so that it is delicious. It's important to start with very fresh fish—frozen fish may be cheaper, but the flavor is usually not the same. And then it's imperative not to overcook the fish or you will get a rough texture. Techniques of recipes in this book will show you simple ways to poach, broil, and bake fish to your heart's content.

Skim-milk products, such as skim-milk yogurt (you'll learn how to make your own), low-fat cottage cheese, all low-fat cheeses, and skim-milk shakes will be encouraged. Eggs should be used with moderation, but dressings that are made with yolks and oil (such as mayonnaise and hollandaise sauces) should be used sparingly.

Hearty homemade vegetable and grain soups should take the place of creamed soups. But homemade pseudo-creamed soups have been included in the recipe section. Canned and dehydrated soups are too high in sodium to be used in the Aerobic Nutrition way of eating.

A preventive medicine health regime such as Aerobic Nutrition should also include the restriction of sodium intake. Salt retains fluid in the body, raises the blood pressure, and is unnecessary in the amounts now used in the American diet. One teaspoon of salt contains 2,300 mg of sodium, so you can readily see how the sodium count can add up during the day. So much sodium is added to the American diet by way of fabricated food that the statistics are out of control. Food has natural sodium in it, enough to satisfy the body's need for sodium: about 2,500 mg in a normal variety of natural food selections is enough for the average person. And that's the goal of this book. Salt is not added to any recipe except in small amounts in some baked goods. The other recipes have been skillfully seasoned with herbs and spices to wean your taste buds away from salt.

Besides avoiding the salt shaker when cooking and at the table, avoid all packaged prefabricated foods. Frozen vegetables (not in any kind of sauce), frozen unsweetened fruit, frozen concentrated fruit juice, and some canned staple items, such as canned tomatoes or tomato sauce, may be used. A large variety of dried herbs and spices, and fresh herbs when in season, can be used to add delicious flavor to your food.

Aerobic Nutrition followers must learn to read labels carefully for accurate ingredient content. The first ingredient on the list comprises the largest component of the package, and it continues in decreasing order. So if sugar is listed first, you know that most of the product is made of sugar.

You will have to become a food detective because sugar can appear in several places on a product in varying amounts. For instance, it can be listed as sugar, then later in the listing there may be some "sucrose" and/or corn syrup, honey, maple syrup, or other sweetener. So if you are on a sugar search when reading a label, take heed of all the sweet words.

Salt is more difficult to recognize. But look for the word *sodium.* Some of the words in ingredient lists are monosodium glutamate (MSG), brine, disodium phosphate, sodium alginate, sodium benzoate, sodium hydroxide, sodium propionate, sodium sulfite—to name a few of those added to our fabricated foods. That's why it's best to use fresh real food whenever possible.

If you are concerned with economy, you'll probably save money by marketing this way. And old-fashioned real food does not have to take any more time than convenience foods, if you learn how to be a short-order cook the gourmet way. Many of the recipes in this book will be ready to eat in fifteen or twenty minutes, or less.

Working men and women can learn how to use a novel method of back-to-back mass-production cooking to stretch the actual time spent in the kitchen, and still be sure that the family is eating healthful food. The following section will tell you how to do it well and fast. The chart, "Strategy for Your Dietary Change," will give you a firm grasp of the goals of the Aerobic Nutrition diet plan.

THE COOK'S VOCABULARY

BAKE.   To bake food means to put it in the oven and cook it with indirect dry heat. 350°F. is considered medium heat, 250°F. is low, and 450°F. is high. Your oven should have an indicator on it with degrees shown for accurate baking temperatures.

BARBECUE.   Usually means to cook over an open fire, but also can refer to the spicy seasoning used on roasted or broiled meats.

BASTE.   Refers to the process of spooning gravy or wine over baking or roasting food that is in the oven. Basting prevents food from drying out if it is uncovered. Avoid using fat for basting.

STRATEGY FOR YOUR DIETARY CHANGE

CURRENT AMERICAN DIET	RECOMMENDED U.S. DIETARY GOALS	AEROBIC NUTRITION
42% ⎡ 16% saturated fat ⎣ 26% unsaturated fat	30% ⎡ 10% saturated fat ⎣ 20% unsaturated fat	20% ⎡ 10% saturated fat ⎣ 10% unsaturated fat
12% protein	12% protein	12% protein
46% ⎡ 22% complex carbohydrate ⎣ 24% sugar	58% ⎡ 43% complex carbohydrate ⎣ 15% sugar	68% ⎡ 63% complex carbohydrate ⎣ 5% sugar
600–700 mg cholesterol	300 mg cholesterol	200 mg cholesterol
8 g fiber	8 g fiber	11 g fiber
8,000 mg salt	5,000 mg salt	2,500 mg salt

BEAT.   Stir food together until smooth; to do it right, think of a fast-moving tune. A waltz just won't do!

BLANCH.   The process you use to remove the skin of fruit, vegetables, or nuts. Immerse the food in boiling water for a minute—then quickly into icy water to stop the cooking action and shed the skin. With this technique it slips off at the flick of a sharp knife.

BLEND.   Stir two or more ingredients together until they become one. Do it with a cooking spoon, or better still, with an electric blender. No need to beat air in —just beat identity out!

BOIL.   If it's liquid and it bubbles while it's cooking—it's boiling. Gentle bubbles are called a low boil, and vigorous bubbles are called a rapid boil. If you are directed to bring something to a boil, cook it until it bubbles.

BRAISE.   This refers to a method of cooking in which you brown the meat on all sides, and then add a small amount of liquid, cover the pot, and simmer over low heat for long, slow cooking. This method is usually used for less tender cuts of meat. Use a nonstick skillet and no fat.

BREAD.   When used as a verb it means to dip food in crumbs until it is completely covered. An easy way to do this is to put the crumbs in a plastic bag and then shake the food inside the bag, one piece at a time, until coated.

BREW.   This refers to a method of extracting flavor from food by letting it stand in hot water until the water is flavored.

BROIL.   Put the food on an open pan under direct heat, gauging the distance from the heat by the thickness of the food. The thinner the food, the closer to the source of heat you can put it. Watch out for fat flare-ups, but if you suddenly see your steak in flames—reach for the salt and throw a handful in: salt is one of the few things that will put a fat fire out fast. Avoid by trimming excess fat before cooking.

CHOP.   To cut food in fine pieces either with a food chopper in a wooden bowl or in an electric blender or food processor. A slower way is to use a knife—and keep your fingers away from the blade!

CREAM.   Don't add cream unless it's called for—this is a verb that means to mix fat until it is fluffy. It can be done with the back of a spoon, but an electric mixer is better.

CUBE.   Cut the ingredient into small squares.

CUT.   Use a knife and divide food as directed. Also used to describe a method of making pastry, where the fat is "cut" into the flour until small particles of the mixture result.

DEVIL.   You just know it's going to be hot! It refers to the addition of condiments to food to give it a spicy taste.

DICE.   Similar to cube, except it's on a smaller scale.

DREDGE.   Sounds like hard work, but it isn't. Just refers to coating food with flour until the entire surface is covered. Use a plastic bag, as in *Bread*.

DUST.   Sprinkle food lightly with flour, just enough to cover with a fine film. The food will definitely not be as well covered as in *Bread* or *Dredge*.

FILLET.   If it's a verb—remove the bones. If it's a noun—they're already out.

FLAKE. Using a fork, break a solid piece of food into flat pieces. Flake off means the same thing, so don't leave!

FLAMBÉ. Set the food ablaze with spirits high in alcohol. Follow directions carefully or there will be a fireman in your future.

FOLD. This method of combining foods is used when it is important not to destroy air bubbles, as with a soufflé or sponge-cake batter. Mix the food from the bottom of the bowl to the top by bringing a cooking spoon down the back of the bowl, through the ingredients at the bottom of the bowl in a direction toward you, and then up the front of the bowl, across the top toward the back of the bowl, then down the back of the bowl again. Repeat in slow motion until the ingredients are combined. Don't stir, mix, or beat, as the mixture will flatten as the air escapes.

FRICASSEE. When you stew meat in gravy for a long time, in a covered pot over low heat—you're doing it!

FRY. Refers to cooking in melted fat. Aerobic Nutrition uses no frying.

GLAZE. A cooking technique that is used when you want to cover food with a mixture that will create a shiny surface.

GRATE. In order to reduce a food to tiny particles, you must rub it against a rough cutting surface with tiny wires or holes—the process is called "grating," the heap of particles are "grated," and the gadget you are using is a "grater."

GRILL. When you cook by broiling on a rack, or over an open fire, you are grilling.

GRIND. A way of reducing food to small particles with a food chopper or blender.

JULIENNE. This refers to food that is cut in slender strips—if it's in cubes or balls, it is not julienne!

KNEAD. The action required to fold and stretch dough until it becomes smooth and elastic. It may be done with your hands, or if you are lucky, with the dough hook on an electric mixer or food processor. An electric beater won't do it.

MARINATE. Think of "soak" and you'll understand. This refers to a technique used to tenderize and flavor meat, and the mixture it is soaking in is called the "marinade."

MINCE. It means chop it very fine.

MIX. As a verb, combine foods together. As a noun referring to "mix" or "mixture," it is already combined.

MOLD. This is the way to get food to retain a particular shape—pour it into a shaped container until chilled, frozen, or set according to directions, and then remove it from the container.

PAN-BROIL. Cook in an uncovered skillet, pouring off fat as it accumulates so you are not frying.

PARBOIL. This refers to a method of cooking food partway in boiling water to prepare for cooking further by another method.

PARE. When you cut the skin off fruits and vegetables, you are doing it.

PEEL. Removal of the skin of a fruit that can be stripped by hand.

POACH. A method of cooking that refers to simmering over low heat in a hot liquid. An excellent technique for Aerobic Nutrition.

PURÉE.   When food is reduced to a smooth sauce in a blender or through a food mill, the sauce is called a "purée."

REDUCE.   To boil a liquid down to a smaller quantity and stronger intensity.

ROAST.   Can be done over an open fire, but in the home it means to cook in the oven.

SAUTÉ.   Another word for fry, in a small amount of fat or liquid, over low heat for a short amount of time.

SCALD.   Heat liquid to a point just below boiling—you've scalded it just before the bubbles break.

SCORE.   Cut lines across the surface of food just before roasting, or around the edges of a steak just before broiling.

SEAR.   Seal in the juices of meat by browning fast either over high heat or in a very hot oven. When you have "seared" in the juices, the heat is reduced for further cooking.

SIMMER.   Cook in liquid over low heat that is just below the boiling point. Used for delicate results.

SKEWER.   As a verb, it is the piercing of food onto a long pin before cooking. As a noun, it is the long pin itself.

SKIM.   Take a spoon and remove fatty or other substances that are floating in your cooking liquid. When it refers to milk, the fatty substances have already been removed.

SLIVER.   Cut food in slender pieces of small size.

STEAM.   A method of cooking food suspended over boiling water.

STEW.   If it's a verb, cook food in liquid over low heat for a long time. If it's a noun, it refers to ingredients already cooked that way.

STIR.   Combine ingredients together with a slow circular motion until blended.

WHIP.   Beat ingredients rapidly, to add air and inflate the volume of the mixture. If you are whipping cream, be sure to stop the moment the shiny mixture breaks into a thick dull one—one moment too much and you will have the beginnings of butter.

WEIGHTS AND MEASURES

WEIGHTS AND MEASURES	EQUIVALENT
⅓ of ½ teaspoon	A pinch
½ of ¼ teaspoon	⅛ teaspoon
3 teaspoons	1 tablespoon
2 tablespoons	⅛ cup
4 tablespoons	¼ cup
5 tablespoons plus 1 teaspoon	⅓ cup
8 tablespoons	½ cup
10 tablespoons plus 2 teaspoons	⅔ cup

12 tablespoons	¾ cup
16 tablespoons	1 cup
1 cup	8 fluid ounces
2 cups	1 pint
2 pints	1 quart
4 cups	1 quart
2 quarts	½ gallon
4 quarts	1 gallon
16 ounces, dry measure	1 pound
32 ounces, fluid measure	1 quart
¼ pound of butter	½ cup
1 pound of butter	2 cups
½ pound Cheddar cheese	2 cups grated
3 ounces of cream cheese	6 tablespoons
1 pound flour	4 cups sifted
1 pound cake flour	4¾ cups sifted
1 medium lemon	3 tablespoons juice
1 medium lemon rind	1 tablespoon grated rind
1 medium orange	⅓ cup juice
1 medium orange	2 tablespoons grated rind
1 pound unshelled walnuts	1⅔ cups chopped nuts
1 pound granulated sugar	2½ cups
1 pound brown sugar	2⅓ cups
1 pound confectioners' sugar	3½ cups
1 cup raw rice	3 cups cooked

PERCENTAGE OF CALORIES AS FAT IN COMMON FOODS*

MEAT	FAT	MEAT (CONT'D)	FAT
Pork sausage	85	Canadian bacon	58
T-bone steak	82	Fish sticks	50
Hot dogs	80	Chuck beef	
Lamb chops	80	(pot roast)	50
Spareribs, pork	80	Lean hamburger	46
Liverwurst sausage	78	Beef liver (fried)	42
Bacon	77	Halibut	37
Ham	75	Haddock	36
Corned beef	74	Turkey (dark meat)	32
Sardines, drained	49	Chicken (dark meat)	32
Bologna	70	Cod, broiled	28
Regular hamburger	64	Turkey, light meat	20
Salmon	54	Chicken, light meat	20
Pork chops (broiled)	52		

*Data from the U. S. Department of Agriculture Handbook Number 8.

PERCENTAGE OF CALORIES AS FAT IN COMMON FOODS (CONT'D)

VEGETABLES	FAT	DAIRY (CONT'D)	FAT
Green/yellow beans	10	Roquefort/blue cheese	80
Lettuce	9	Cheddar cheese	72
Average	1–13	American cheese	66
		Swiss cheese	66
LEGUMES		Mozzarella cheese	
Soybeans	37	(part skim)	50
Chickpeas	13	Cottage cheese	36
Kidney beans	3	Low-fat yogurt	31
Lentils	3	Cottage cheese	
		uncreamed	3
GRAINS		Ice cream	54
Oatmeal	15	Milk, whole 3.7%	50
Corn	11	2%	30
White/whole-		Skim	3
wheat bread	9		
Wheat	5	HIGH OIL CONTENT	
Brown rice	4	Olives, green/ripe	98/98
Average	2–14	Avocado	92
		Almonds	83
DRESSINGS AND SAUCES		Sesame seeds	78
Mayonnaise	90	Peanut butter	75
Salad dressing	88–100	Peanuts in shell	74
low-fat	40–54	Nuts/seeds average	70–80
Broccoli	8		
hollandaise sauce	73	MISCELLANEOUS	
with butter sauce	44	Egg (1 medium)	66
		Tuna in oil	64
FRUIT		drained	40
Grapes	12	in water	5
Apple	8	Caviar, sturgeon	57
Apricots, dried	6	Cheese pizza	34
Orange	3	Lobster tails	18
Banana	1	Popcorn, plain	8
Nectarines	1–2	buttered	50
Average	2–13	Potatoes	1
		French fries	43
DAIRY		chips	64
Cream cheese	90		
Cream (light)	87		

BACK-TO-BACK COOKING TECHNIQUES

Even though you may take pride in being a working person, there may also be times when you envy your stay-at-home friends. Like dinner time, when the pressure to produce a good meal all too often makes you wish you had longer to prepare. The trick is to make whatever time you do spend in the kitchen work double for you, without resorting to convenience foods.

The way to do it is to prepare two or more dinners in the same time you usually cook one. How? By cooking one large, more-than-enough main course that will provide leftovers for the next night's meal. Another way is to broil one meal for immediate use while you simmer or bake another for dinner the following night. The whole idea is to have one night of cooking and one night of "coasting."

Once you have experienced the pleasure of coasting, you will begin to see ways of making that one night in the kitchen more productive. A clever person with a good freezer can get away with cooking main dishes just two times a week—and still serve the family delicious homemade dinners every night.

COOKING SESSION #1:

Instead of purchasing 1 pound of ground beef for patties, buy 5 pounds. Also, buy enough chicken parts for 2 dinners.

1. Prepare hamburgers for broiling, using 1 pound of the ground beef. Form the patties and season as desired. Set aside until ready to broil for tonight's dinner.
2. Prepare two Fluffy Meatloaves by doubling the recipe. Freeze raw in aluminum foil loaf pans until ready to use. On the morning of the day of use, place a frozen meatloaf in the refrigerator to thaw safely during the day. Bake for one hour, as directed in the recipe. There should also be some leftovers from each of these meatloaves, so you may have managed some coasting for lunchboxes too.
3. Next, arrange the chicken parts in two baking pans. Season according to Baked Orange Chicken. Bake while you are having dinner. After dinner, store one pan of baked chicken in the refrigerator to be heated the following night. Wrap and store the other pan in the freezer.

Results of cooking session #1:

TONIGHT:	Hamburgers
TOMORROW:	Baked Chicken
IN THE FREEZER:	2 Meatloaves
	1 Pan Baked Chicken

5 Main Courses

COOKING SESSION #2:

Instead of purchasing 2 pounds of stew meat, triple it and buy 6 pounds. Also, buy enough extra fish for leftover cold fish salad.

1. Prepare a triple recipe of Curried Beef Stew and let it simmer slowly through the dinner and cleanup hours. Refrigerate one-third of the stew for reheating for tomorrow's dinner. Freeze the rest in two containers. On the morning of the day of use, place a container of frozen stew in the refrigerator to thaw safely during the day. Heat for dinner.
2. While the stew is simmering, broil fish for tonight's dinner. Mash the extra fish into cold fish salad for lunch sandwiches for tomorrow.

Results of cooking session #2:

TONIGHT:	Broiled Fish
TOMORROW:	Fish Salad Sandwiches (Lunch)
	Beef Stew (Dinner)
IN THE FREEZER:	2 Beef Stews

4 Main Courses plus 1 Lunch

In each cooking session, you have managed to prepare a variety of delicious meals in a minimum of time. In between, you will have hugged a child or two, doled out a scraped carrot intended for the stew, and probably stirred up some gelatin for tomorrow's dessert. Mass production in limited time can become a game once you discover how to accomplish it with ease.

A good casserole recipe can be money in the bank in an emergency or when your budget doesn't "fit." Leftover meat, chicken, or fish, combined with less expensive ingredients, turns into a nourishing main dish with a "gourmet touch." Pasta, rice, and vegetables can really stretch leftovers, too.

If you have a freezer, put it to work by planning a larger quantity of leftovers, so that you can double recipes and prepare extra dishes to be frozen. Reminder: You can freeze main dishes containing meat, chicken, or fish once raw and once cooked. Do not refreeze any of these dishes after it has thawed.

If your able-to-freeze baking dishes are in short supply, line the ones intended for the freezer with aluminum foil, using a large enough piece to be able to seal over the top of the contents. Freeze and, when solid, remove contents from container for other use. To use, remove the frozen block of food from foil and fit it back into the original container for reheating.

To cut down on reheating time for a frozen main course, place the dish in refrigerator to thaw on the morning of the day you plan to serve it.

Just as you have previously learned to streamline your life style to accommodate your many roles as working person, spouse, and parent, so you can now revamp the chore of cooking dinner every night to suit your schedule—as well as your creativity. If your mood calls for cooking, then cook up a storm of meals at one time. They will be ready and waiting when your day has been particularly harried and your creativity level is at zilch.

THE AEROBIC NUTRITION WEIGHT-LOSS DIET

The object of Aerobic Nutrition is to improve the oxygen delivery system in your body. When your body is at optimum weight you will be at optimum health. What better way to lose weight than to go on a well-balanced variety of low-calorie foods that add up to fewer than 1,000 calories a day? That's the point where most people can shed unwanted pounds easily and still manage to eat well and feel well.

This is not a fad diet. The meals are patterned as normally as possible, so you can continue the diet for as long as you wish. All the items are easy to cook or easy to order in a restaurant. When you have to make substitutions, make sensible ones. If you can't have Veal Paprikash as suggested for dinner one day, have one small broiled veal chop, or a very lean hamburger of no more than four ounces. If turkey isn't available, substitute a similar portion of plain roasted or poached chicken. If you'd prefer to eat a whole raw apple in place of a baked apple, do so.

The Aerobic Nutrition Weight-Loss Diet is intended to be a sensible assortment of palatable meals. It is not healthful to try to lose more than two or three pounds a week. The weight did not go on in a week and it should not come off any faster than it went on, if you gradually want to accustom your body to shed the weight without jolting the metabolism into a severe imbalance.

If you find that you are losing much more than two or three pounds a week, you might want to add some more vegetables and another slice of whole-wheat bread each day. If you are not losing more than a pound a week, you might want to cut the diet by another 100 calories each day to find the exact level at which your body will let go of that excess poundage.

The menu plan of the Aerobic Nutrition Weight-Loss Diet takes advantage of foods that you already know how to prepare. The following week of menus is a plan to show you how the rest of the book may be used. Every recipe in this book has nutritional data that includes calorie counts for the entire recipe and for each portion.

To keep calorie counts within the set goal of 1,000 calories or less, use no butter or oleomargarine, no salt in cooking or at the table (there is enough natural sodium in foods to keep your body in perfect sodium balance), and no sugar in your tea or decaffeinated coffee. To keep fat intake down, use only skim milk and nonfat or low-fat milk products, aiming for 1 percent to 2 percent fat in cheeses, yogurt, and all other dairy foods.

Use only fresh fruit or water-packed canned fruit. You may also use any frozen fruit that does not have sugar added. Use fresh vegetables or frozen vegetables that do not have sodium added. Use only water-packed tuna. Trim all meats very well, but start with the leaner cuts of beef, veal, and lamb. Do not use pork, ham, or bacon products, which are generally higher in fat.

When cooking chicken, pull off all excess fat from the bird before cooking. Fat is usually visible at the rear cavity. If time allows, cook poultry and chill it to let the fat solidify in the gravy. Then remove the block of fat and reheat the chicken. Always remove poultry skin before eating, to avoid the fat that lurks underneath it.

Be sure to drink several glasses of water each day, along with other fluids that are listed in the menus.

Use the Mannerberg Method of Movement, keeping your body in constant activity—bending, reaching, stretching, and walking.

Be sure to diet under your doctor's supervision. Don't be surprised to find that you will lose weight comfortably with this easy-to-prepare Aerobic Nutrition Weight-Loss Diet. Because the menus are sensible, you will find it easy to make substitutions and to continue to formulate menus that will get the weight off and keep it off. Use the same basic weekly menu and write in substitutions of other recipes that you find in this book that have similar calorie counts and are similar types of food.

SEVEN-DAY WEIGHT-LOSS DIET

MONDAY

BREAKFAST
½ cup orange juice
1 cup cooked oatmeal
1 teaspoon raisins
½ cup skim milk
Coffee or tea*

LUNCH
Chef salad: Shredded lettuce, tomato,
   ¼ cup diced cooked chicken,
   ¼ cup diced Swiss cheese,
   1 tablespoon corn oil,
   unlimited vinegar and herbs
Fresh peach, or ½ cup canned water-packed peaches
Coffee or tea

DINNER
½ cup tomato juice
Broiled fillet of sole, 4 ounces
2 stalks broccoli
½ baked potato
1 baked apple
Coffee or tea

TUESDAY

BREAKFAST
½ sliced orange
1 egg omelet, filled with 2 tablespoons low-fat cottage cheese
1 slice whole-wheat toast
Coffee or tea

LUNCH
Salmon platter: 3¾-ounce can salmon,
   bed of lettuce,
   1 tomato,
   ½ cup coleslaw
2 apricots, or ½ cup canned water-packed apricots
Coffee or tea

*Decaffeinated coffee and weak tea or herb tea are better choices.

DINNER

    1 cup bouillon
    Veal Paprikash
    ½ cup cooked brown rice
    ½ cup cooked carrots
    ½ cup unsweetened applesauce
    Coffee or tea

WEDNESDAY

BREAKFAST

    ½ grapefruit
    1 cup cooked Wheatena, or cold whole-grain cereal
    ½ cup skim milk
    Coffee or tea

LUNCH

    1 cup vegetable soup
    Broiled butterfly shrimp or cold shrimp
    1 broiled tomato
    ½ cup cooked green beans
    1 fresh pear, or ½ cup canned water-packed pears
    Coffee or tea

DINNER

    ½ cup tomato juice
    Broiled Chicken Parmesan
    ½ cup cooked zucchini
    ½ boiled potato
    Spinach and sliced mushroom salad, with lemon juice
    ½ cup canned water-packed mandarin oranges, with a
       pinch of shredded coconut
    Coffee or tea

THURSDAY

BREAKFAST

    ½ cup unsweetened pineapple juice
    ½ cup low-fat cottage cheese
    ½ sliced banana
    Coffee or tea

LUNCH
½ grapefruit
Sliced turkey sandwich on whole-wheat toast
Coffee or tea

DINNER
1 cup onion soup
1 4-ounce slice roast beef
½ cup cooked kasha or brown rice
½ cup cooked spinach
½ cup fresh or frozen blueberries or strawberries
Coffee or tea

FRIDAY

BREAKFAST
½ cup orange juice
1 slice whole-wheat toast, topped with
   1 slice American cheese
Coffee or tea

LUNCH
½ cup tomato juice
Chicken salad sandwich: ½ cup diced cooked chicken;
   ¼ cup diced celery,
   1 tablespoon mayonnaise,
   1 slice rye bread
½ cup coleslaw
Coffee or tea

DINNER
1 cup bouillon
Baked haddock or any broiled fish, no butter
½ medium baked acorn squash
½ cup cooked green beans
1 fresh apple, or ½ cup Waldorf Salad
Coffee or tea

SATURDAY

BREAKFAST
½ small melon or ½ sliced orange
2 slices Whole-wheat French Toast
Coffee or tea

LUNCH

Tuna salad platter: ½ cup water-packed tuna,
¼ cup diced celery,
1 tablespoon mayonnaise,
shredded lettuce,
tomato
Coffee or tea

DINNER

½ cup tomato juice
Broiled Chicken à l'Orange
½ cup cooked brown rice
½ cup cooked carrots
Romaine lettuce with lemon juice
1 fresh peach, or ½ cup water-packed sliced peaches
Coffee or tea

SUNDAY

BREAKFAST

½ grapefruit
1 poached egg on 1 slice whole-wheat toast
Coffee or tea

LUNCH

Oatmeal Meatloaf
Shredded lettuce
1 tomato
½ green pepper, sliced
½ cup raw cauliflower
½ cup canned water-packed pineapple tidbits
Coffee or tea

DINNER

½ cup cranberry juice
5 ounces roast turkey
½ baked potato
6 stalks asparagus or other low-calorie green vegetable
1 slice Orange Sponge Cake or angel-food cake
Coffee or tea

GENERAL CALORIE COUNTS

DAIRY PRODUCTS
CHEESES
American,

Cheddar type	115	1 oz.
	70	1" cube
	225	½ cup, grated
Process American,		
Cheddar type	105	1 oz.
Blue-mold (Roquefort)	105	"
Cottage, not creamed	25	2 tbs.
Cottage, creamed	30	"
Cream cheese	105	"
Parmesan, dry, grated	40	"
Swiss	105	1 oz.

FLUID MILK

Whole	165	1 cup
Skim	90	"
Buttermilk	90	"
Evaporated (undiluted)	170	½ cup
Condensed, sweetened (undiluted)	490	"
Half-and-half (milk and cream)	330	1 cup
	20	1 tbs.

MILK BEVERAGES

Cocoa (all milk)	235	1 cup
Chocolate-flavored milk drink	190	"
Chocolate milk shake	520	12 oz.
Malted milk	280	1 cup

OTHERS

Butter	100	1 tbs.
Cream, light	35	"
Cream, heavy whipping	55	"
Ice cream, plain	130	3½ oz.
Ice cream soda, chocolate	455	1 glass
Ice milk	140	½ cup
Yogurt (partially skimmed milk)	120	1 cup

MEATS AND POULTRY
(Cooked, without bone)
BEEF
Pot roast or braised

Lean and fat	245	3 oz.
Lean only	140	2½ oz.
Oven roast		
Lean and fat	220	3 oz.
Lean only	130	2½ oz.
Steak, broiled		
Lean and fat	330	3 oz.
Lean only	115	2 oz.
Hamburger		
Regular ground beef	245	3 oz. patty
Lean ground round	185	"
Corned beef, canned	180	3 oz.
Corned beef hash, canned	120	"
Dried beef, chipped	115	2 oz.
Meatloaf	115	"
Beef and vegetable stew	90	½ cup
Beef potpie, baked	460	1 pie, 4¼" dia.

VEAL
Cutlet, broiled

(meat only)	185	3 oz.

CHICKEN

Broiled	185	3 oz.
Fried	215	½ breast
	245	thigh and drumstick
Canned	190	½ cup

LAMB
Chop

Lean and fat	405	4 oz.
Lean only	140	2⅗ oz.
Roast leg		
Lean and fat	235	3 oz.
Lean only	130	2½ oz.

PORK

Chop		
Lean and fat	260	2⅓ oz.
Lean only	130	2 oz.
Roast Loin		
Lean and fat	310	3 oz.
Lean only	175	2⅖ oz.
Ham, cured		
Lean and fat	290	3 oz.
Lean only	125	2⅕ oz.
Bacon, broiled	95	2 thin slices

SAUSAGE AND VARIETY MEATS

Bologna sausage	170	2 oz.
Liver sausage	175	"
Vienna sausage, canned	135	"
Pork sausage, bulk	170	2 oz. patty
Beef liver, fried	120	2 oz.
Beef tongue, boiled	205	3 oz.
Frankfurter	155	each
Boiled ham	170	2 oz.
Spiced ham, canned	165	"

FISH AND SHELLFISH

Bluefish, baked	135	3 oz.
Clams, shelled		
Raw, meat only	70	"
Canned, clams and juice	45	"
Crab meat	90	"
Fish Sticks	200	4 oz.
Haddock, fried	135	3 oz.
Mackerel		
Broiled	200	"
Canned	155	"
Ocean perch, fried	195	"
Oysters, raw	80	6 to 10
Salmon		
Broiled	205	4 oz.
Canned (pink)	120	3 oz.
Sardines, canned in oil	180	"
Shrimp, canned	110	"
Tuna, canned in oil	170	"

EGGS

Fried	100	1 large
Boiled	80	"
Scrambled or omelet	110	"
Poached	80	"

NUTS

Almonds, shelled	105	15 nuts
Brazil nuts, broken	115	2 tbs.
Cashew nuts, roasted	95	5 nuts
Coconut, shredded	40	2 tbs.
Peanuts, roasted shelled	105	"
Peanut butter	90	1 tbs.
Pecans, shelled	90	12 halves
Walnuts, shelled		
Black	100	2 tbs.
English	80	10 halves

VEGETABLES

Asparagus	20	6 spears
Beans, fresh		
Lima	75	½ cup
Snap, green, or wax	15	"
Beans, dried		
Red kidney, cooked	115	"
Lima, cooked	130	"
Baked		
With pork	165	"
Without pork	160	"
Beets	35	"
Beet greens, cooked	20	"
Broccoli	20	"
Brussels sprouts	30	"
Cabbage		
Raw	10	"
Coleslaw (with dressing)	50	"
Cooked	20	"
Carrots	20	"
Cauliflower	15	"
Celery	10	2 large stalks
Chard	25	½ cup
Collards	40	"
Corn on cob	65	1 ear

Corn, cooked	85 ½ cup	Apple juice	60 ½ cup
Cress, garden	35 "	Applesauce	
Cucumbers	5 6 slices	Sweetened	90 "
Kale	20 ½ cup	Unsweetened	50 "
Kohlrabi	25 "	Apricots	
Lettuce	5 3 leaves	Raw	55 3
Mushrooms, canned	15 ½ cup	Canned, water pack	45 ½ cup
Mustard greens	15 "	Canned, syrup pack	110 "
Okra, cooked	15 4 pods	Dried, cooked,	
Onions		unsweetened	120 "
Raw	50 1	Frozen, sweetened	125 "
	medium	Avocados	185 ½ 10 oz.
Cooked	40 ½ cup	Bananas, raw	85 1
Parsnips, cooked	50 "		medium
Peas, green	60 "	Berries	
Peppers, green	15 1	Blackberries, raw	40 ½ cup
	medium	Blueberries, raw	45 "
Potatoes		Raspberries, raw	35 "
Baked or boiled	90 "	Frozen, sweetened	120 "
Chips	110 10	Strawberries, raw	30 "
	medium	Frozen, sweetened	120 "
French fried	155 10 pieces	Cantaloupe, raw	40 ½
Hash browned	235 ½ cup		melon,
Mashed with milk	70 "		5" dia.
Pan fried	240 "	Cherries	
Radishes	10 4 small	Raw	30 ½ cup
Sauerkraut, canned	15 ½ cup	Canned red, sour,	
Spinach	20 "	pitted	55 "
Squash		Cranberry sauce,	
Summer	20 "	sweetened	30 1 tbs.
Winter, baked	50 "	Cranberry juice	
Sweet Potatoes		cocktail	70 ½ cup
Baked	155 1	Dates	250 "
	medium	Figs	
Canned	120 ½ cup	Raw	90 3 small
Tomato juice	25 "	Canned, heavy syrup	110 ½ cup
Tomatoes		Dried	60 1 large
Raw	30 1	Fruit cocktail,	
	medium	canned in syrup	100 ½ cup
Cooked or canned	25 ½ cup	Grapefruit	
Turnips, cooked	20 "	Raw	50 ½
Turnip greens	20 "		medium
		Canned water pack	35 ½ cup
		Canned syrup pack	80 "
FRUITS		Grapefruit juice	
Apples, raw	70 1	Unsweetened	50 "
	medium	Sweetened	65 "

Grapes	45	3½ oz.
Grape juice, bottled	75	½ cup
Honeydew melon	50	2" × 7" wedge
Lemon juice	30	½ cup
	5	1 tbsp.
Lemonade	65	½ cup
Oranges, raw	70	1 orange
Orange juice	60	½ cup
Peaches		
Raw	35	1 medium
Canned, water pack	40	½ cup
Canned, syrup pack	100	"
Dried, cooked, unsweetened	110	"
Frozen, sweetened	105	"
Pears		
Raw	100	1 pear
Canned in heavy syrup	100	½ cup
Pineapple		
Raw	35	½ cup, diced
Canned, syrup pack	100	½ cup or 2 slices
Pineapple juice	60	½ cup
Plums		
Raw	30	1 plum
Canned syrup pack	90	½ cup
Prunes, dried cooked		
Unsweetened	150	9 prunes
Sweetened	260	"
Prune juice, canned	85	½ cup
Raisins, dried	230	"
Rhubarb, cooked, sweetened	190	"
Tangerine, raw	40	1 medium
Tangerine juice, canned	50	½ cup
Watermelon, raw	120	4" × 8" wedge

BREADS AND CEREALS

Cracked wheat	60	slice
Raisin	60	"
Rye	55	"
White	60	"
Whole wheat	55	"

OTHER BAKED GOODS

Baking powder biscuit	130	each
Graham crackers	55	2 medium
Saltines	35	2
Soda crackers	45	2
Plain muffins	135	each
Bran muffins	125	"
Corn muffins	155	"
Pancakes, wheat	60	4" dia.
Buckwheat cakes	45	"
Pizza (cheese)	180	⅛, 14" pie
Pretzels	20	5 sticks
Plain pan rolls	115	each
Hard round rolls	160	"
Sweet pan rolls	135	"
Rye wafers	45	2
Waffles	240	4½" × 5½"

CEREALS AND OTHER GRAIN PRODUCTS

Bran flakes (40% bran)	85	1 oz.
Corn, puffed, presweetened	110	"
Corn and soy shreds	100	"
Corn flakes	110	"
Corn grits, cooked	90	¾ cup
Farina, cooked	80	"
Macaroni, cooked	115	"
Macaroni and cheese	240	½ cup
Noodles, cooked	150	¾ cup
Oat cereal	115	1 ounce
Oatmeal, cooked	110	¾ cup
Rice, cooked	150	"
Rice Flakes	115	1 cup
Rice, puffed	55	"
Spaghetti, cooked	115	¾ cup
Spaghetti with meat sauce	215	"

Spaghetti in tomato sauce, with cheese	160	"
Wheat, puffed	100	1 oz.
Wheat, puffed, presweetened	105	"
Wheat, rolled, cooked	130	¾ cup
Wheat, shredded, plain	100	1 oz.
Wheat flakes	100	¾ cup
Wheat flours		
Whole wheat	300	"
All-purpose flour	300	¾ cup sifted
Wheat germ	185	¾ cup

FATS, OILS, AND RELATED PRODUCTS

Margarine	100	1 tbs.
Cooking Fats		
Vegetable	110	"
Lard	135	"
Salad or Cooking Oils	125	"

SALAD DRESSINGS

French	60	1 tbs.
Blue cheese, French	90	"
Home-cooked, boiled	30	"
Low-calorie	15	"
Mayonnaise		
Home-cooked	110	"
Commercial	60	"
Thousand Island	75	"

CANDY, SYRUPS, JAMS, JELLY

Caramels	120	1 oz.
Chocolate creams	110	"
Chocolate, milk, sweetened	145	1-oz. bar
Chocolate, milk, sweetened, with almonds	150	"
Chocolate mints	110	1 oz.
Fudge, chocolate	115	"
Gumdrops	95	"
Hard candy	110	1 oz.
Jelly beans	65	"
Marshmallows	90	"

Peanut brittle	125	"
Chocolate syrup	40	1 tbs.
Honey	60	"
Molasses, cane, light	50	"
Syrup, table blends	55	"
Jelly	50	"
Jam, marmalade, preserves	55	"
Sugar	15	1 tsp.

DESSERTS

Apple Betty	175	½ cup
Angel food cake	110	2" sector
Butter cake, plain	180	3" × 2" × 1½" slice, or
	130	cupcake
Chocolate cake, with fudge icing	420	2" piece
Doughnut	135	each
Fruitcake, dark	105	2" × 2" × ½" slice
Gingerbread	180	"
Pound cake	130	1" slice
Sponge cake	115	2" piece
Cookies, plain	110	3" dia.
Cornstarch pudding	140	½ cup
Custard, baked	140	"
Fig bars, small	55	each
Fruit ice	75	½ cup
Gelatin dessert, plain	80	"
Pies		
Apple	330	4" piece
Cherry	340	"
Custard	265	"
Lemon Meringue	300	"
Mince	340	"
Pumpkin	265	"
Prune whip	100	½ cup
Rennet dessert pudding	125	"
Sherbet	120	"

BEVERAGES

Ginger ale	80	8 oz.
Cola type	105	"

Low-calorie type	10 "	90-proof	110 "
Postum	5 1 cup	86-proof	105 "
Coffee or tea	0 "	80-proof	100 "
Beer, 4% alcohol	175 12 oz.	70-proof	85 "
Whisky, gin, rum:		Wines, table use	70 3 oz.
100-proof	125 1½ oz.	Sweet wines	120 "

SEASONINGS TO ENHANCE FLAVOR

Since salt is rarely used in Aerobic Nutrition, it is important that you master the use of herbs and spices to complement the ingredients of your meal. The recipes in this book will show you how a dash of this and a dash of that will enhance your cooking.

Buy herbs and spices in small quantities and keep them in a cool, dry place. Be sure that the containers are tightly closed, especially the ones with shaker holes that you may carelessly leave open when you are in a hurry. Try to keep your spices together—if they are lined up on a rack, place them in alphabetical order so you can find them quickly as you cook. If you keep them in an upper cabinet near the range, place them on a circular rack with some system so you can revolve the rack and pluck out the spice you need with ease.

In the beginning, there is a great temptation to use too much of one spice, or too many different kinds of seasonings in one dish. The great puzzle with herbs and spices is to find out which ones go well together and which are not compatible. Following recipes carefully is one way to learn the proper amounts to use and the tasty combinations that may be made. If you are "winging it" and cooking as you go, just remember to use small pinches of seasonings—they do go a long way.

Here is a list of popular seasonings that describes their taste and how best to use them to improve the flavor of your cooking. Since each spice and herb has an affinity with certain vegetables and fruits, here is a helping-hand checklist for you to use to help you determine compatibility. It's like having your own computer-dating list for each seasoning!

ABOUT HERBS AND SPICES

ALLSPICE.   A sharply flavored berry that is dried and ground into a powder that tastes like a combination of cinnamon and cloves. Another product called all-spice —notice the hyphen—is a blend of many spices, including cinnamon, cloves, and nutmeg. Both can be used to enhance the flavor of fruit, such as in pies; and in some meat dishes. Use with beets, cabbage, carrots, eggplant, spinach, tomatoes, yellow squash, apples, cherries, cranberries, figs, peaches, and rhubarb.

BASIL, SWEET.   Although a member of the mint family, this leaf has a sweetish flavor. It enhances tomato dishes, soups and salads, and Italian-style sauces. Use with asparagus, beans, beets, broccoli, Brussels sprouts, cabbage, carrots, cauliflower, celery, onions, peas, potatoes, spinach, summer squash, tomatoes, white turnips, yellow turnips, and zucchini.

BAY LEAF.   A dried leaf of the laurel family, it has a strong aromatic flavor and is especially good with potted meats and hearty meat soups. Use with beets, cabbage, carrots, potatoes, and tomatoes.

CARAWAY.   The small aromatic seeds of a parsley-type plant, it is used to flavor bread, cheese, cabbage dishes, and some meat dishes. Use with cabbage, potatoes, and white turnips.

CARDAMOM.   A seed that is sold both ground and whole, it is a member of the ginger family and has a sweet, pungent taste. It is also spelled cardamum and cardamon. It is frequently used in Indian and Scandinavian cooking, in curries, and in pastries. Use with carrots, onions, peas, sweet potatoes, apples, cherries, cranberries, figs, grapefruit, oranges, peaches, pears, pineapple, and rhubarb.

CAYENNE PEPPER.   This is also called red pepper or chili pepper. It is ground into a powder from the fruit of the capsicum plant. The powder is very hot with a biting taste and may be used sparingly in some meat dishes, cheese dishes, and spicy sauces. Use with beans, tomatoes, and corn.

CHERVIL.   Has an anise flavor and is a member of the parsley family. It may be used in soups, egg dishes, and some vegetable dishes. Use with carrots, peas, and spinach.

CHILI POWDER.   A powdered blend of spices that has been created to enhance the flavor of Mexican cooking. The basic ingredients are chili pepper, oregano, cumin, and garlic, sometimes with cloves and allspice added. Use in sauces, stews, and meats for south-of-the-border flavor. Use with carrots, eggplant, onions, potatoes, and white turnips.

CHIVES.   Hollow green tips of an onion-family plant that have a subtle onion taste. Use in salads, with sour cream for baked potatoes, in delicate sauces, and in some cheese dishes. Use with beans, cauliflower, mushrooms, peas, potatoes, and tomatoes.

CINNAMON.   Has an aromatic, sweet-pungent taste and is available in stick form or ground into a fine powder. Made from the bark of several trees, including the cassia in the United States, it is used to complement fruit in pastries and compotes, and in meat dishes in many Middle Eastern countries. Use with sweet potatoes, yellow squash, apples, apricots, blueberries, cherries, cranberries, figs, grapefruit, peaches, pears, pineapple, plums, prunes, and rhubarb.

CLOVES.   An aromatic, pungent-tasting, dried bud that is available both whole and ground. It has a warm spicy flavor that can enhance pickled dishes, ham, tongue, desserts, mulled wines, and teas. Use with beets, cabbage, carrots, yellow squash, apples, apricots, blueberries, cherries, cranberries, lemon, lime, peaches, pears, plums, prunes, and rhubarb.

CORIANDER.   A member of the parsley family; its leaves are used in salads, soups, stews. The seeds of the plant are also used and have a lemon-sage flavor that is used in curries, pastries, and some meat dishes. Use with artichokes and tomatoes.

CUMIN.   A nutty-flavored seed that is related to the parsley family. It is available whole or ground and is an ingredient of chili powder and curry powder. It adds a pungent flavor to Middle Eastern recipes for soups, cabbage dishes, and fish and meat dishes. Use with cabbage, corn, and cucumbers.

CURRY POWDER.   A blend of many spices ground together, it has a hot, spicy flavor. It usually contains cayenne, coriander, cumin, turmeric, and sometimes allspice, cinnamon, ginger, and pepper. It is used in Indian-style cooking, for soups, sauces, stews, and seafood dishes. Use with beans, broccoli, Brussels sprouts, cabbage, corn, onions, potatoes, and summer squash.

DILL.   A member of the parsley family, this herb has a recognizable odor and flavor. The stem and leaves of the plant are available as "dillweed" and the seeds as "dillseed." They are used in pickling, soups, seafood and chicken dishes, and are especially tasty in cream sauces. Use with beans, beets, Brussels sprouts, cabbage, carrots, eggplant, potatoes, spinach, tomatoes, white turnips.

GARLIC.   Has a strong and distinct odor and flavor, and is available as a bulb with many cloves, or in powder form. Rub a cut clove on a salad bowl for subtle flavor, or use it to season meats, seafood, chicken, and sauces. Very nice mixed with butter and spread on Italian or French bread before heating. Use with onions, mushrooms, potatoes, and tomatoes.

GINGER.   Has a sweet and spicy flavor and is obtained from the root of a tropical plant. It is available ground or in slivers, and is used to flavor cooked fruits, pastry, sauces, some Far Eastern–style meat dishes, and some vegetable dishes. Use with carrots, onions, peas, sweet potatoes, apples, cherries, cranberries, figs, grapefruit, peaches, pears, pineapple, and rhubarb.

MACE.   A powder ground from the membrane of the fruit of the nutmeg tree. It has a flavor similar to nutmeg—warm and spicy but a little more pungent. It is lighter in color than nutmeg and is frequently used in light-colored dishes. Can be used in baking, sauces, pumpkin dishes, and in some meat, vegetable, and fish dishes. Use with carrots, potatoes, spinach, sweet potatoes, apples, peaches, and pineapple.

MARJORAM.   A member of the mint family, this leaf has a sweet, tangy taste and is available whole or ground. It is used in some vegetables, soups, lamb dishes, and in stuffings. Use with asparagus, beets, Brussels sprouts, carrots, celery, onions, peas, spinach, summer squash, tomatoes, and zucchini.

MINT.   An aromatic herb whose most popular variety is spearmint. This leaf is used in jellies, sauces, candies, meat dishes, and some desserts. Use with beans, beets, carrots, peas, potatoes, spinach, melon, oranges, and pineapple.

MUSTARD.   Prepared from the mustard seed in powdered or paste form. It has a hot, sharp flavor and is used in cheese, meat, and fish dishes, and as a condiment for sandwiches. Use with cucumber pickles, spinach, peas, cabbage, celery.

NUTMEG.   A seed that has a sweet, spicy flavor, and is available in whole or ground form. It is used in baking, puddings, sauces, some vegetables, and some meat dishes. Use with asparagus, beans, beets, broccoli, Brussels sprouts, cabbage, carrots, cauliflower, onions, peas, spinach, summer squash, sweet potatoes, yellow squash, apples, blueberries, cherries, cranberries, grapefruit, lemon, lime, pineapple, and rhubarb.

OREGANO.   A member of the mint family, this leaf has a strong but pleasantly bitter taste. It is used frequently in Italian and Mexican cooking and is especially good in tomato sauces, eggs, cheese, and meat dishes. Use with beans, broccoli, eggplant, mushrooms, onions, peas, spinach, tomatoes, and zucchini.

PAPRIKA.   A fine, red powder with a slightly sweet taste, made from the fruit of a variety of red pepper, it is used both to decorate and to flavor food. It is especially popular in Hungarian cuisine, and may be used as a garnish, on roasts, on poultry, and in soups. Use with cauliflower, corn, onions, and potatoes.

PARSLEY.   An herb with distinctly aromatic-tasting leaves. Available fresh, or dried and chopped. Used as a garnish for its lacy leaves, and as a seasoning for fish, meat, soups, and sauces. Use with asparagus, beets, eggplant, mushrooms, potatoes, tomatoes, and zucchini.

PEPPER.   A dried, pungent berry that is available in whole form, known as "pepper-corns," or ground. Black pepper is obtained from the entire berry and has a more intense taste, while white pepper is ground after the outer covering of the seed is removed. White pepper is used where a more subtle flavor is desired, and where the food is light in color. It is used to flavor soups, sauces, meat of all kinds, and vegetables. Use with beans, cabbage, celery, eggplant, onions, peas, potatoes, spinach, tomatoes, and zucchini.

ROSEMARY.   The dried or fresh leaf of a mint-family plant, this has a sweet flavor and is especially good in lamb dishes, vegetables, sauces, and soups. Use with carrots, cauliflower, eggplant, mushrooms, onions, peas, potatoes, spinach, summer squash, white turnips, and yellow turnips.

SAFFRON.   A spice that is made from the dried golden stigmas of a variety of crocus, it is used sparingly for its slightly bitter taste and as a yellow coloring agent for food. Very popular in Spanish, French, and Italian dishes that contain rice. Also used in some sauces and soups. Use with rice.

SAGE.   The leaves of this pungent, slightly bitter-tasting member of the mint family are usually dried and ground. Use to season stuffings, some soups, sauces, and meat dishes. Adds distinction to vinegar marinades. Use with Brussels sprouts, eggplant, onions, potatoes, summer squash, and tomatoes.

SAVORY.   Available in two varieties. Summer savory is more subtle in taste than winter savory, which has a thymelike flavor. Savory is a member of the mint family and is used in vegetables, sauces, and egg cookery. Use with asparagus, beans, Brussels sprouts, eggplant, and yellow turnips.

TARRAGON. Aromatic leaves that have a slightly licoricelike flavor. Used to enhance sauces, chicken, eggs, and some meat dishes. Use with asparagus, beets, cabbage, mushrooms, and tomatoes.

THYME. A member of the mint family that has a warm, aromatic flavor. It is frequently used in chowders, poultry stuffings, with tomatoes, and in some cheese and fruit dishes. Use with asparagus, beans, beets, carrots, eggplant, mushrooms, onions, potatoes, spinach, tomatoes, white turnips, yellow turnips, and zucchini.

TURMERIC. A member of the ginger family, this is an important ingredient of curry powder. It is used in curries, fish dishes, sauces, and for pickling. Use with cauliflower, peas, and tomatoes.

APPETIZERS

What can you serve as a prelude to the main course when you plan to follow a more healthful food plan? Anything that is low-fat, low-sugar, and low-sodium. Check the ingredients of your own favorite recipes with the calorie chart in the previous chapter to see whether you want to continue using them. Some recipes can be changed to conform to the Aerobic Nutrition way of eating. Sometimes it can be done by substituting a low-fat yogurt for the heavier-fatted sour cream, or by skipping a step that calls for deep-fat frying and perhaps steaming the food instead.

You have learned how much the food you eat affects your oxygen delivery system. The little nibbles and pickup foods at parties can add up to very high-fat, high-sugar, and high-sodium ingestion. The fancy first courses at the company table can do likewise. Without insulting your hosts, you have to be able to analyze what is in the food you are about to fork into your system. It's best to look for the crudité tray of raw fresh vegetables with a dip. Eat the crudités, if you're not on friendly enough terms to ask about the ingredients in the dip. Sauces should always be under suspicion until proved fat-free.

Practice and develop appetizing ways to serve fresh fruit. No need to serve a plain melon wedge when you can slip a knife under the entire segment, slice it into bite-size pieces, then give each alternate piece a push off-center. Place a lemon wedge at the end of the "boat" with perhaps a sprig of mint, and you suddenly have a fancy first course.

If you're tired of serving plain grapefruit halves, dab them with a bit of

111

honey, slip them under the broiler for a few minutes, and serve broiled grapefruit instead.

Or if you planned to use the fresh grapefruit half as the fruit container, turn it into a basket by slicing a thin piece at each end almost to the middle. Then lift up the two pieces toward the middle and tie with a bit of ribbon to make a basket handle. Do the same with a half orange and fill it with an assortment of fresh fruit pieces.

If you are using a can of tuna for a quick spread, be sure that it is the kind packed in water instead of in oil. There are several hundred calories to be saved and they are all in *fat*.

Here is an assortment of appetizer recipes that can be used for parties at the cocktail hour or for family and friends as a first course at the table. They will help you to recognize what a healthier appetizer should be.

AVOCADO DIP

Although avocado is a high-fat food, most of its fat is unsaturated, and the amount you pick up when dipping is small. Here it is mashed with low-fat yogurt to make an exquisite mouthful at a mere 14 calories per tablespoon.

1 ripe avocado	½ teaspoon dried dillweed
1 tomato, skinned	¼ teaspoon pepper
1 small onion, minced fine	2 tablespoons wine vinegar
1 cup plain low-fat yogurt	

Peel and mash the avocado. Chop the tomato fine and add to avocado. Add onion, yogurt, dillweed, pepper, and vinegar. Mix well. Cover tightly and refrigerate until ready to serve. Serve with crackers or fresh vegetables. Makes 2 cups of spread.

	PROTEIN (grams)	FAT UNSATURATED (grams)	FAT SATURATED (grams)	CARBOHYDRATES (grams)	CALORIES
TOTAL RECIPE	8	21	7	30	450
EACH TBS.	.25	.67	.23	.95	14

CRUDITÉ DIP

Here's the way to make a zippy low-calorie dip for crisp chilled vegetable pieces. Figure that three pieces will add up to 1 tablespoon of adhering dip.

1 cup low-fat cottage cheese
¼ cup plain low-fat yogurt
½ teaspoon prepared white horseradish

½ teaspoon garlic powder
¼ teaspoon white pepper
⅛ teaspoon ground thyme

Place all ingredients in an electric blender or food processor and process until mixture is creamy. Serve with a platter of raw vegetables as a dip. Makes 1¼ cups.

	PROTEIN (grams)	FAT UNSATURATED (grams)	FAT SATURATED (grams)	CARBOHYDRATES (grams)	CALORIES
TOTAL RECIPE	27	.4	.6	7	156
EACH TBS.	1.4	.02	.03	.35	8

CLAM DIP

Dips don't have to be rich and fattening when you use low-fat dairy ingredients. The horseradish gives it zing.

½ cup plain nonfat yogurt
½ cup low-fat cottage cheese
6 medium clams, cooked and chopped fine
1 tablespoon grated onion

1 teaspoon lemon juice
½ teaspoon dried oregano
½ teaspoon prepared white horseradish

Combine yogurt and cottage cheese; blend well. Add chopped clams, onion, lemon juice, oregano, and horseradish; mix thoroughly. Makes 1 cup of dip for crackers or raw vegetables.

	PROTEIN (grams)	FAT UNSATURATED (grams)	FAT SATURATED (grams)	CARBOHYDRATES (grams)	CALORIES
TOTAL RECIPE	29	Trace	Trace	10	176
EACH TBS.	2	Trace	Trace	.65	11

CURRIED CHEESE DIP

If you have a fancy for curry, here's a way to enjoy its spicy flavor in a dip. The cheese is puréed into a creamy substance that defies detection.

1 cup low-fat cottage cheese
1 tomato, cut up
1 scallion, sliced

1 teaspoon curry powder
1 teaspoon lemon juice

Place all ingredients in an electric blender or a food processor and process until smooth. Serve with a platter of raw vegetables as a dip. Makes 1¼ cups.

	PROTEIN (grams)	FAT UNSATURATED (grams)	FAT SATURATED (grams)	CARBOHYDRATES (grams)	CALORIES
TOTAL RECIPE	27	Trace	Trace	14	170
EACH TBS.	1.3	Trace	Trace	.7	8.5

CHOPPED VEGETABLE SPREAD

This is a wonderful low-calorie spread with garbanzo beans adding a punch of protein. Serve several tablespoonfuls on a bed of lettuce for a tasty first course.

2 onions, sliced thin
¼ small head cabbage
2 carrots, scraped
1 stalk celery, trimmed

1 small green pepper, seeded
¼ cup garbanzo beans, drained
⅛ teaspoon pepper

Place onions in a small saucepan; add a little water and simmer until tender. Drain. Grind cabbage, carrots, celery, green pepper, and garbanzo beans, using a fine blade. Add cooked onions and pepper. Mix well. If mixture does not stick together, add some of the onion cooking liquid to the mixture. Chill. Makes 1½ cups of vegetable spread.

	PROTEIN (grams)	FAT UNSATURATED (grams)	FAT SATURATED (grams)	CARBOHYDRATES (grams)	CALORIES
TOTAL RECIPE	17	2.67	.22	70	355
EACH TBS.	.71	.11	.01	3	15

CHOPPED CHICKEN LIVERS

Chicken livers are high in protein and iron. This is a healthier method of simmering in water rather than the usual way of sautéing in fat. A bit of sherry gives it a pleasant kick.

1 pound fresh chicken livers	2 tablespoons dry sherry
1 onion, sliced thin	⅛ teaspoon pepper
2 hard-cooked eggs	

Place chicken livers and onions in a large skillet; barely cover the bottom of the skillet with water. Cover and simmer for five minutes, turning the livers occasionally. Add more water if needed. Remove livers and onions with a slotted spoon. Chop livers, onion, and eggs together, or place all in a food processor and blend for 1 second. Add sherry and pepper; mix through by hand. Chill until ready to serve as a spread. Makes 1½ cups of chopped liver.

	PROTEIN (grams)	FAT UNSATURATED (grams)	FAT SATURATED (grams)	CARBOHYDRATES (grams)	CALORIES
TOTAL RECIPE	134	10	8	24	970
EACH TBS.	6	.43	.34	1	40

CHOPPED EGGPLANT

If you use a food processor for this, it will be ready with a flick of the wrist. Serve it with tiny slices of pumpernickel bread.

1 medium eggplant	¼ teaspoon pepper
1 small onion, diced	¼ teaspoon garlic powder
2 tablespoons lemon juice	2 teaspoons salad oil
1 teaspoon brown sugar	

Bake the whole eggplant, uncovered, in a 350°F. oven until the skin turns dark brown and is wrinkled. Remove from oven, cut the skin away, and then cut eggplant into several thick slices. Place eggplant slices in a large chopping bowl; add onion and chop very fine. Add lemon juice, brown sugar, pepper, garlic, and salad oil; mix well. Chill. Makes about 2 cups of spread.

	PROTEIN (grams)	FAT UNSATURATED (grams)	FAT SATURATED (grams)	CARBOHYDRATES (grams)	CALORIES
TOTAL RECIPE	6	7	.91	31	218
EACH TBS.	.19	.23	.03	1	7

SALMON CHEESE DIP

Let a bit of cooked salmon turn your cheese dip pink and peppy. Don't forget that dillweed has an affinity with fish.

1 cup low-fat cottage cheese
½ cup flaked cooked salmon
½ teaspoon dried dillweed

½ teaspoon paprika
¼ cup plain low-fat yogurt
1 teaspoon chopped chives

Place all ingredients in an electric blender or food processor and process until mixture is creamy smooth. Serve with a platter of raw vegetables or crackers as a dip. Makes 1¾ cups.

	PROTEIN (grams)	FAT UNSATURATED (grams)	FAT SATURATED (grams)	CARBOHYDRATES (grams)	CALORIES
TOTAL RECIPE	49	4	3.8	7	343
EACH TBS.	1.75	.14	.13	.2	12

PICKLED MUSHROOMS

This is the kind of a nibble that dieters love. The mushrooms will keep in the refrigerator for several days.

1 pound tiny raw mushrooms	1 teaspoon paprika
½ cup red wine vinegar	¼ teaspoon ground cumin
2 tablespoons salad oil	⅛ teaspoon ground cloves

Trim mushrooms of stems by cutting across at the bottom of the cap rather than removing the complete stem. (Reserve remaining stems for another use.) Combine vinegar, oil, paprika, cumin, and cloves. Shake well and pour over mushrooms. Let stand in refrigerator overnight, tightly covered, until ready to serve. Drain and serve with picks. Makes about 3 dozen.

	PROTEIN (grams)	FAT UNSATURATED (grams)	FAT SATURATED (grams)	CARBOHYDRATES (grams)	CALORIES
TOTAL RECIPE	12	22	2.72	20	367
EACH SERVING	.34	.61	.08	.56	10

STUFFED CELERY

Celery is one of those almost-minus-calorie foods. You use more energy to chew it than the celery contains.

10 deep-curved stalks celery, trimmed	½ teaspoon garlic powder
⅔ cup low-fat cottage cheese	½ teaspoon onion powder
½ teaspoon dried dillweed	¼ teaspoon paprika

Cut celery stalks in half, crosswise, to get smaller pieces. Combine cottage cheese, dillweed, garlic, onion powder, and paprika; mix well. Spread lightly into curves of celery stalks. Dust with additional paprika, if desired. Makes 20 appetizers.

	PROTEIN (grams)	FAT UNSATURATED (grams)	FAT SATURATED (grams)	CARBOHYDRATES (grams)	CALORIES
TOTAL RECIPE	27	Trace	Trace	20	186
EACH SERVING	1.35	Trace	Trace	1	9

CRAB PUFFS

If you are not counting calories, slip all onto melba rounds. Either way, these crab puffs look deceivably rich and naughty.

1 egg white
2 tablespoons Mayonnaise
¼ teaspoon dried tarragon
½ cup flaked cooked crab meat

18 cucumber slices, unpeeled, ¼ inch thick
Paprika

Beat egg white until stiff peaks form. Combine mayonnaise, tarragon, and cooked crab meat; mix well. Fold mixture into egg whites. Pile teaspoonfuls onto each slice of cucumber. Place on a cookie sheet and broil until lightly browned. Makes 18 servings.

	PROTEIN (grams)	FAT UNSATURATED (grams)	FAT SATURATED (grams)	CARBOHYDRATES (grams)	CALORIES
TOTAL RECIPE	17.5	16	4	11	322
EACH SERVING	1	.9	.2	.6	18

PETITE BEAN SPROUT PATTIES

You can make these patties larger and serve for lunch or supper. Use a ¼-cup ice-cream scoop for uniform portions and flatten with the back of the scoop before baking.

1 cup bean sprouts, chopped
¾ cup wheat germ
½ cup plain nonfat yogurt
½ cup grated Swiss cheese
1 egg, slightly beaten

1 clove garlic, minced fine
½ teaspoon dried oregano
¼ teaspoon onion powder
⅛ teaspoon pepper

Combine chopped sprouts, wheat germ, yogurt, Swiss cheese, and egg. Mix well. Add garlic, oregano, onion powder, and pepper, and mix through. Place by teaspoonfuls an inch apart on a nonstick-surface baking sheet. Bake in a 350°F. oven for 15 minutes, or until lightly browned and firm. Serve warm. (Can be made ahead and then warmed through.) Makes 4 dozen appetizers.

	PROTEIN (grams)	FAT UNSATURATED (grams)	FAT SATURATED (grams)	CARBOHYDRATES (grams)	CALORIES
TOTAL RECIPE	63	20	20	46	819
EACH SERVING	1.32	.42	.43	1	17

PETITE PIZZAS

There's something virtuous about a wheat-germ crust. Be sure to use low-fat mozzarella cheese made from skim milk to keep the saturated fat level down.

¾ cup unbleached flour
¼ cup soft shortening
¼ cup wheat germ
¼ teaspoon dried thyme
5–6 teaspoons cold water
    8-ounce can tomato sauce

½ teaspoon dried oregano
½ teaspoon dried basil
¼ teaspoon garlic powder
4 ounces low-fat mozzarella
    cheese
¼ cup grated Parmesan cheese

Combine flour and shortening until mixture looks like fine meal. Add wheat germ and thyme, working through the dough well. Add just enough cold water to make a firm dough. Roll out on a lightly floured board to ⅛-inch thickness. Cut into rounds with a floured 2-inch cutter. Place on an ungreased baking sheet. Bake at 425°F. for 4 to 6 minutes, or until golden brown. Remove from oven, remove from pan, and cool on a rack. Combine tomato sauce, oregano, basil, and garlic powder; spoon over each pastry round. Cut mozzarella cheese into enough small slices to cover each round with one slice (about 24). Sprinkle Parmesan over each. Place on an ungreased baking sheet. Broil 2 to 3 minutes, until cheese melts. Serve warm. Makes 2 dozen.

	PROTEIN (grams)	FAT UNSATURATED (grams)	FAT SATURATED (grams)	CARBOHYDRATES (grams)	CALORIES
TOTAL RECIPE	50	40	16	114	1193
EACH SERVING	2	1.68	.69	4.76	50

ZUCCHINI CHEESE SQUARES

This is a quick baked appetizer that has a gourmet flair. Freezes well after baking, so have a party any time. Appetizer squares may be warmed just before serving.

3 cups thinly sliced zucchini
1 cup grated Parmesan cheese
¾ cup wheat germ
4 eggs, slightly beaten
2 tablespoons corn oil

½ cup finely chopped onion
½ cup chopped fresh parsley
1 clove garlic, minced
1 teaspoon dried marjoram
¼ teaspoon pepper

Combine zucchini, Parmesan cheese, and wheat germ. Combine eggs and corn oil, beating well; pour over zucchini mixture. Add onion, parsley, garlic, marjoram, and pepper. Mix well. Spread mixture in a greased 13-by-9-inch baking pan. Bake at 350°F. for 15 to 20 minutes, or until set and lightly browned. Cool about 5 minutes. Cut into squares. Makes 5 dozen appetizers.

	PROTEIN (grams)	FAT UNSATURATED (grams)	FAT SATURATED (grams)	CARBOHYDRATES (grams)	CALORIES
TOTAL RECIPE	91	49	25	66	1353
EACH SERVING	1.52	.81	.43	1	23

CRUSTLESS YOGURT MUSHROOM QUICHE

If you prefer a crust, use the pastry shell on page 296. It boosts the calories and really isn't necessary.

4 eggs, slightly beaten
1 cup plain low-fat yogurt
1 tablespoon cornstarch
¾ cup skim milk
Dash of pepper

⅛ teaspoon ground nutmeg
1 small onion, diced fine
4 ounces Swiss cheese, diced
¼ pound sliced mushrooms
2 tablespoon Parmesan cheese

Preheat oven to 375°F. Combine eggs, yogurt, cornstarch, milk, pepper, and nutmeg; beat well. Add diced onion, Swiss cheese, and mushrooms. Pour into a greased 9-inch pie pan. Sprinkle grated Parmesan cheese on top. Bake 35 minutes, or until lightly browned. Let stand 10 minutes before serving. Makes 8 servings.

	PROTEIN (grams)	FAT UNSATURATED (grams)	FAT SATURATED (grams)	CARBOHYDRATES (grams)	CALORIES
TOTAL RECIPE	79	27	30	33	1043
EACH SERVING	10	3	4	4	130

GRAPE JUICE SANGRÍA

When is sangría not made with wine? When it's made with unfermented grape juice. Add lemons, limes, or other fruits in season.

1 quart unsweetened grape juice
1 pint unsweetened pineapple juice

1 pint club soda
1 orange, thinly sliced
1 apple, cut in small wedges

Combine grape juice, pineapple juice, and club soda. Add orange and apple. Pour into glasses over ice cubes. Makes 8 servings.

	PROTEIN (grams)	FAT UNSATURATED (grams)	FAT SATURATED (grams)	CARBOHYDRATES (grams)	CALORIES
TOTAL RECIPE	5.6	0	0	275	1102
EACH SERVING	.7	0	0	34	138

HOT CINNAMON APPLE DRINK

You can stretch these servings if you use small punch cups. Add cinnamon sticks to swizzle the flavor further, if desired.

1 quart unsweetened apple juice   ¼ teaspoon ground cloves
½ teaspoon ground cinnamon   4 slices lemon

Heat apple juice with cinnamon and cloves. Pour into 4 mugs, and add a slice of lemon to each. Makes 4 servings.

	PROTEIN (grams)	FAT UNSATURATED (grams)	FAT SATURATED (grams)	CARBOHYDRATES (grams)	CALORIES
TOTAL RECIPE	1.3	0	0	126	492
EACH SERVING	.3	0	0	31	123

SOUP

Whatever happened to old-fashioned homemade soup? Real soup—the kind that simmered on the back of the range, wafting fragrant aromas throughout the house, letting everyone know that somebody cared enough to get some good food going? Are we too busy to cook soup? It takes about ten minutes to fill up a huge soup pot with bones and a wide assortment of vegetables, a few seasonings, and a lot of water. The rest of the cooking time you are free to do whatever is demanding your attention. The soup can be stored in the refrigerator for a week, it can be altered with a handful of rice or pasta or some leftover vegetables, or it can be stored in small containers in the freezer. Even a person who lives alone can make a big pot of vegetable soup and store single portions in the freezer to coast on for months. Make a few different soups and you'll never resort to cans of high-sodium condensed soups again.

When making chicken bouillon, be sure to refrigerate it and let the chicken fat solidify on the top. Remove the fat and do yourself a favor and dispose of it. This is saturated animal fat and you get enough of it in your meats without deliberately using it to flavor up your food. Store excess bouillon in the freezer. If you freeze it in ice cube trays first and then store it in heavy plastic bags, you'll be able to reach in and have a soup cube whenever you need it.

Get in the habit of conducting a "refrigerator roundup" every few weeks. Gather up those carrots that are beginning to wilt, the half stalk of celery, the turnip that you forgot to cook, that half a head of cabbage you meant to turn into slaw, and turn everything into a great soup. It's the most economical way to salvage your good intentions, and it has a special hospitality that shows you care.

This large group of recipes will show you how easy it is to make your own low-sodium, low-sugar, and low-fat soup.

SUPER SOUP

It's a one-pot meal with the kind of cooked-soft meat that Mama used to make. Add other vegetables as the spirit moves you.

1 large onion, sliced
4 carrots, scraped and cut into chunks
4 stalks celery, cut into chunks
1 large yellow turnip, peeled and cut into chunks
3 large parsnips, peeled and cut into chunks
1 cup small white lima beans

1 pound lean beef chuck
16-ounce can tomatoes
2 quarts water
1 cup macaroni
2 bay leaves
2 cloves
½ teaspoon pepper
¼ teaspoon dried oregano

Place everything in a large soup pot. Bring to a boil, then reduce heat and simmer, covered, for 2 to 3 hours. Skim residue off top occasionally. When vegetables and meat are tender, the soup is done. Makes 16 servings.

	PROTEIN (grams)	FAT UNSATURATED (grams)	FAT SATURATED (grams)	CARBOHYDRATES (grams)	CALORIES
TOTAL RECIPE	108	16	16	262	1801
EACH SERVING	6.7	1	1	16	112

CHICKEN BOUILLON

Freeze extra soup in ice cube trays. Then store in plastic bags in the freezer to use as needed. Be sure to remove fat as directed in the recipe.

1 chicken, about 4 pounds	1 large parsnip, scraped
2 quarts water	3 sprigs parsley
2 large onions	3 sprigs fresh dill
2 stalks celery, including leaves	½ teaspoon salt
4 scraped carrots	⅛ teaspoon white pepper

Place chicken in a deep pot and cover with water. Add neck, gizzard, and even feet if you have them. Add remaining ingredients. Bring to a boil and then turn the heat low and simmer for 1½ to 2 hours, covered. Remove chicken from soup. (Use it for the base of a hot dish or cut it up into chicken salad.) Pour soup through a strainer into a large clean container. Put whole cooked carrots into the strained soup. Chill until fat rises and solidifies. Remove fat. Heat just before serving. Makes 8 servings.

	PROTEIN (grams)	FAT UNSATURATED (grams)	FAT SATURATED (grams)	CARBOHYDRATES (grams)	CALORIES
TOTAL RECIPE	7	Trace	Trace	46	201
EACH SERVING	.8	Trace	Trace	5.7	25

TOMATO BOUILLON

Add some rice or a bit of pastina. Who needs high-sodium canned soup when you can perform a trick like this?

1 quart tomato juice	1 teaspoon sugar
2 cups chicken bouillon	½ teaspoon dried dillweed
1 tablespoon lemon juice	

Combine tomato juice with chicken bouillon; add lemon juice, sugar, and dillweed. Simmer for 10 minutes and serve hot. Makes 8 servings.

	PROTEIN (grams)	FAT UNSATURATED (grams)	FAT SATURATED (grams)	CARBOHYDRATES (grams)	CALORIES
TOTAL RECIPE	9	Trace	Trace	47	203
EACH SERVING	1	Trace	Trace	6	25

ONION SOUP

It's so easy to make your own healthful low-sodium onion soup. Bake it in individual crocks with a topping of low-fat bland cheese, if desired.

1 quart Chicken Bouillon
4 large onions, sliced thin
¼ teaspoon Worcestershire sauce

2 tablespoons grated Parmesan cheese

Pour chicken bouillon into a large saucepan; add onions and Worcestershire sauce. Simmer, covered, for 20 minutes. Serve with a sprinkling of Parmesan cheese. Makes 6 servings.

	PROTEIN (grams)	FAT UNSATURATED (grams)	FAT SATURATED (grams)	CARBOHYDRATES (grams)	CALORIES
TOTAL RECIPE	9	.8	1.4	30	170
EACH SERVING	1.4	.15	.2	5	28

FISH CHOWDER

A salad would complete this for a great Sunday supper. Serve fresh fruit for dessert and you've made an easy meal.

2 peeled and cubed potatoes
1 onion, thinly sliced
1 sprig dill, finely chopped
2 cups water
1 pound fish fillets

2 cups skim milk
1 tablespoon soft margarine
¼ teaspoon dried thyme
¼ teaspoon white pepper

Simmer potatoes, onions, and dill in water, covered, until potatoes are soft, about 15 minutes. Cut fish fillets into small chunks and add to the potatoes. Stir in the milk, margarine, thyme, and pepper. Simmer, covered, for an additional 15 to 20 minutes, stirring occasionally. Serve at once. Makes 8 servings.

	PROTEIN (grams)	FAT UNSATURATED (grams)	FAT SATURATED (grams)	CARBOHYDRATES (grams)	CALORIES
TOTAL RECIPE	101	2.6	2.6	97	932
EACH SERVING	12.6	.3	.3	12	116

OYSTER CHOWDER

Be sure to use the oyster liquid for more intense flavor. This is also the time to use thyme, a most savory herb.

1 potato, pared and cut into chunks
1 onion, diced
1 carrot, pared and finely chopped
½ cup chopped celery
1 tablespoon chopped green pepper

¼ teaspoon ground thyme
¼ teaspoon pepper
½ cup water
1 quart skim milk
12 small oysters

Place potato, onion, carrot, celery, green pepper, thyme, pepper, and water in a medium saucepan. Cover and simmer for 15 minutes, or until vegetables are tender. Add milk, oysters, and oyster liquid. Heat only until the edges of the oysters curl, about 5 minutes. Serve at once. Makes 6 servings.

	PROTEIN (grams)	FAT UNSATURATED (grams)	FAT SATURATED (grams)	CARBOHYDRATES (grams)	CALORIES
TOTAL RECIPE	54	Trace	Trace	104	670
EACH SERVING	9	Trace	Trace	17	112

VEGETABLE SOUP

You'll want to double this and freeze it for the many soup-filled days ahead. It's the way to cook and coast on a single effort.

4 beef marrow bones
2 quarts water
2 onions, sliced
½ cup barley
2 carrots, scraped and sliced
2 celery stalks, sliced
3 tomatoes, cut up
1 large potato, peeled and diced

½ pound trimmed green beans, cut up
½ pound shelled peas
1 bay leaf
2 whole cloves
1 sprig parsley
¼ teaspoon dried thyme
¼ teaspoon pepper

Place bones in a large pot and cover with water. Add onions and barley. Bring to a boil, then turn down heat and simmer about 30 minutes, occasionally skimming residue off the top. Add the rest of the ingredients and cook for 30 minutes over low heat, or until all vegetables are tender. Makes 10 servings.

	PROTEIN (grams)	FAT UNSATURATED (grams)	FAT SATURATED (grams)	CARBOHYDRATES (grams)	CALORIES
TOTAL RECIPE	42	0	0	218	1015
EACH SERVING	4.2	0	0	22	102

LIMA BEAN BARLEY SOUP

It may not seem like much barley, but remember that it expands like rice. A little can go a long way to give texture and nourishment. Extra soup may be frozen for future use.

1 cup dried small lima beans
½ cup barley
2 cups chopped tomatoes
4 carrots, scraped and sliced
2 stalks celery, sliced thin
2 onions, sliced

1 garlic clove, minced fine
¼ pound mushrooms, sliced
1 large sprig dill
1 large sprig parsley
1 tablespoon lemon juice
¼ teaspoon pepper

In a heavy soup pot, soak beans in 6 cups water for several hours or overnight. Drain. Add remaining ingredients and 2 quarts fresh water. Bring to a boil, reduce heat, cover pot, and simmer 3 hours, or until all is tender. Makes 10 servings.

	PROTEIN (grams)	FAT UNSATURATED (grams)	FAT SATURATED (grams)	CARBOHYDRATES (grams)	CALORIES
TOTAL RECIPE	62	0	0	275	1345
EACH SERVING	6.2	0	0	28	135

WHITE BEAN SOUP

Soaking the beans makes them cook much faster. And it's also a nice energy-saving economy. Serve this soup with grated Parmesan cheese, if desired.

2½ cups dried white beans
2 tablespoons corn oil
1 clove garlic, minced fine
1 onion, chopped fine
1 carrot, scraped and chopped
  fine

1 stalk celery, chopped fine
Several meat bones
½ teaspoon dried rosemary
¼ teaspoon white pepper

Soak beans overnight in 1 quart of water. Heat corn oil in the bottom of the soup kettle; sauté garlic, onion, carrot, and celery until lightly browned. Pour off oil. Add beans and water for soaking. Add bones, rosemary, and white pepper. Add 1 quart more of water. Simmer gently for 2 hours, or until beans are tender. Remove bones. Rub half the beans through a sieve back into the soup. Makes 10 servings.

	PROTEIN (grams)	FAT UNSATURATED (grams)	FAT SATURATED (grams)	CARBOHYDRATES (grams)	CALORIES
TOTAL RECIPE	35	22	2.72	102	791
EACH SERVING	3.5	2	.3	10	79

BARLEY BEAN SOUP

The combination of a grain and a legume adds up to an excellent protein source. Takes only minutes to fill the pot, then let it simmer while you putter elsewhere.

1 cup dried lima beans	2 sprigs fresh dill
3 meaty neck bones	¼ cup pearl barley
1 onion	¼ teaspoon pepper
2 sprigs fresh parsley	2 bay leaves

Soak dried lima beans for a few hours, or overnight. Drain and add to 2 quarts of water in a heavy saucepan. Add neck bones, onion, parsley, dill, barley, pepper, and bay leaves. Bring to a boil and then turn the heat low and simmer for 2 hours, or until beans and meat are tender. Remove bones and cut up chunks of meat; return meat to the soup. Remove bay leaves. Chill and remove solidified fat. Reheat when ready to serve. Makes 10 servings.

	PROTEIN (grams)	FAT UNSATURATED (grams)	FAT SATURATED (grams)	CARBOHYDRATES (grams)	CALORIES
TOTAL RECIPE	58	14	15	81	848
EACH SERVING	6	1.4	1.5	8	85

BEEF, BEAN, AND BARLEY SOUP

Here carrot gives a natural sweetness to a hearty combination. Would you believe that a salt-free soup could taste so downright good?

2 cups Great Northern beans
3 quarts water
½ cup barley
4 meaty beef neck bones
1 cup sliced fresh mushrooms
½ cup finely diced celery
1 medium onion, diced fine
1 carrot, diced fine
1 bay leaf
4 peppercorns

Combine beans and water in a heavy soup pot. Bring to a boil, then turn off and let stand 1 hour. Add barley and beef bones. Bring to a boil and skim residue off the top. Add remaining ingredients. Cover and simmer 3 hours, or until beans are tender. Remove bones, cut up meat, and return to soup. Remove bay leaf. Serves 16.

	PROTEIN (grams)	FAT UNSATURATED (grams)	FAT SATURATED (grams)	CARBOHYDRATES (grams)	CALORIES
TOTAL RECIPE	124	27	29	319	2336
EACH SERVING	8	1.7	1.8	20	146

BEAN, BARLEY, AND VEGETABLE SOUP

Here's a vegetarian version of a bean and barley soup. Great protein with no meat.

1 cup Great Northern beans
½ cup barley
1 onion, sliced thin
2 carrots, scraped and sliced
2 stalks celery, sliced
2 parsnips, scraped and sliced
1 turnip, peeled and cut into chunks
2 cloves garlic, minced
1 sprig dill, chopped
1 sprig parsley, chopped
2 bay leaves
1 teaspoon dried basil
½ teaspoon pepper

Soak beans for 1 hour. Pour off water. Add remaining ingredients and cover with 2 quarts water. Cover and cook over low heat for 3 hours, or until beans are tender. Stir occasionally. Makes 10 servings.

	PROTEIN (grams)	FAT UNSATURATED (grams)	FAT SATURATED (grams)	CARBOHYDRATES (grams)	CALORIES
TOTAL RECIPE	58	0	0	266	1302
EACH SERVING	5.8	0	0	26	130

CABBAGE SOUP

Do you pine for old-fashioned cabbage soup? Here it is with a sweet-and-sour tang.

3 soup bones
1 head cabbage, shredded
1½ quarts water
3 tomatoes, chopped
2 onions, sliced thin
1 apple, peeled and diced fine
1 potato, peeled and diced fine

¼ cup white seedless raisins
¼ cup lemon juice
2 tablespoons brown sugar
¼ teaspoon ground cloves
¼ teaspoon pepper
¼ teaspoon powdered ginger

Put the soup bones in a heavy saucepan. Add the shredded cabbage and water. Stir in remaining ingredients. Bring to a boil, reduce heat, and simmer for 1½ hours, stirring occasionally. Discard bones. Makes 8 servings.

	PROTEIN (grams)	FAT UNSATURATED (grams)	FAT SATURATED (grams)	CARBOHYDRATES (grams)	CALORIES
TOTAL RECIPE	20	0	0	181	758
EACH SERVING	2.5	0	0	22	95

MUSHROOM-BARLEY SOUP

Did you know that a bit of uncooked farina cereal thickens soup nicely? One instance when a bit of a refined grain is an asset.

2 beef marrow bones	2 sprigs dill, chopped
¾ pound sliced fresh mushrooms	2 sprigs parsley, chopped
⅓ cup barley	¼ teaspoon white pepper
1 onion, diced	3 tablespoons farina cereal
1 carrot, finely diced	1 cup skim milk
1½ quarts water	

Place bones, mushrooms, barley, onion, and carrot into a deep pot. Add water, dill, parsley, and pepper. Bring to a boil, then reduce heat and cover. Simmer for 1 hour. Stir farina into milk and add to the soup, stirring constantly. Let soup thicken and then serve. Makes 10 servings.

	PROTEIN (grams)	FAT UNSATURATED (grams)	FAT SATURATED (grams)	CARBOHYDRATES (grams)	CALORIES
TOTAL RECIPE	33	0	0	146	729
EACH SERVING	3.3	0	0	15	73

LENTIL SOUP

Taste this good example of how herbs and spices flavor a salt-free soup. Add some cooked rice if you want to have a meatless meal. Again, legumes and grain form a complete protein combo.

1 cup dried lentils	3 beef bones
1 onion	1 carrot, scraped
1 bay leaf	½ teaspoon dried tarragon
2 cloves	⅛ teaspoon pepper

Soak lentils for a few hours, or overnight. Drain and add to 2 quarts of water in a heavy saucepan. Add remaining ingredients. Bring to a boil, then turn the heat low and simmer about 2 hours, covered, until lentils are soft. Remove bones, bay leaf, and cloves. Force all else through a food mill. Makes 10 servings.

	PROTEIN (grams)	FAT UNSATURATED (grams)	FAT SATURATED (grams)	CARBOHYDRATES (grams)	CALORIES
TOTAL RECIPE	49	0	0	128	709
EACH SERVING	4.9	0	0	13	71

CURRIED SPLIT PEA AND RICE SOUP

If you're a curry craver, here's a soup with just your flavor. Serve with a dollop of yogurt if company's coming.

2 cups dried split peas	1 large onion, grated
2½ quarts cold water	1 teaspoon curry powder
1 large carrot, grated	½ teaspoon pepper
2 medium potatoes, grated	1 cup cooked rice

Wash split peas, drain, and place in a large kettle with tight-fitting lid. Add water, carrot, potatoes, onion, curry powder, and pepper. Cover kettle and bring to a boil; then lower heat and simmer for about 2 hours, or until peas are soft. Stir until peas fall apart, or press soup through a strainer. Add cooked rice and serve. Makes 10 servings.

	PROTEIN (grams)	FAT UNSATURATED (grams)	FAT SATURATED (grams)	CARBOHYDRATES (grams)	CALORIES
TOTAL RECIPE	17	0	0	170	748
EACH SERVING	1.7	0	0	17	75

SPINACH SOUP

A food processor or blender makes this dish a cinch. It's easy to cook well when you have the right equipment.

10-ounce package frozen
chopped spinach, thawed
3 cups Chicken Bouillon
1 hot boiled potato, peeled

½ teaspoon onion powder
⅛ teaspoon pepper
⅛ teaspoon ground nutmeg

Put thawed spinach and 1 cup chicken bouillon into a food processor or electric blender. Add the boiled potato. Blend until smooth. Pour into a heavy saucepan; add remaining chicken bouillon, onion powder, pepper, and nutmeg. Heat and serve. Makes 6 servings.

	PROTEIN (grams)	FAT UNSATURATED (grams)	FAT SATURATED (grams)	CARBOHYDRATES (grams)	CALORIES
TOTAL RECIPE	12	0	0	42	210
EACH SERVING	2	0	0	7	35

GAZPACHO

This chilled soup of Spanish origin is the perfect hot-day meal. This version uses nothing but fresh tomatoes as the base, reduced to a fine froth in the food processor.

4 large tomatoes, cut up
1 clove garlic, peeled
2 tablespoons wine vinegar
1 egg
¼ teaspoon pepper

2 tablespoons dry sherry
1 cucumber, peeled and diced
1 green pepper, seeded and
diced
3 finely sliced scallions

Purée tomatoes in an electric blender or food processor until smooth. Add garlic, vinegar, egg, pepper, and sherry; blend again until smooth. Pour into a bowl. Add cucumber, green pepper, and scallions. Refrigerate until ready to serve. Serve chilled. Makes 4 servings.

	PROTEIN (grams)	FAT UNSATURATED (grams)	FAT SATURATED (grams)	CARBOHYDRATES (grams)	CALORIES
TOTAL RECIPE	17	Trace	Trace	49	325
EACH SERVING	4	Trace	Trace	12	81

TOMATO YOGURT SOUP

Here's a way to give a kick to tomato juice. Fast food is better at home.

3 cups tomato juice
1 cup plain low-fat yogurt
1 tablespoon fresh lemon juice

1 teaspoon Worcestershire sauce
½ celery stalk, cut up

Place all ingredients in an electric blender. Blend on high speed until smooth. Chill. Makes 4 servings.

	PROTEIN (grams)	FAT UNSATURATED (grams)	FAT SATURATED (grams)	CARBOHYDRATES (grams)	CALORIES
TOTAL RECIPE	6.9	Trace	Trace	33	146
EACH SERVING	1.7	Trace	Trace	8	36

CUCUMBER YOGURT SOUP

Here's a Middle Eastern dish that's sure to find a lot of admirers. Super for supper on a hot summer day.

2 large cucumbers
1 cup plain low-fat yogurt
½ cup skim milk

1 teaspoon finely grated onion
½ teaspoon dried dillweed

Pare cucumbers; split lengthwise and remove seeds. Grate cucumbers. Combine yogurt, milk, onion, and dillweed. Stir cucumbers into yogurt mixture. Cover and chill. Makes 4 servings.

	PROTEIN (grams)	FAT UNSATURATED (grams)	FAT SATURATED (grams)	CARBOHYDRATES (grams)	CALORIES
TOTAL RECIPE	10	Trace	Trace	27	135
EACH SERVING	2.5	Trace	Trace	7	34

BORSCHT

Don't throw the beet tops away—they're a good source of nondairy calcium. Serve this borscht chilled with chopped cucumber, a hot boiled potato, and/or a dollop of plain low-fat yogurt.

2 bunches beets (about 2 pounds)
1 large onion, sliced
2 quarts water

Juice of 1 lemon
2 tablespoons brown sugar
1 whole clove

Wash beets thoroughly. Cut off tops (they may be steamed and served like spinach). Place beets in a heavy saucepan with onion and water. Add lemon juice, sugar, and clove. Bring to a boil; reduce heat and cover. Simmer for 1 hour. Cool. Remove beets, peel, cut up, and return to soup. If desired, beets may be placed in the food processor and reduced to a purée before adding to the soup. Chill. Makes 10 servings.

	PROTEIN (grams)	FAT UNSATURATED (grams)	FAT SATURATED (grams)	CARBOHYDRATES (grams)	CALORIES
TOTAL RECIPE	16	0	0	120	505
EACH SERVING	1.6	0	0	12	50

SORREL SOUP

This is an unusual grass soup that is popular in Europe. A lovely summer snack when you're watching your weight. Serve this soup cold with a dollop of plain yogurt if you like.

2 cups chopped sorrel leaves	¼ teaspoon cayenne
1 small onion, sliced	1 tablespoon lemon juice
2 tablespoons corn oil	1 tablespoon sugar
2 cups water	1 egg
½ teaspoon salt	

Cook sorrel and onion in oil until limp; then add water, salt, cayenne, lemon juice, and sugar. Bring to a boil, reduce heat, and simmer for 35 minutes. Strain. Beat egg, and slowly pour into the sorrel soup while stirring constantly to prevent curdling. Chill. Makes 8 servings.

	PROTEIN (grams)	FAT UNSATURATED (grams)	FAT SATURATED (grams)	CARBOHYDRATES (grams)	CALORIES
TOTAL RECIPE	12	25	4	22	425
EACH SERVING	1.5	3	.5	2.7	53

MEAT

There's a big calorie and fat spread among the many choices of meat. The trick is to choose only the leanest cuts and to limit your portions to four or five ounces per meal. Schedule less meat and more chicken and fish dinners into your weekly menu. Face all meat dishes well armed with a sharp knife to trim off all visible fat before eating.

The American who sits down to eat a sixteen-ounce steak is not only gluttonous and extravagant but foolhardy and unhealthy. There are roughly 320 calories in a quarter pound of regular ground beef. To get those calories down, choose a leaner cut such as round, or grind your own.

The Aerobic Nutrition program limits your saturated fat content to 10 percent each day of your total caloric intake. You will undoubtedly get this in the meat and other protein that you eat, and even then you will have to trim, trim, trim that fat away before eating.

Suggested techniques for cooking include broiling, braising, sautéing in a nonstick-surface skillet, baking in a covered container, and roasting. Sometimes it is necessary to sear the surface of meat to keep the juices in and the meat tender. In these cases, the recipes in this book will use very small amounts of unsaturated oil and will require you to sear the meat quickly and pour off any extra oil that is not needed.

When you plan a meat meal, select only low-fat accompanying dishes so you can minimize your fat intake. The nutritional data given with the recipes should make this easy for you to do. The fat in meat often comprises up to 30 percent of the calories, even when you think you are choosing the leanest cuts and cooking the leanest ways. If you choose all other foods from the lowest fat counts, you can average that high-fat content of meat down to Aerobic Nutrition's required 10 percent of your day's total caloric intake.

Select the leanest cuts of beef, veal, and lamb. Lamb is a fattier type of meat than beef or veal, so you must be very careful about the cuts you do select or eat lamb only on rare occasions. Pork is extremely high in fat and so is not offered in recipes in this book. The use of bacon and ham for breakfast and sandwiches is also not recommended for this reason.

But the good news is that you can cook many delicious low-fat, low-sodium meat meals. Here is a wide assortment of delicious recipes to help you to eat the healthier way.

BROILED FLANK STEAK

This is by nature a lean cut of beef. Slice as for London Broil.

1 lean flank steak, about 1½
   pounds
½ teaspoon garlic powder

½ teaspoon onion powder
2 teaspoons prepared mustard

Arrange flank steak in a broiling pan. Sprinkle with garlic and onion powders. Spread a thin layer of mustard over the top. Broil 5 minutes, then turn and broil other side until degree of doneness is attained. Slice thin on the diagonal. Makes 6 servings.

	PROTEIN (grams)	FAT UNSATURATED (grams)	FAT SATURATED (grams)	CARBOHYDRATES (grams)	CALORIES
TOTAL RECIPE	147	18	18	.60	989
EACH SERVING	24	3	3	.10	165

FLANK STEAK TERIYAKI

This flank steak has a decidedly Far Eastern flair. Marinate steak in seasoned sherry for several hours before broiling if you desire a more intense flavor.

1 flank steak, about 2 pounds, lean and well trimmed of fat
¼ cup dry sherry wine

½ teaspoon powdered ginger
1 clove garlic, crushed

Place flank steak on a broiling rack. Combine sherry, ginger, and garlic. Brush half the mixture on top of steak; broil in a preheated broiler for 10 minutes. Turn and brush remaining sauce on top of steak; broil 5 to 10 minutes more, depending on desired degree of rareness. Slice steak diagonally as for London Broil. Makes 8 servings.

	PROTEIN (grams)	FAT UNSATURATED (grams)	FAT SATURATED (grams)	CARBOHYDRATES (grams)	CALORIES
TOTAL RECIPE	196	24	25	.9	1310
EACH SERVING	24.5	3	3	.11	164

STUFFED FLANK STEAK

These swirled slices of beef and stuffing make a pretty platter. Looks like more calories than it has.

1 flank steak, about 1½ pounds
2 teaspoons prepared mustard
1 onion, diced fine
¾ cup wheat germ

¼ cup chopped fresh parsley
½ teaspoon dried thyme
½ teaspoon dried rosemary
⅛ teaspoon pepper

Spread flank flat; cut in half horizontally, starting at the long side and stopping within ½ inch of the other side. Open the cut steak and press flat. Cover surface with a thin coating of mustard. Combine onion, wheat germ, parsley, thyme, rosemary, and pepper; sprinkle mixture over the mustard. Roll up, jelly-roll fashion, starting at the longest side. Tie with string in several places. Place in a large roasting pan. Bake in a 375°F. oven for 30 to 40 minutes, or until cooked through but still rare. Slice into 1-inch diagonal pieces and serve. Makes 6 servings.

	PROTEIN (grams)	FAT UNSATURATED (grams)	FAT SATURATED (grams)	CARBOHYDRATES (grams)	CALORIES
TOTAL RECIPE	170	23	20	45	1294
EACH SERVING	28	4	3.3	7	216

PEPPER STEAK

Low-sodium soy sauce may be hard to find. Look for it in your local health food store.

1 pound sirloin steak, cut into ⅛-inch strips
2 teaspoons paprika
1 clove garlic, minced fine
1 tablespoon corn oil
½ cup sliced scallions, including tops

2 green peppers, cut into 1-inch squares
2 tomatoes, chopped
½ cup beef bouillon
2 teaspoons cornstarch
1 teaspoon low-sodium soy sauce
2 cups cooked brown rice

Sprinkle sirloin strips with paprika, covering all sides. Sauté garlic in corn oil, using a wok or skillet; add steak strips and brown on all sides, stirring constantly. Add onions, green peppers, and tomatoes; mix through. Add bouillon, cover, and cook until vegetables are soft, about 15 minutes. Blend cornstarch with a small amount of water to make a thin paste; add soy sauce and mix through. Spoon some of the hot gravy into the cornstarch mixture, then return all to the beef mixture, stirring constantly. Let mixture cook and thicken for 2 minutes, stirring constantly. Serve over hot cooked rice. Makes 6 servings.

	PROTEIN (grams)	FAT UNSATURATED (grams)	FAT SATURATED (grams)	CARBOHYDRATES (grams)	CALORIES
TOTAL RECIPE	163	27	18	136	1691
EACH SERVING	27	4.5	3	23	282

SWISS STEAK

Long cooking over low heat is the secret to Swiss steak success. When you sear the surface, the juices stay inside.

3 pounds round steak, cut 1½ inches thick
1 garlic clove, finely chopped
¼ cup flour
¼ teaspoon paprika
⅛ teaspoon pepper

2 tablespoons corn oil
1 onion, sliced
¼ cup thinly sliced celery
½ cup thinly sliced carrots
1 sprig dill, finely chopped
2 coarsely chopped tomatoes

Rub round steak with chopped garlic on both sides. Combine flour, paprika, and pepper; pound this mixture into the surface of the meat, using a meat mallet or heavy saucer. Heat oil in a heavy skillet and sauté onion until translucent; push aside. Brown meat in the skillet, turning to sear all sides. Lower heat and add celery, carrots, dill, and chopped tomatoes. Add a little water. Cover and cook over low heat for 2 to 3 hours, or until tender, adding additional boiling water if needed. Makes 10 servings.

	PROTEIN (grams)	FAT UNSATURATED (grams)	FAT SATURATED (grams)	CARBOHYDRATES (grams)	CALORIES
TOTAL RECIPE	285	99	80	60	3198
EACH SERVING	28	10	8	6	320

CURRIED BEEF STEW

If you have an electric slow cooker, this is a good recipe to start early in the day. It'll be ready for dinner when you are.

1 pound lean beef stew meat, cut in chunks
4 fresh tomatoes, cut in quarters
1 teaspoon chili powder
1 teaspoon curry powder
2 onions, sliced thin

1 yellow turnip, diced
1 green pepper, trimmed and diced
1 carrot, grated
1 cup water or red wine

Place beef chunks in a heavy Dutch oven. Add tomatoes, chili powder, and curry powder. Mix well, mashing tomato pieces as you work. Add onion, turnip, green pepper, and grated carrot; mix through. Add water or wine. Cover tightly and bake in a 350°F. oven for 1½ hours. Makes 6 servings.

	PROTEIN (grams)	FAT UNSATURATED (grams)	FAT SATURATED (grams)	CARBOHYDRATES (grams)	CALORIES
TOTAL RECIPE	77	13	14	86	985
EACH SERVING	12.7	2.2	2.3	14	164

BAKED BRISKET AND SWEET POTATOES

Add more carrots to the pot if you wish to have a meal-in-one. A crisp green salad would round out the nutritional offering.

1 piece beef brisket, about 3 pounds
2 onions, sliced thin
1 clove garlic, minced fine
½ teaspoon paprika
2 bay leaves

2 cups water
4 medium sweet potatoes, peeled and cut in half
4 carrots, scraped and cut into chunks

Choose a fresh beef brisket from the flat first cut of the section. (This cut does not have a wedge of fat through the middle.) Trim most of the fat away from the exterior of the meat. Place in a Dutch oven or roasting pan.

Add onions and garlic. Sprinkle beef with paprika. Add bay leaves to the pan and then pour water around the beef. Cover tightly and bake in a 350°F. oven for 2 hours. Add sweet potatoes and carrots for the last hour of cooking time. When brisket is tender, remove and slice across the grain. Serve with the pan gravy (remove the bay leaves) and vegetables. Makes 10 servings.

	PROTEIN (grams)	FAT UNSATURATED (grams)	FAT SATURATED (grams)	CARBOHYDRATES (grams)	CALORIES
TOTAL RECIPE	427	48	50	180	3490
EACH SERVING	43	5	5	18	349

BEEF, POTATO, AND PRUNE CASSEROLE

Orange juice and prunes with meat? In this case it has a definite advantage.

1½ pounds lean beef cubes
4 sweet potatoes
4 white potatoes
4 carrots
½ cup prunes, pitted

¾ cup orange juice
¼ teaspoon ground nutmeg
⅛ teaspoon pepper
⅛ teaspoon dried thyme

Place beef cubes in a Dutch oven or heavy casserole. Peel and quarter sweet and white potatoes; place in with the beef. Scrape and cut carrots into 1-inch chunks; add to beef. Add prunes and mix through. Add orange juice, nutmeg, pepper, and thyme. Cover tightly with a lid or with aluminum foil. Bake in a 325°F. oven for 1 hour, or until beef is tender. Makes 8 servings.

	PROTEIN (grams)	FAT UNSATURATED (grams)	FAT SATURATED (grams)	CARBOHYDRATES (grams)	CALORIES
TOTAL RECIPE	130	20	21	588	3210
EACH SERVING	16	2.5	2.6	74	401

SAUERBRATEN

When you yearn for old-fashioned pot roast, here's the recipe to use. Well worth the time and trouble.

4-pound beef top round roast	2 bay leaves
⅛ teaspoon pepper	½ teaspoon ground ginger
½ clove garlic	6 whole peppercorns
2 cups red wine vinegar	¼ cup flour
1 cup water	2 tablespoons corn oil
1 onion, chopped	

Sprinkle beef roast with pepper and rub on all sides with the cut side of garlic clove. Place roast on end in a large plastic bag and set in a deep bowl. Heat vinegar, water, onion, bay leaves, ginger, and peppercorns together in a saucepan; simmer for about 5 minutes. Cool slightly and pour into plastic bag over the roast; fasten the bag with a wire tie. Refrigerate for a day or two, turning the bag occasionally to redistribute the marinade. When ready to cook, remove the meat and wipe dry. Pat meat with flour. Heat oil in a Dutch oven; brown meat on all sides over high heat, searing the juices in. Reduce heat and add the remaining marinade. Simmer, covered, for 2 hours or until meat is tender. Serve in thick slices with gravy. Makes 12 servings.

	PROTEIN (grams)	FAT UNSATURATED (grams)	FAT SATURATED (grams)	CARBOHYDRATES (grams)	CALORIES
TOTAL RECIPE	588	86	70	27	4125
EACH SERVING	49	7	5.8	2.2	344

MOUSSAKA WITH YOGURT TOPPING

Who says that moussaka has to have a high-fat topping? Try this yogurt trick for rave reviews.

½ pound lean ground beef
1 onion, diced fine
1 clove garlic, crushed
½ teaspoon dried basil
½ teaspoon dried oregano
½ teaspoon ground cinnamon
2 cups tomato sauce

1 large eggplant, peeled and
   sliced thin
¼ cup grated Parmesan cheese
2 eggs
1 cup plain low-fat yogurt
1 teaspoon cornstarch

Sauté ground beef in a nonstick skillet until it is browned and crumbled. Add onion, garlic, basil, oregano, cinnamon, and tomato sauce. Simmer uncovered for 20 minutes. Spread a layer of sauce on the bottom of a baking dish. Top with a single layer of eggplant slices. Cover with another layer of sauce; sprinkle with Parmesan cheese. Repeat, finishing with a layer of sauce. Beat eggs slightly; add yogurt and cornstarch. Spoon over top of sauce; sprinkle with remaining Parmesan cheese. Bake in a 350°F. oven for 35 minutes. Makes 6 servings.

	PROTEIN (grams)	FAT UNSATURATED (grams)	FAT SATURATED (grams)	CARBOHYDRATES (grams)	CALORIES
TOTAL RECIPE	93	20	20	93	1142
EACH SERVING	15.5	3.4	3.4	15.5	190

MEATBALLS IN CRANBERRY SAUCE

What a terrific tang results from the marriage of tomatoes and cranberries. In this case, it makes a zesty sauce.

1 pound lean ground beef
1 egg
⅓ cup unseasoned bread crumbs
⅛ teaspoon pepper

¼ teaspoon dried oregano
2 tomatoes
½ cup fresh cranberries
Juice of ½ lemon

Combine ground beef with egg, bread crumbs, pepper, and oregano. Place the tomatoes, cranberries, and lemon juice in an electric blender and purée.

Form meatballs, about 1 inch diameter, and brown in a nonstick skillet. Add tomato-cranberry mixture. Cover and simmer for 45 minutes. Makes 4 servings.

	PROTEIN (grams)	FAT UNSATURATED (grams)	FAT SATURATED (grams)	CARBOHYDRATES (grams)	CALORIES
TOTAL RECIPE	109	25	24	49	1133
EACH SERVING	27	6	6	11	283

MEATBALLS IN PLUM SAUCE

If fresh plums are out of season, use canned water-packed plums. Either way, they add a delightfully different flavor.

1½ pounds lean ground beef
1 egg white, slightly beaten
¼ cup grated potato
1 tablespoon grated onion
1 tablespoon chopped fresh parsley
½ pound fresh plums, pitted

2 tomatoes, quartered
2 tablespoons red wine vinegar
½ cup Burgundy wine
½ teaspoon chili powder
¼ teaspoon garlic powder
¼ teaspoon ground ginger

Combine beef, egg white, potato, onion, and parsley; form into small meatballs and place in a heavy saucepan. Place plums and tomatoes into an electric blender; purée. Add enough water to the puréed plums to make 2 cups. Add vinegar, wine, chili powder, garlic powder, and ginger. Pour sauce over meatballs. Cover and simmer slowly for about 30 minutes. Makes 6 servings.

	PROTEIN (grams)	FAT UNSATURATED (grams)	FAT SATURATED (grams)	CARBOHYDRATES (grams)	CALORIES
TOTAL RECIPE	153	33	34	62	1550
EACH SERVING	25	5.6	5.7	10	258

MEATLOAF

It's good to use a grain extender to get more servings from ground beef. This meatloaf is excellent when leftovers are sliced cold the next day.

1 slice whole-wheat bread
2 pounds lean ground beef
1 egg
½ cup raw oatmeal
1 onion, grated
¼ cup chopped fresh parsley

1 tablespoon grated Parmesan cheese
¼ teaspoon pepper
1 tomato
¼ teaspoon dried oregano

Preheat oven to 350°F. Soak bread in water, squeeze out excess, and tear bread into tiny pieces. Combine with beef, egg, oatmeal, onion, parsley, Parmesan cheese, and pepper. Mix well. Chop tomato fine; add oregano and mix through meat. Spoon mixture into a loaf pan, pressing to shape firmly. Bake in oven for 1 hour. Makes 8 servings.

	PROTEIN (grams)	FAT UNSATURATED (grams)	FAT SATURATED (grams)	CARBOHYDRATES (grams)	CALORIES
TOTAL RECIPE	208	48	47	56	2017
EACH SERVING	26	6	6	7	252

OATMEAL MEATLOAF

Here's a simpler version of the previous meatloaf—no tomato to chop and no Parmesan cheese. For a juicier loaf pour extra tomato juice over the top before baking.

2 pounds lean ground beef
1 egg
½ cup raw oatmeal
1 onion, grated

¼ cup chopped fresh parsley
½ cup tomato juice
¼ teaspoon pepper
¼ teaspoon dried oregano

Preheat oven to 350°F. Combine beef, egg, oatmeal, onion, and parsley; stir in tomato juice, pepper, and oregano. Mix well. Spoon into a loaf pan, pressing to shape firmly. Bake for 1 hour. Makes 8 servings.

	PROTEIN (grams)	FAT UNSATURATED (grams)	FAT SATURATED (grams)	CARBOHYDRATES (grams)	CALORIES
TOTAL RECIPE	203	47	46	42	1924
EACH SERVING	25	6	6	5	240

FLUFFY MEATLOAF

The secret is the grated potato. No one will ever accuse you of making a dense meatloaf again.

1½ pounds lean ground beef
½ cup tomato juice
1 egg
2 slices whole-wheat bread

1 small potato, peeled
½ teaspoon dried oregano
¼ teaspoon pepper

Preheat oven to 350°F. Place ground beef in a bowl. Add tomato juice and egg and mix through meat. Soak bread in water, squeeze, and tear into bits; add to meat and work through. Grate potato finely into meat mixture. Add oregano and pepper. Mix well. Pack into a loaf pan and bake 1½ hours. Makes 6 servings.

	PROTEIN (grams)	FAT UNSATURATED (grams)	FAT SATURATED (grams)	CARBOHYDRATES (grams)	CALORIES
TOTAL RECIPE	155	35	34	46	1520
EACH SERVING	25	6	6	7	253

MUFFIN BURGERS

Here's how to bring portion control into your kitchen. Applesauce is the surprise taste teaser.

1½ pounds ground beef	½ teaspoon dry mustard
1½ cups bread crumbs	1 cup unsweetened applesauce
1 teaspoon minced onion	

Combine ground beef, bread crumbs, onion, and mustard in a large bowl. Add the applesauce and mix thoroughly with a wooden spoon. Let stand until the applesauce has moistened the ingredients thoroughly. Divide the meat mixture into 12 equal portions and pack into ungreased muffin cups. Bake in a 350°F. oven for 25 minutes. Makes 12 burgers.

	PROTEIN (grams)	FAT UNSATURATED (grams)	FAT SATURATED (grams)	CARBOHYDRATES (grams)	CALORIES
TOTAL RECIPE	160	36	34	137	1909
EACH SERVING	13	3	3	11	159

HERBED BURGERS

When you want a special burger, here's the way to spice it up. Add a bit of cold water if you prefer your burgers soft.

1 pound ground beef	⅛ teaspoon dried thyme
¼ teaspoon pepper	1 tablespoon chopped fresh
1 tablespoon minced onion	parsley
¼ teaspoon dried marjoram	

Combine all ingredients. Shape into patties. Cook on a grill or broil. Makes 4 servings.

	PROTEIN (grams)	FAT UNSATURATED (grams)	FAT SATURATED (grams)	CARBOHYDRATES (grams)	CALORIES
TOTAL RECIPE	94	21	22	1.20	818
EACH SERVING	23	5	5	.30	204

STUFFED PEPPERS

Raisins give a sweet and tangy touch. Baste peppers with sauce once or twice during baking.

4 large green peppers
1 pound lean ground beef
½ cup cooked rice
1 egg
1 small onion, grated
¼ cup tomato purée

½ teaspoon dried thyme
¼ teaspoon pepper
    28-ounce can Italian tomatoes in sauce
    Juice of 1 lemon
1 cup seedless raisins

Wash green peppers and cut in half lengthwise. Remove seeds and membranes. Combine ground beef, cooked rice, egg, grated onion, and tomato purée. Season with thyme and pepper. Stuff halves of peppers with this mixture. In a large Dutch oven, combine the tomatoes with the lemon juice and raisins. Place stuffed peppers in this sauce. Cover tightly and bake in a 350°F. oven for 40 minutes. Makes 8 servings.

	PROTEIN (grams)	FAT UNSATURATED (grams)	FAT SATURATED (grams)	CARBOHYDRATES (grams)	CALORIES
TOTAL RECIPE	124	24	24	217	1793
EACH SERVING	15.5	3	3	27	224

STUFFED PEPPERS II

The flavoring is Middle Eastern and appetizingly different—a nice change from having plain hamburger. Extra portions may be frozen.

½ pound lean ground beef
½ pound ground veal
½ apple, grated
1 egg, lightly beaten
¼ teaspoon ground cinnamon

⅛ teaspoon ground nutmeg
4 well-shaped green peppers
2 cups chopped tomatoes
2 tablespoons grated onion
1 tablespoon lemon juice

Combine beef and veal; add grated apple, egg, cinnamon, and nutmeg. Mix well. Cut green peppers in half, remove membranes and seeds, and wash well. Lightly stuff pepper halves with meat mixture. Place peppers in a flat baking dish. Combine tomatoes, onion, and lemon juice. Pour over and around peppers. Cover dish lightly with foil. Bake in a 350°F. oven for 1 hour. Makes 8 servings.

	PROTEIN (grams)	FAT UNSATURATED (grams)	FAT SATURATED (grams)	CARBOHYDRATES (grams)	CALORIES
TOTAL RECIPE	115	47	48	55	1614
EACH SERVING	14	6	6	7	201

SKILLET BEEF HASH

Put it all together and make a meal-in-one. Add leftover vegetables if you want to stretch it further.

2 tablespoons corn oil
1 onion, sliced thin
½ green pepper, diced small
½ pound lean ground beef
½ teaspoon chili powder

2 tomatoes, chopped coarsely
1 teaspoon Worcestershire sauce
1 teaspoon prepared mustard
½ cup raw rice
1 cup tomato juice

In skillet, heat oil. Add onion and green pepper and cook over low heat until vegetables are limp. Add beef, breaking it into bits with a fork, and let cook until lightly browned. Add chili powder, chopped tomatoes, Worcestershire sauce, and mustard; stir well. Stir in rice and tomato juice. Cover skillet and simmer over low heat for 25 minutes, or until rice is tender. Makes 3 servings.

	PROTEIN (grams)	FAT UNSATURATED (grams)	FAT SATURATED (grams)	CARBOHYDRATES (grams)	CALORIES
TOTAL RECIPE	62	31	14	115	1171
EACH SERVING	20	10	5	38	390

HERBED BEEF AND NOODLE SKILLET

Why use an additive- and sodium-laden mix when you can start from scratch?

2 coarsely chopped tomatoes	1 cup chopped onions
½ cup water	1 clove garlic, crushed
1½ teaspoons dried oregano	1 green pepper, diced
¼ teaspoon dried thyme	1 cup sliced celery
¼ teaspoon pepper	½ cup chopped fresh parsley
1 pound lean ground beef	8 ounces cooked broad noodles

Combine tomatoes, water, oregano, thyme, and pepper; set aside. Heat a heavy nonstick skillet; add meat and stir constantly, breaking meat apart, until browned. Remove meat with a slotted spoon and set aside. Sauté onion, garlic, green pepper, and celery in the drippings in the skillet, until tender. Cover the skillet and cook mixture about 7 minutes over low heat, stirring occasionally. Stir in parsley. Add the meat, the tomato mixture, and the hot cooked noodles to the skillet and toss lightly. Cook for several minutes until heated through. Makes 6 servings.

	PROTEIN (grams)	FAT UNSATURATED (grams)	FAT SATURATED (grams)	CARBOHYDRATES (grams)	CALORIES
TOTAL RECIPE	131	26	25	198	1851
EACH SERVING	22	4.3	4	33	308

BEEF AND YOGURT ON PITA BREAD

You can stir up a great pita bread stuffing in just a few minutes. These thin round Middle Eastern breads are perfect pockets for other stuffings too. Choose the whole-wheat pita breads, if available.

½ pound ground beef	⅛ teaspoon pepper
1 clove garlic, crushed	2 tablespoons plain low-fat yogurt
1 cup tomato sauce	2 large pita breads
1 teaspoon dried oregano	Plain yogurt for topping
1 teaspoon dried thyme	Chopped onion

Brown meat and garlic in a nonstick skillet. Add tomato sauce, oregano, thyme, and pepper. Simmer 10 minutes, stirring occasionally. Remove from heat. Stir a little of the mixture into the 2 tablespoons yogurt, then stir all back together. Cut pita breads in half. Open pockets. Fill with meat mixture. Top with a dollop of plain yogurt and a sprinkling of chopped onion. Makes 4 servings.

	PROTEIN (grams)	FAT UNSATURATED (grams)	FAT SATURATED (grams)	CARBOHYDRATES (grams)	CALORIES
TOTAL RECIPE	56	12	12	50	652
EACH SERVING	14	3	3	12.5	163

CHILI TACOS

If you like your chili hot, add some extra chili powder to taste. For a better-balanced meal, top the tacos with sprouts, shredded lettuce, and grated cheese.

1 pound ground beef	½ cup water
½ cup cooked pinto beans	½ teaspoon garlic powder
1 onion, diced fine	½ teaspoon dried basil
1½ teaspoons chili powder	10 taco shells
4-ounce can tomato paste	

Sauté ground beef in a nonstick skillet, breaking meat apart with fork as it browns. Add pinto beans, onion, chili powder, tomato paste stirred with water, garlic powder, and basil. Mix well. Cook until thick and tender, about 15 minutes. Spoon mixture into taco shells. Makes 10 servings.

	PROTEIN (grams)	FAT UNSATURATED (grams)	FAT SATURATED (grams)	CARBOHYDRATES (grams)	CALORIES
TOTAL RECIPE	117	30	25	136	1541
EACH SERVING	11.7	3	2.5	13.6	154

VEAL MARSALA

The nicest thing about cooking with wine is that the calories evaporate while the flavor remains. Dry sherry is a suitable substitute for marsala if your wine cellar has limited variety.

2 pounds veal scallopini	1 tablespoon dried dillweed
¼ cup unbleached flour	½ cup dry marsala wine
2 tablespoons corn oil	

Pound veal slices thin. Dip each slice into flour and shake off excess so slice is only lightly dusted. Heat oil in a large skillet; brown veal slices lightly on each side. Sprinkle with dillweed and pour marsala wine over all. Cover. Reduce heat and simmer for 5 to 10 minutes, or until veal is cooked through. Makes 8 servings.

	PROTEIN (grams)	FAT UNSATURATED (grams)	FAT SATURATED (grams)	CARBOHYDRATES (grams)	CALORIES
TOTAL RECIPE	180	60	42	28	1896
EACH SERVING	22	7.5	5	3.5	237

HERBED VEAL

Pounding the veal slices both flattens and tenderizes at the same time. Here's a way to get a creamy gravy with nonfat dried milk.

2 pounds thin veal slices	½ cup water
3 tablespoons unbleached flour	½ teaspoon dried thyme
2 tablespoons corn oil	½ teaspoon dried tarragon
¼ teaspoon pepper	¼ teaspoon paprika
¼ cup nonfat dried milk	

Cover each veal slice with waxed paper and pound with the flat side of a cleaver or wooden mallet until ⅛ inch thick. Dredge the cutlets in flour. Heat oil in a skillet; add veal, sprinkle with pepper, and brown lightly on both sides. Remove veal to a warm platter. Stir dried milk into water; add thyme, tarragon, and paprika and mix until smooth. Stir this mixture into the skillet; heat slowly over low heat, stirring in the brown crusty residue in the pan. Pour sauce over veal and serve. Makes 8 servings.

	PROTEIN (grams)	FAT UNSATURATED (grams)	FAT SATURATED (grams)	CARBOHYDRATES (grams)	CALORIES
TOTAL RECIPE	187	68	51	34	2080
EACH SERVING	23	8.5	6	4	260

VEAL SCALLOPINI OREGANO

Lightly dredge means to dip the meat into the flour mixture and shake off the excess. Don't forget the mushrooms—they do make a difference.

1 pound veal scallopini, leg cut	¼ pound sliced mushrooms
¼ cup flour	1 teaspoon dried oregano
2 tablespoons corn oil	½ teaspoon dried thyme
2 cups tomato juice	¼ teaspoon pepper

Lightly dredge the veal slices in flour. Heat oil in a large skillet. Brown veal slices on both sides. Pour tomato juice over all. Add mushrooms, oregano, thyme, and pepper. Cover skillet and simmer for 15 minutes, or until veal is tender. Makes 4 servings.

	PROTEIN (grams)	FAT UNSATURATED (grams)	FAT SATURATED (grams)	CARBOHYDRATES (grams)	CALORIES
TOTAL RECIPE	99	43	24	52	1274
EACH SERVING	25	11	6	16	318

VEAL PICCATA

Fast food can have a gourmet's touch. Be sure to slice that lemon paper-thin for the most subtle flavor.

2 pounds veal scallopini
¼ cup unbleached flour
3 tablespoons corn oil
¼ teaspoon pepper

2 lemons
2 tablespoons chopped fresh parsley

Pound veal slices thin. Dip each slice into flour and shake off excess so slice is only lightly dusted. Heat oil in a large skillet; brown veal slices lightly on each side. Sprinkle with pepper. Add the juice of 1 lemon. Slice the second lemon thin and add slices to the skillet. Add chopped parsley. If needed, add a small amount of water. Cover and cook for 5 to 10 minutes, or until veal is cooked through. Makes 8 servings.

	PROTEIN (grams)	FAT UNSATURATED (grams)	FAT SATURATED (grams)	CARBOHYDRATES (grams)	CALORIES
TOTAL RECIPE	182	75	48	41	2107
EACH SERVING	22.7	9.4	6	5	263

VEAL PAPRIKASH

This veal dish can be stretched by serving on cooked rice or noodles. This is a perfect recipe to double and tuck extra servings in the freezer.

2 pounds cubed lean shoulder of veal
2 tablespoons paprika
3 onions, sliced thin
2 tablespoons minced fresh parsley

1 green pepper, seeded and diced fine
½ teaspoon dried thyme
2 cups beef bouillon
½ cup white wine (optional)
1½ tablespoons cornstarch

Put veal into a small Dutch oven or casserole that has a tight-fitting cover. Add paprika, and stir through to coat the meat. Add onion slices, parsley, green pepper, and thyme. Pour bouillon and wine (if you wish) around the meat. Cover tightly and bake in a 325°F. oven for about 2 hours, or until fork tender. Stir cornstarch with a small amount of water until dissolved into a thin paste; add some of the hot gravy to this paste and stir until smooth. Return this mixture to the cooked meat and gravy on top of the range, stirring constantly, until the gravy is slightly thickened. Makes 8 servings.

	PROTEIN (grams)	FAT UNSATURATED (grams)	FAT SATURATED (grams)	CARBOHYDRATES (grams)	CALORIES
TOTAL RECIPE	181	41	43.5	39	1774
EACH SERVING	22.6	5	5.4	4.8	222

VEAL STEAKS WITH BARBECUE SAUCE

Pineapple and green pepper marry nicely with chili powder to give a low-calorie barbecue sauce that is lip-smacking good. Turn oven to its lowest setting after 30 minutes if dinner has to be held.

6 thin shoulder veal steaks
½ cup flour
½ teaspoon dried thyme
¼ teaspoon garlic powder
1 tablespoon corn oil
8-ounce can tomato sauce

8¾-ounce can unsweetened pineapple tidbits
1 green pepper, seeded and cut in chunks
½ teaspoon chili powder
¼ teaspoon powdered ginger

Dredge veal steaks in a mixture of the flour, thyme, and garlic powder. Heat corn oil in a skillet; quickly brown the veal steaks on both sides and remove from pan to a flat casserole. Combine tomato sauce, pineapple tidbits including juice, green pepper, chili powder, and ginger in a small saucepan; simmer for 5 minutes. Pour sauce over veal steaks. Bake in a 350°F. oven for 30 minutes, or until veal is tender. Makes 6 servings.

	PROTEIN (grams)	FAT UNSATURATED (grams)	FAT SATURATED (grams)	CARBOHYDRATES (grams)	CALORIES
TOTAL RECIPE	145	42	34	101	1747
EACH SERVING	24	7	5.6	16.8	291

OSSO BUCCO

Ask for the hind shanks only, to avoid the muscular development that toughens the forelegs. Be sure to savor the extra bonus of delectable marrow.

2 tablespoons corn oil
2 cloves garlic, minced fine
1 onion, sliced thin
8 slices veal shank, bone in
¼ cup unbleached flour
2 large tomatoes, chopped
1 small carrot, scraped and grated

1 celery stalk, chopped fine
2 tablespoons tomato paste
1 cup dry white wine
2 bay leaves
1 teaspoon dried rosemary
¼ teaspoon pepper

Heat oil in a heavy saucepan; sauté garlic and onion until golden. Dredge veal pieces in flour and shake off excess. Brown on all sides in the oil. Pour off any remaining oil. Add tomatoes, carrot, celery, tomato paste, and wine; mix well. Add bay leaves, rosemary, and pepper. Cook over low heat, covered, for 45 minutes, or until veal is tender. Makes 8 servings.

	PROTEIN (grams)	FAT UNSATURATED (grams)	FAT SATURATED (grams)	CARBOHYDRATES (grams)	CALORIES
TOTAL RECIPE	216	65	48	253	2355
EACH SERVING	27	8	6	9	294

BAKED VEAL AND PEPPERS

Use a Dutch oven and bake the stew the French way. You'll never cook stew on top of the range again. Beef cubes may be substituted for veal, if desired. Notice that the meat is not browned in oil first. You may prepare bite-size meatballs with this same method of baking in sauce in a tightly covered casserole.

35-ounce can tomatoes in sauce
2 tablespoons tomato paste
1 onion, sliced
4 sweet green peppers, seeded and cubed

2 pounds veal, cubed
½ teaspoon dried thyme
¼ teaspoon pepper
¼ teaspoon dried rosemary
¼ teaspoon dried basil

Empty tomatoes into a Dutch oven or similar covered casserole. Add tomato paste and stir. Add onion, green peppers, veal, thyme, pepper, rosemary, and basil. Mix well. Cover tightly and bake 1 hour, or until tender, in a 350°F. oven. Makes 8 servings.

	PROTEIN (grams)	FAT UNSATURATED (grams)	FAT SATURATED (grams)	CARBOHYDRATES (grams)	CALORIES
TOTAL RECIPE	192	42	44	70	1902
EACH SERVING	24	5	5	9	238

CURRIED VEAL STEW

Don't overdo the curry powder if you're not used to it. The combination of spices will produce a piquant flavor when measured carefully.

1 pound veal stew meat, cut in chunks
2 cups chopped tomatoes
1 tablespoon chili powder

1 teaspoon curry powder
12 small whole white onions
2 cups cooked green beans

Place veal, tomatoes, chili powder, curry powder, and onions in a heavy saucepan. Cover and simmer until beef is tender, about 1 to 1½ hours. Add green beans. Continue to simmer until heated through. Makes 4 servings.

	PROTEIN (grams)	FAT UNSATURATED (grams)	FAT SATURATED (grams)	CARBOHYDRATES (grams)	CALORIES
TOTAL RECIPE	87	17	17	77	980
EACH SERVING	22	4	4	19	245

VEAL BALLS IN ORANGE SAUCE

You don't have to brown the veal balls first to sear the juices inside. This method produces juicy meat and keeps the fat content to a minimum.

1½ pounds ground veal	1 cup orange juice
1 cup oatmeal	1 tablespoon frozen apple juice
2 eggs	concentrate
⅛ teaspoon ground cloves	1 cup water
⅛ teaspoon ground nutmeg	2 tablespoons lemon juice
4 tablespoons cornstarch	1 orange, peeled, sectioned, and
2 teaspoons grated orange peel	cut up

Combine veal, oatmeal, eggs, cloves, and nutmeg. Shape into 1-inch balls. Place in a nonstick-surface skillet. Combine cornstarch, orange peel, and orange juice and stir until smooth. Add apple juice concentrate, water, and lemon juice. Pour mixture over veal balls. Cook about 45 minutes, covered, over low heat. Gently stir in orange pieces; heat until warm, then serve. Makes 8 servings.

	PROTEIN (grams)	FAT UNSATURATED (grams)	FAT SATURATED (grams)	CARBOHYDRATES (grams)	CALORIES
TOTAL RECIPE	160	41	37.6	135	1981
EACH SERVING	20	5	4.7	17	248

APRICOT-GLAZED LAMB CHOPS

When you have to make dinner in a hurry, there's no need to skimp on flavor. Here's a fast food trick that will bring applause.

4 thin shoulder lamb chops	¼ teaspoon ground ginger
⅓ cup canned unsweetened	
apricot nectar	

Trim shoulder chops of all excess visible fat. Arrange on a broiling rack. Combine apricot nectar with ginger; spoon half of the mixture over the chops. Broil 4 minutes, turn chops, and spoon remaining mixture over them. Broil 4 minutes longer or until desired doneness is achieved. Makes 4 servings.

	PROTEIN (grams)	FAT UNSATURATED (grams)	FAT SATURATED (grams)	CARBOHYDRATES (grams)	CALORIES
TOTAL RECIPE	59	29	41	12	960
EACH SERVING	15	7	10	3	240

BRAISED LAMB SHOULDER CHOPS

If you have a hankering for soft-cooked meat, this is the technique that can make it possible. Cook it low and slow for best results.

6 shoulder lamb chops, about
  ½ inch thick
1½ cups chopped onion
1 garlic clove, minced
2 cups sliced celery
1 green pepper, chopped

¼ cup water
3 tomatoes, cut up
2 bay leaves
¼ teaspoon dried basil
¼ teaspoon pepper

Broil chops until lightly browned on both sides. In a skillet, place onions, garlic, celery, and green pepper. Add water, tomatoes, bay leaves, basil, and pepper; cover and cook over low heat for 15 minutes. Add lamb chops and cover; cook over low heat for 15 minutes, or until lamb is tender. Stir occasionally. Makes 6 servings.

	PROTEIN (grams)	FAT UNSATURATED (grams)	FAT SATURATED (grams)	CARBOHYDRATES (grams)	CALORIES
TOTAL RECIPE	102	54	77	62	1902
EACH SERVING	17	9	13	10	317

BROILED LAMB WITH HERB MARINADE

The longer you soak the meat in marinade the more tender it will be. Herbs are an essential for fine-tasting food.

4 thin shoulder lamb chops
½ cup Burgundy wine
½ teaspoon pepper
1½ tablespoons chopped fresh parsley

1 garlic clove, minced fine
1 small bay leaf
¼ teaspoon dried thyme
¼ teaspoon dried rosemary

Place lamb chops flat in a baking dish. Combine wine, pepper, parsley, garlic, bay leaf, thyme, and rosemary. Pour mixture over the lamb chops and cover. Refrigerate for several hours or overnight, turning the chops occasionally in the marinade. Remove chops from marinade when ready to cook; place on a broiler pan. Pour marinade over the chops, and broil for 5 minutes on each side, basting occasionally with marinade. Makes 4 servings.

	PROTEIN (grams)	FAT UNSATURATED (grams)	FAT SATURATED (grams)	CARBOHYDRATES (grams)	CALORIES
TOTAL RECIPE	59	29	41	1.35	920
EACH SERVING	14.7	7	10	.33	230

CURRIED FRUITED LAMB CHOPS

Apricots, like other dried fruits, have high amounts of natural sugar and consequently are high in caloric content. Here half a cupful has great flavoring power, which is shared among four lucky diners.

½ cup dried apricots
4 thin shoulder lamb chops
½ cup pineapple juice
1 teaspoon curry powder

⅛ teaspoon pepper
2 carrots, scraped and cut into ½-inch chunks

Soak apricots in a small bowl with just enough water to cover; let soak for at least 3 hours. Pour fruit and liquid into a casserole. Add lamb chops, pineapple juice, curry powder, and pepper. Cover tightly and bake in a 350°F. oven for 2 hours. Add carrots during the last hour of cooking time. Makes 4 servings.

	PROTEIN (grams)	FAT UNSATURATED (grams)	FAT SATURATED (grams)	CARBOHYDRATES (grams)	CALORIES
TOTAL RECIPE	64	29	41	73	1208
EACH SERVING	16	7	10	18	302

LAMB CHOPS WITH PEACH TOPPING

If fresh peaches are out of season, drain sliced water-packed canned peaches and proceed with the recipe. Use sage wisely—a little gives a lot of flavor.

4 thin shoulder lamb chops
½ teaspoon powdered sage
1 fresh peach, chopped

1 teaspoon frozen apple juice concentrate

Rub each chop with sage. Broil chops 8 minutes on one side. Turn. Combine chopped peach and apple juice. Spread on top of chops in a thin layer. Broil 5 minutes. Makes 4 servings.

	PROTEIN (grams)	FAT UNSATURATED (grams)	FAT SATURATED (grams)	CARBOHYDRATES (grams)	CALORIES
TOTAL RECIPE	59	28	41	20	994
EACH SERVING	15	7	10	5	248

SKILLET LAMB STEW

You can cook great things on just one burner, and this is the way to do it. Follow the gravy directions for lumpless perfect sauce.

1 pound lean lamb cubes
1 cup water
4 carrots, scraped and cut in chunks
4 potatoes, peeled and quartered
½ pound green beans, trimmed

2 onions, sliced thin
½ teaspoon dried rosemary
½ teaspoon dried thyme
1 bay leaf
2 teaspoons flour

Trim excess fat from lamb cubes. Brown lamb in a nonstick skillet. Add water, carrots, potatoes, beans (whole or cut up), onion, rosemary, thyme, and bay leaf. Cover and simmer for 1 hour, or until tender. Combine flour with a small amount of water to make a thin paste; spoon some of the gravy into this paste and then return all of the mixture to the skillet. Cook and stir until gravy thickens. Makes 6 servings.

	PROTEIN (grams)	FAT UNSATURATED (grams)	FAT SATURATED (grams)	CARBOHYDRATES (grams)	CALORIES
TOTAL RECIPE	148	18	25	191	1775
EACH SERVING	25	3	4	32	296

SHISH KEBAB

Pieces of pineapple, whole cherry tomatoes, and other broilable vegetables take kindly to this cooking technique. Add them on as your desire for taste and color dictates.

1 pound lean lamb cubes
1 green pepper, cut into cubes
12 medium mushroom caps

¼ teaspoon garlic powder
¼ teaspoon dried oregano
⅛ teaspoon pepper

Place lamb cubes, green pepper, and mushroom caps alternately on 4 long skewers. Sprinkle with garlic powder, oregano, and pepper. Broil for 15 minutes, turning once during broiling. Makes 4 servings.

	PROTEIN (grams)	FAT UNSATURATED (grams)	FAT SATURATED (grams)	CARBOHYDRATES (grams)	CALORIES
TOTAL RECIPE	66	9.2	13.2	6.6	518
EACH SERVING	16.5	2.3	3.3	1.6	129.5

BRAISED LAMB SHANKS

Trim all excess fat from around the lamb shanks. If you've never had lamb shanks before, you're going to be surprised at what you've been missing.

4 lamb shanks
1 clove garlic, minced fine
1 onion, chopped
1 teaspoon dried rosemary

⅛ teaspoon pepper
1 cup tomato juice
½ cup dry white wine

Rub lamb shanks with minced garlic. Place in a heavy pot and add onion, rosemary, and pepper. Pour tomato juice and wine around shanks. Cover and simmer over low heat for 1½ hours, or until shanks are tender. Makes 4 servings.

	PROTEIN (grams)	FAT UNSATURATED (grams)	FAT SATURATED (grams)	CARBOHYDRATES (grams)	CALORIES
TOTAL RECIPE	71	19	28	19	828
EACH SERVING	18	5	7	5	207

HERBED LEG OF LAMB

Each person should be served two thin slices to keep the fat and calorie intake down. Extra portions can be refrigerated or frozen for another time.

1 leg of lamb, about 4 pounds, boned and tied
1 clove garlic, crushed
2 tablespoons unbleached flour
1 teaspoon dried marjoram, crushed
1 teaspoon dried thyme, crushed

1 teaspoon dried rosemary, crushed
¼ teaspoon pepper
¼ teaspoon ground nutmeg
1 cup dry white wine
1 cup water

Place lamb in a roasting pan. Rub garlic over lamb. Combine flour, marjoram, thyme, rosemary, pepper, and nutmeg. Pat over lamb surface. Add wine and water around lamb. Bake in a 325°F. oven for 2 hours, basting often. After first 30 minutes of baking, cover with a lid or with foil. Makes 12 servings.

	PROTEIN (grams)	FAT UNSATURATED (grams)	FAT SATURATED (grams)	CARBOHYDRATES (grams)	CALORIES
TOTAL RECIPE	324	94	135	14	3614
EACH SERVING	27	8	11	1.2	301

ROASTED BONED STUFFED LEG OF LAMB

Tiny pignolia nuts pack a big wallop of flavor when tucked into this lamb dish. When combined with raisins and herbs, they turn plain leg of lamb into a Greek offering.

1 boned leg of lamb, 4 pounds
¼ teaspoon pepper
¼ cup raisins
¼ cup unsalted pignolia nuts
1 tablespoon chopped fresh parsley

1 teaspoon chopped fresh dill
1 tablespoon corn oil
1 tablespoon lemon juice

Preheat oven to 325°F. Sprinkle the inside cavity of leg of lamb with pepper. Combine raisins, pignolia nuts, parsley, and dill. Place in cavity. Secure opening with skewers and string. Brush lamb with combined oil and lemon juice. Place in a shallow roasting pan and roast for 30 to 35 minutes per pound, or until meat thermometer registers 175°F. for medium doneness. Makes 12 servings.

	PROTEIN (grams)	FAT UNSATURATED (grams)	FAT SATURATED (grams)	CARBOHYDRATES (grams)	CALORIES
TOTAL RECIPE	316	57	67	30	2640
EACH SERVING	26	4.7	5.6	2.5	220

ROAST LAMB AND EGGPLANT

Here the lamb roasts in the center of a vegetable stew. Each serving gets a share of the succulent vegetables.

1 leg of lamb, about 4 pounds, boned, rolled, and tied
2 onions, sliced thin
2 green peppers, seeded and diced
2 tomatoes, chopped

1 large eggplant, peeled and diced
½ teaspoon dried thyme
½ teaspoon dried oregano
¼ teaspoon pepper
1 cup dry sherry wine

Place lamb roast in a Dutch oven or roasting pan. Place onions, green peppers, tomatoes, and eggplant around the roast. Sprinkle with thyme, oregano, and pepper. Pour sherry over all. Cover tightly with a lid or aluminum foil. Bake in a 350°F. oven for 2 to 2½ hours, or until lamb is tender. Makes 12 servings.

	PROTEIN (grams)	FAT UNSATURATED (grams)	FAT SATURATED (grams)	CARBOHYDRATES (grams)	CALORIES
TOTAL RECIPE	335 ·	93	134	58	3811
EACH SERVING	28	7.8	11	4.8	317

MOUSSAKA

Lamb is the traditional meat to use for this dish, but it works well with ground veal or lean ground beef. Don't forget the cinnamon—it's the Middle Eastern flavor that makes moussaka such a special treat.

1½ pounds very lean ground lamb
2 onions, diced
4 tomatoes, chopped fine
3 tablespoons chopped fresh parsley
½ teaspoon powdered cinnamon
½ teaspoon ground nutmeg
¼ teaspoon white pepper
1 cup water
3 tablespoons tomato paste (no added sodium)
1 large eggplant
½ cup fine bread crumbs

Cook the ground meat in a large nonstick skillet, breaking the meat apart with a fork as it cooks. Pour off any excess fat after meat is browned and crumbled. Add onions, chopped tomatoes, parsley, cinnamon, nutmeg, and pepper. Combine water and tomato paste; add to meat mixture. Cover and simmer for 30 minutes. Peel and slice eggplant into thin slices. Cover the bottom of an 8-by-12-inch baking pan with some of the sauce. Arrange a layer of eggplant slices side by side; cover with more sauce. Continue to fill the pan with layers of eggplant and thin layers of sauce, ending with a layer of sauce. Sprinkle bread crumbs over top. Bake in a 350°F. oven for 1 hour. Makes 6 servings.

	PROTEIN (grams)	FAT UNSATURATED (grams)	FAT SATURATED (grams)	CARBOHYDRATES (grams)	CALORIES
TOTAL RECIPE	117	22	22	115	1368
EACH SERVING	20	3.7	3.7	19	228

ROAST SHOULDER OF LAMB WITH BEAN SAUCE

Here's a way to get dried beans into the dinner act with flavorful results. The soaking and parboiling are necessary for best results.

½ pound dried white beans
3 pounds boneless shoulder of
   lamb, rolled and tied
¼ teaspoon pepper
¼ teaspoon paprika
1 onion, chopped

1 clove garlic, minced
2 tablespoons chopped fresh
   parsley
½ teaspoon dried thyme
½ bay leaf
2 cups chopped tomatoes

Soak the beans overnight, drain and parboil them, then simmer covered in fresh water until tender. Drain. Arrange lamb roast in a flat casserole; sprinkle with pepper and paprika. Place in a 325°F. oven for 2½ hours. Meanwhile, cook onion, garlic, parsley, thyme, and bay leaf in ¼ cup water in a skillet until onion is tender. Add tomatoes and simmer for 15 minutes longer. Add cooked beans and simmer 15 minutes longer. Pour mixture around lamb roast; return to oven for last 15 minutes. Makes 10 servings.

	PROTEIN (grams)	FAT UNSATURATED (grams)	FAT SATURATED (grams)	CARBOHYDRATES (grams)	CALORIES
TOTAL RECIPE	246	27	39	169	2357
EACH SERVING	25	2.7	3.9	17	236

POULTRY

Chicken is a good choice for many meals throughout the week. So are Rock Cornish hens and sliced turkey, particularly the leaner cuts of white meat. Duckling is generally a high-fat bird, but you can melt off the fat and leave the succulent meat if you follow the recipe directions with care.

Methods of oven frying are offered in recipes in this chapter. High-fat frying is unhealthful and unnecessary—one of those instances when what tastes wonderfully good is just not good for your physical well-being at all. But you don't have to give up fried chicken. You can bake a crust on chicken and avoid frying altogether.

Remember to remove the plastic wrappings from your package of poultry and wrap loosely in wax paper before refrigerating. Cook poultry as soon as possible. After cooking, it will keep fresh for several days in the refrigerator, and the leftovers are excellent for soups, salads, and casseroles.

It's best to cook poultry low and slow for tender results. High and fast cooking tends to give you a tough bird with poor taste.

Most ready-to-cook poultry is at least partially cleaned, but some birds need an extra amount of preparation. Remove any remaining pinfeathers and wash away any clinging interior particles. Rub a lemon half over the surfaces, both inside and out, to remove any offending odor. Then season and cook according to the recipe directions.

Frozen poultry may be cooked without thawing if it has been cleaned before freezing. It is easier to handle frozen poultry if it is cut into parts before freezing. If the bird has been frozen whole without the giblets, you'll be able to proceed with all roasting and braising recipes without thawing. Do add extra time needed to cook the bird thoroughly.

Stuff poultry just before roasting for safety's sake. Remove stuffing to a separate bowl before storing leftovers in the refrigerator. If the stuffing is left in the bird for storage, the cold may not penetrate the bird to the center cavity and there is danger of bacteria growth that can cause illness.

When choosing a turkey for roasting, keep in mind that the bone structure stops growing at about the 10-pound size, so every pound over that is proportionately more meat and less bone for the price.

Here is a roasting guide to help you determine how long your poultry selection should cook in the oven:

KIND OF POULTRY	WEIGHT			ROASTING TIME (AT 325°F.)			
Chickens	1½	to	2¼ lbs.	1	to	2	hrs.
	2½	to	4½ lbs.	2	to	3½	hrs.
Ducks	4	to	6 lbs.	2	to	3	hrs.
Turkeys	6	to	8 lbs.	3	to	3½	hrs.
	8	to	12 lbs.	3½	to	4½	hrs.
	12	to	16 lbs.	4½	to	5½	hrs.
	16	to	20 lbs.	5½	to	6½	hrs.
	20	to	24 lbs.	6½	to	7	hrs.

BROILED CHICKEN À L'ORANGE

Instead of slathering your broiled chicken with butter, use this concentrated orange juice trick. It tastes better and is better for you.

1 broiler chicken, quartered
½ teaspoon dried thyme
¼ teaspoon paprika
¼ teaspoon onion powder

3 tablespoons frozen orange juice concentrate
1 teaspoon dried parsley
½ teaspoon honey

Sprinkle chicken with thyme, paprika, and onion powder; arrange in a broiling pan and broil for 10 minutes, skin side down. Meanwhile, combine orange juice concentrate, parsley, and honey in a small saucepan; heat and stir until juice is melted. Brush chicken lightly with half the mixture during the first 10 minutes of broiling, then turn and broil other side about 10 minutes more or until done. Brush with remaining orange mixture about 3 minutes before removing from broiler. Makes 4 servings.

	PROTEIN (grams)	FAT UNSATURATED (grams)	FAT SATURATED (grams)	CARBOHYDRATES (grams)	CALORIES
TOTAL RECIPE	85	9	13	22	571
EACH SERVING	21	2	3	5.5	143

BROILED CHICKEN MANDARIN

If you haven't a can of these delicate orange segments on hand, use a small fresh tangerine instead. Both have a tang slightly different from that of regular oranges.

1	broiler chicken, quartered	1	teaspoon cornstarch
¼	teaspoon paprika	⅛	teaspoon dried rosemary
	8-ounce can water-packed mandarin oranges	⅛	teaspoon dried marjoram

Arrange chicken parts in a broiler pan. Sprinkle with paprika. Broil skin side down for 10 minutes, then turn and broil another 10 minutes or until cooked through. Drain juice from canned oranges into a small saucepan. Stir in cornstarch, rosemary, and marjoram, until mixture is smooth. Heat and stir until mixture thickens and clears. Add orange segments and heat through. Pour over broiled chicken just before serving. Makes 4 servings.

	PROTEIN (grams)	FAT UNSATURATED (grams)	FAT SATURATED (grams)	CARBOHYDRATES (grams)	CALORIES
TOTAL RECIPE	85	9	13	10	521
EACH SERVING	21	2.2	3.3	2.5	130

HAWAIIAN CHICKEN

This plastic bag trick is the easiest way to control the distribution of marinade. Just turn the bag this way and that every hour or so, and you'll soak all parts of the chicken with ease.

2 broiler chickens, cut in parts
½ cup pineapple juice
1 tablespoon corn oil
1 teaspoon Worcestershire sauce
½ clove garlic, crushed
½ teaspoon powdered ginger

Place chicken parts in a large plastic bag, set into a deep bowl. Combine pineapple juice, corn oil, Worcestershire sauce, garlic, and ginger; pour into the bag over chicken and fasten the bag closed. Place in refrigerator for at least 3 hours, turning the bag occasionally to redistribute the marinade. When ready to cook, place chicken parts in a flat baking pan and pour the remaining marinade over all. Bake in a 350°F. oven for 1 hour, or until tender. Makes 8 servings.

	PROTEIN (grams)	FAT UNSATURATED (grams)	FAT SATURATED (grams)	CARBOHYDRATES (grams)	CALORIES
TOTAL RECIPE	168	30	28	17	1150
EACH SERVING	21	4	3.5	2	144

CURRIED COUNTRY CHICKEN

When you want to pep up a plain country chicken dish, use this recipe which has a good helping of curry. Cook longer at lower heat, if desired.

1 onion, sliced thin
1 green pepper, sliced thin
1 clove garlic, minced
2 tablespoons vegetable oil
1 broiler chicken, cut up
4 cups chopped tomatoes
¼ cup chopped fresh parsley
2 teaspoons curry powder
½ teaspoon dried thyme
½ teaspoon pepper
1 cup water

In the bottom of a Dutch oven sauté onion, green pepper, and garlic in oil. Add chicken parts, tomatoes, parsley, curry, thyme, and pepper. Add water. Cover and bake in a 350°F. oven for 1 hour. Makes 4 servings.

	PROTEIN (grams)	FAT UNSATURATED (grams)	FAT SATURATED (grams)	CARBOHYDRATES (grams)	CALORIES
TOTAL RECIPE	99	31	16	65	1019
EACH SERVING	25	8	4	16	255

CHICKEN JAMBALAYA

If you add some shrimp and clams to this dish, you'll have a reasonable facsimile of a Spanish paella. With or without them, it's a tasty treat.

2 small fryer chickens, cut up
2 tablespoons corn oil
1 clove garlic, minced
2 stalks celery, diced fine
2 teaspoons chopped fresh parsley
1 bay leaf
⅛ teaspoon pepper
½ teaspoon dried thyme
1 quart water
1 cup raw brown rice
1 cup fresh shelled peas, or thawed frozen peas

Wash chicken pieces and pat dry with paper toweling. Brown chicken in oil, using a heavy nonstick saucepan. Pour off excess oil. Add garlic, celery, parsley, bay leaf, pepper, and thyme. Pour in water, cover, and simmer for 45 minutes, or until chicken is tender. Remove chicken from broth, discard bay leaf, and remove skin and bones from chicken. Return chicken to broth in large pieces. Add rice and peas. Bring to a boil, then reduce heat and simmer, covered, for 15 minutes, or until rice is tender. Makes 8 servings.

	PROTEIN (grams)	FAT UNSATURATED (grams)	FAT SATURATED (grams)	CARBOHYDRATES (grams)	CALORIES
TOTAL RECIPE	192	31	30	176	2046
EACH SERVING	24	4	3.7	22	256

CHICKEN ITALIENNE

Use a garlic press for quick mincing of garlic. Fresh tomatoes do make a difference in this dish, but be sure that they are completely ripe to get the best flavor.

1 fryer chicken, cut into small parts
1 tablespoon corn oil
1 zucchini, sliced
1 green pepper, seeded and sliced into strips
1 onion, sliced thin
1 clove garlic, minced fine
3 tomatoes, chopped coarsely
1 cup white or red dry wine, or 1 cup tomato juice
¼ teaspoon dried oregano
⅛ teaspoon pepper

In a large nonstick skillet, brown chicken parts in oil. Pour off any remaining oil. Add remaining ingredients. Cover skillet and cook over low heat for 45 minutes, or until chicken parts are tender. Makes 4 servings.

	PROTEIN (grams)	FAT UNSATURATED (grams)	FAT SATURATED (grams)	CARBOHYDRATES (grams)	CALORIES
TOTAL RECIPE	92	20	15	34	756
EACH SERVING	23	5	3.7	8.4	189

CHICKEN CACCIATORE

This is a fat-controlled version of an old-time favorite. Pull visible fat from chicken before you start to cook.

½ pound mushrooms, sliced
½ green pepper, diced fine
2 onions, sliced thin
2 cloves garlic, minced
2 tablespoons vegetable oil
1 broiler chicken, cut up

2 cups chopped tomatoes
½ teaspoon dried basil
½ teaspoon dried oregano
¼ teaspoon pepper
½ cup water or red wine

In a heavy saucepan, sauté mushrooms, green pepper, onions, and garlic in oil. Add chicken parts, tomatoes, basil, oregano, and pepper. Add water or wine. Cover and cook over low heat for 1½ hours, or until chicken is tender. Serves 4.

	PROTEIN (grams)	FAT UNSATURATED (grams)	FAT SATURATED (grams)	CARBOHYDRATES (grams)	CALORIES
TOTAL RECIPE	99	32	16	54	984
EACH SERVING	25	8	4	14	246

BURGUNDY CHICKEN

Who says that only white wine goes with chicken? Serious students of fine dining prefer the heartier Burgundy flavor for a zestier chicken.

1 chicken, about 3½ pounds, quartered
1 clove garlic, minced fine
1 small onion, minced fine
½ teaspoon paprika
⅛ teaspoon pepper

1 teaspoon curry powder
½ cup Burgundy wine
1 cup fat-free Chicken Bouillon
¼ pound button mushrooms, cleaned and trimmed

Arrange chicken parts in a single layer in a Dutch oven or covered baking dish. Rub chicken with garlic and onion, then place remaining garlic and onion around chicken. Sprinkle with paprika and pepper. Stir curry powder into wine; add bouillon. Pour mixture over chicken. Cover and bake in a 350°F. oven for 30 minutes. Add mushrooms, cover, and bake 30 minutes more, or until tender. Makes 4 servings.

	PROTEIN (grams)	FAT UNSATURATED (grams)	FAT SATURATED (grams)	CARBOHYDRATES (grams)	CALORIES
TOTAL RECIPE	89	9	13	13	548
EACH SERVING	22	2	3	3	137

BAKED ORANGE CHICKEN

Never underestimate the seasoning power of orange. If you reduce the heat to the lowest degree, you can hold this dish for an hour or more when done.

2 broiler chickens, cut in parts
½ cup water
½ cup orange juice
½ teaspoon garlic powder

½ teaspoon ground ginger
1 teaspoon honey
1 orange, peeled and sliced into round disks

Place chicken parts in a casserole. Combine water, orange juice, garlic powder, ginger, and honey; pour over chicken. Cover tightly and bake in a 350°F. oven for 1 hour, or until tender. Add orange slices about 10 minutes before chicken is done. Makes 8 servings.

	PROTEIN (grams)	FAT UNSATURATED (grams)	FAT SATURATED (grams)	CARBOHYDRATES (grams)	CALORIES
TOTAL RECIPE	170	19	27	152	1532
EACH SERVING	21	2.3	3.3	19	192

BAKED CHICKEN STEW

This French method of cooking stew uses the technique of bombarding the pot on all sides with heat, for a moister and more tender meal.

1 broiler chicken, about 3 pounds
½ teaspoon garlic powder
¼ teaspoon white pepper
1 teaspoon dried dillweed
1 onion, sliced
4 celery stalks, cut into 1-inch chunks
4 carrots, scraped and cut into 1-inch chunks

4 potatoes, peeled and quartered
2 fresh tomatoes, quartered
10-ounce package frozen cut green beans
½ pound fresh whole mushrooms
1 cup tomato juice

Wash, dry, and place chicken in a roaster with a tight lid. Sprinkle chicken with garlic, pepper, and dillweed. Arrange onion slices, celery, carrots, and potatoes around chicken. Add tomatoes, beans, and mushrooms. Pour tomato juice around chicken. Cover with lid and bake in oven at 350°F. for 1½ hours, or until chicken is fork tender. Cut chicken into quarters and serve with vegetables. Makes 4 servings.

	PROTEIN (grams)	FAT UNSATURATED (grams)	FAT SATURATED (grams)	CARBOHYDRATES (grams)	CALORIES
TOTAL RECIPE	120	9	13	196	1372
EACH SERVING	30	2	3.3	49	343

OVEN-FRIED CHICKEN

No need to use high-sodium packaged baking coatings when you can stir up your own. Just a dip into skim milk will hold the coating on.

⅓ cup flour
2 tablespoons grated Parmesan cheese
½ teaspoon garlic powder

⅛ teaspoon paprika
1 broiler chicken, cut in parts
½ cup skim milk

Combine flour, cheese, garlic powder, and paprika. Dip chicken parts in milk and then in flour mixture. Place in a greased casserole. Bake at 350°F. for 20 minutes; turn and bake 15 to 20 minutes longer, or until tender. Makes 4 servings.

	PROTEIN (grams)	FAT UNSATURATED (grams)	FAT SATURATED (grams)	CARBOHYDRATES (grams)	CALORIES
TOTAL RECIPE	97	10	15	41	729
EACH SERVING	24	2.5	3.7	10	182

LEMON FRIED CHICKEN

Lemon does enhance the taste of chicken. Here it joins with a variety of herbs and seasonings and then bakes into simulated fried chicken.

1 chicken, about 3 pounds, cut up
2 tablespoons lemon juice
2 tablespoons corn oil
¼ teaspoon garlic powder
¼ teaspoon ground thyme
¼ teaspoon ground marjoram
⅓ teaspoon pepper
½ teaspoon grated lemon rind
¼ cup flour
½ teaspoon paprika

Preheat oven to 350°F. Wash and skin chicken; dry well and place in large shallow pan. Mix together lemon juice, oil, garlic powder, thyme, marjoram, pepper, and lemon rind. Pour over chicken and marinate in refrigerator at least 3 hours, turning occasionally. Drain chicken on absorbent paper. Mix flour and paprika. Coat chicken pieces with mixture; shake off excess. Place in baking dish. Bake for 30 minutes; turn and bake 30 minutes more, or until chicken is tender. Makes 4 servings.

	PROTEIN (grams)	FAT UNSATURATED (grams)	FAT SATURATED (grams)	CARBOHYDRATES (grams)	CALORIES
TOTAL RECIPE	88	31	16	29	853
EACH SERVING	22	8	4	7	213

LEMON GINGER CHICKEN

No one will guess that a ginger-seasoned yogurt is the base of the interesting coating. It bakes right into a delicious crust.

1 broiler chicken, cut into parts
¼ cup fresh lemon juice
½ teaspoon paprika
½ cup plain low-fat yogurt

2 teaspoons lemon juice
2 teaspoons flour
1 teaspoon ground ginger
1 clove garlic, crushed

Arrange chicken pieces in a baking pan. Pour lemon juice over skin, then sprinkle with paprika. Bake in a 350°F. oven for 40 minutes, or until tender. Combine yogurt, lemon juice, flour, ginger, and garlic; spread over chicken pieces. Bake 5 minutes more. Makes 4 servings.

	PROTEIN (grams)	FAT UNSATURATED (grams)	FAT SATURATED (grams)	CARBOHYDRATES (grams)	CALORIES
TOTAL RECIPE	89	10	14.5	17	581
EACH SERVING	22	2.5	3.6	4	145

POTTED CHICKEN

This is a soft and delicate-flavored chicken dish that takes kindly to a bed of rice or noodles. Rosemary is an herb that should be on your staple shelf to use for chicken, veal, and lamb dishes.

1 whole chicken, about 3 pounds
16-ounce can whole tomatoes
1 onion, sliced
1 green pepper, seeded and diced
½ pound fresh mushrooms, cleaned

½ teaspoon dried rosemary
¼ teaspoon pepper
1 sprig fresh dill, or 1 teaspoon dried dillweed
½ cup white wine (optional)

Place chicken in a Dutch oven or similar covered baking container. Add tomatoes around chicken, breaking up the tomatoes into coarse pieces. Add onion, green pepper, and whole mushrooms. Sprinkle with rosemary and pepper. Add dill and wine. Cover and place in a 350°F. oven for 1 hour, or until chicken is tender. Makes 4 servings.

	PROTEIN (grams)	FAT UNSATURATED (grams)	FAT SATURATED (grams)	CARBOHYDRATES (grams)	CALORIES
TOTAL RECIPE	97	10	13	40	687
EACH SERVING	24	2	3.3	10	172

POTTED CHICKEN WITH ARTICHOKE HEARTS

Some unusual vegetables are most economical and easy to use when canned. This is one rare case when the canned product gets a vote of confidence. It's just too much work and too expensive to prepare your own artichoke hearts from scratch, and the flavor is too interesting to skip altogether.

1 chicken, about 3 pounds, cut up
2 cups chopped tomatoes
1 onion, sliced
1 green pepper, diced
    16-ounce can artichoke hearts, with liquid

1 tablespoon lemon juice
½ teaspoon dried tarragon
½ teaspoon dried basil
½ teaspoon paprika

Place chicken parts in a heavy skillet. Add tomatoes, onion, green pepper, and artichoke hearts with liquid. Add lemon juice, tarragon, and basil; mix well. Sprinkle paprika over chicken. Cover tightly and simmer 45 minutes, or until tender. Makes 4 servings.

	PROTEIN (grams)	FAT UNSATURATED (grams)	FAT SATURATED (grams)	CARBOHYDRATES (grams)	CALORIES
TOTAL RECIPE	91	9	13	33	632
EACH SERVING	23	2	3.3	8	158

BONELESS CHICKEN ON RICE

Brown rice has extra nutrients that are hulled away when it is refined into white rice. It tastes a little nuttier too.

2 fryer chickens, cut up
6 cups water
2 cups sliced celery stalks and leaves
¾ cup parsley sprigs
2 medium onions, sliced

2 bay leaves
¼ teaspoon ground thyme
⅛ teaspoon pepper
6 tablespoons cornstarch
4 cups cooked brown rice

Place chicken in a 6-quart kettle; cover with water. Add celery, parsley, onions, bay leaves, thyme, and pepper. Cover; bring to a boil, reduce heat, and simmer 1¼ hours or until chicken is tender. Remove chicken and cut from bones. Strain broth; measure 6 cups, adding boiling water if necessary. Return 5 cups of the broth to the kettle. Mix together the remaining cup of broth and the cornstarch until smooth. Stir into broth in kettle. Cook and stir until thickened. Add chicken and heat through. Serve over cooked rice. Makes 8 servings.

	PROTEIN (grams)	FAT UNSATURATED (grams)	FAT SATURATED (grams)	CARBOHYDRATES (grams)	CALORIES
TOTAL RECIPE	193	19	27	264	2167
EACH SERVING	24	2	3	33	271

BROILED CHICKEN PARMESAN

No need for high-calorie take-out chicken when you can broil a fast food dish like this. It has a minimum of fat and sodium and a maximum of good taste.

4 boneless chicken breast halves, about 4 ounces each
4 teaspoons lemon juice

4 teaspoons grated Parmesan cheese
Paprika

Arrange chicken breasts in a broiling pan. Sprinkle with lemon juice and then with Parmesan cheese. Dust lightly with paprika. Broil 10 minutes on each side, or until cooked through. Makes 4 servings.

	PROTEIN (grams)	FAT UNSATURATED (grams)	FAT SATURATED (grams)	CARBOHYDRATES (grams)	CALORIES
TOTAL RECIPE	105	14	7	5	668
EACH SERVING	26	3.5	1.7	1.3	167

CHICKEN LUAU

Chicken does have an affinity with fruit. Try to find the low-sodium soy sauce that is sold in health food stores to keep the sodium content of the dish down.

6 boned and skinned chicken breast halves
13½-ounce can pineapple chunks with natural juice

1 tablespoon cornstarch
1 teaspoon honey
¼ teaspoon ground ginger
¼ teaspoon soy sauce

Preheat oven to 350°F. Arrange chicken breasts in a small baking dish. In a small bowl, drain pineapple juice into cornstarch and blend until smooth. Add pineapple chunks, honey, ginger, and soy sauce. Pour over chicken breasts, coating them well. Bake for 25 to 30 minutes, basting occasionally with sauce in the pan. Makes 6 servings.

	PROTEIN (grams)	FAT UNSATURATED (grams)	FAT SATURATED (grams)	CARBOHYDRATES (grams)	CALORIES
TOTAL RECIPE	155	19	9	57	1152
EACH SERVING	26	3	1.4	9.5	192

POACHED CHICKEN AND MUSHROOMS

How could anything so simple to prepare taste so good? Try it and find out that poaching is a technique to use more often.

4 boned and skinned chicken
  breast halves
1 cup water
1 sprig fresh dill, or 1 teaspoon
  dried dillweed

½ pound sliced fresh mushrooms
2 carrots, scraped and sliced
  thinly
1 onion, sliced

Arrange chicken breasts in a large skillet. Pour water around chicken. Add dill, mushrooms, carrots, and onion. Cover and simmer gently for 15 to 20 minutes, or until chicken is cooked through. Makes 4 servings.

	PROTEIN (grams)	FAT UNSATURATED (grams)	FAT SATURATED (grams)	CARBOHYDRATES (grams)	CALORIES
TOTAL RECIPE	112	13	5.8	36	796
EACH SERVING	28	3	1.4	9	199

CHICKEN STROGANOFF

Cornstarch helps to stabilize the yogurt so the sauce doesn't separate. Don't let it boil and you'll become an expert saucier.

4 boned and skinned chicken
  breast halves
¼ cup lemon juice
¼ teaspoon pepper

½ teaspoon paprika
½ cup water
¼ cup plain low-fat yogurt
1 teaspoon cornstarch

Sprinkle chicken with lemon juice and refrigerate for 1 hour. Then arrange in a nonstick skillet, including lemon juice. Sprinkle with pepper and paprika. Add water. Cover tightly and simmer for 15 to 20 minutes, or until tender. Remove chicken to a platter. Combine yogurt and cornstarch; stir into broth, then cook over very low heat to prevent curdling. Pour over chicken and serve at once. Dash paprika over chicken, if desired. Makes 4 servings.

	PROTEIN (grams)	FAT UNSATURATED (grams)	FAT SATURATED (grams)	CARBOHYDRATES (grams)	CALORIES
TOTAL RECIPE	105	13	6	15	695
EACH SERVING	26	4.3	1.6	3.7	174

CHICKEN PARMESAN

This technique gives you the illusion of fried chicken without the high fat that goes with it. Toss bread crumbs, cheese, and parsley into the food processor for a whirl of fine crumbs in an instant.

½ cup whole-wheat bread crumbs
¼ cup grated Parmesan cheese
2 tablespoons chopped fresh parsley

1 fryer chicken, cut in parts
1 clove garlic, minced
½ cup skim milk

Combine bread crumbs, cheese, and parsley. Rub chicken parts with garlic. Dip chicken into milk; roll in crumb mixture. Place pieces, skin side up and not touching, in lightly oiled jelly-roll pan. Bake in a 350°F. oven for 1 hour, or until tender. Serves 4.

	PROTEIN (grams)	FAT UNSATURATED (grams)	FAT SATURATED (grams)	CARBOHYDRATES (grams)	CALORIES
TOTAL RECIPE	104	13	17	45	826
EACH SERVING	26	3	4	11	206

CREAMY CHICKEN SALAD RING

Leftover chicken or turkey takes on a whole new look when propped up in a delectable gelatin salad ring. Fill the center with tiny cherry tomatoes for a colorful offering.

2 envelopes (2 tablespoons)
  unflavored gelatin
½ cup cold water
1 cup tomato juice
⅓ cup lemon juice
½ teaspoon onion powder
2 cups plain low-fat yogurt
⅓ cup crumbled blue cheese

2½ cups diced cooked chicken
1 cup finely chopped celery
½ cup toasted slivered almonds
⅓ cup chopped green pepper
  Salad greens
  Tomato wedges for garnish
  Cucumber spears for garnish

Soften gelatin in cold water. Mix ½ cup of the tomato juice and softened gelatin in a saucepan; heat, stirring constantly, until gelatin is dissolved. Add the remaining tomato juice, lemon juice, and onion powder. Chill until partially set. Stir in yogurt, blue cheese, chicken, celery, almonds, and green pepper; mix well. Pour into a 7-cup ring mold. Chill until firm. To serve, unmold on salad greens and garnish with tomato wedges and cucumber spears. Makes 8 servings.

	PROTEIN (grams)	FAT UNSATURATED (grams)	FAT SATURATED (grams)	CARBOHYDRATES (grams)	CALORIES
TOTAL RECIPE	143	42	15	62	1354
EACH SERVING	18	5	2	8	169

CHICKEN TETRAZZINI

Here's a perfect thing to do with leftover cooked chicken or turkey. It doubles easily for a crowd or for making an extra casserole for the freezer.

1 tablespoon cornstarch
1 cup skim milk
¼ teaspoon dried dillweed
¼ teaspoon paprika
1 teaspoon lemon juice
2 cups cubed cooked chicken

8-ounce package broad
  noodles, cooked
¼ cup crumbs from whole-wheat
  toast
1 tablespoon grated Parmesan
  cheese

Preheat oven to 350°F. Stir cornstarch and milk together; cook, stirring constantly, until mixture thickens. Add dillweed, paprika, and lemon juice. Combine sauce with cooked chicken and noodles; spoon into a lightly buttered baking dish. Top with crumbs and sprinkle with Parmesan cheese. Bake 15 minutes, or until crumbs are browned and ingredients are bubbly hot. Makes 6 servings.

	PROTEIN (grams)	FAT UNSATURATED (grams)	FAT SATURATED (grams)	CARBOHYDRATES (grams)	CALORIES
TOTAL RECIPE	131	12	7	202	1581
EACH SERVING	22	2	1.1	34	264

ROCK CORNISH HENS

Prices are reasonable on these delectable little birds, making them a good choice for family meals or for the single person. Cold leftovers are good enough to plan to have some.

1 Rock Cornish hen, about 1 pound
½ lemon
1 tablespoon corn oil

½ teaspoon paprika
¼ teaspoon pepper
1 tablespoon frozen orange juice concentrate

Rinse and dry hen. Rub inside and out with the lemon; tuck piece of lemon into the cavity of the hen, remembering to remove it before serving. Brush hen with oil. Sprinkle with paprika and pepper. Bake in a 350°F. oven for 45 minutes to 1 hour, depending on size. Brush surface with thawed orange juice concentrate about 15 minutes before hen is done. Makes 2 servings.

	PROTEIN (grams)	FAT UNSATURATED (grams)	FAT SATURATED (grams)	CARBOHYDRATES (grams)	CALORIES
TOTAL RECIPE	30	14	6	9	324
EACH SERVING	15	7	3	4.5	162

ROAST CHICKEN WITH ORANGE-PRUNE STUFFING

When you're tired of the same old stuffing, try this one. No need to let your cooking get boring. Healthier food is stunningly better too.

1 roaster chicken, 4½–5 pounds
1 teaspoon dried thyme
½ teaspoon garlic powder
2 oranges
8 large pitted prunes

1 egg
½ cup bread crumbs
1 tablespoon brown sugar
2 crushed gingersnaps

Rub chicken with thyme and garlic powder, inside and outside. Chop the pulp of the oranges and the prunes; add the egg, bread crumbs, sugar, and gingersnaps. Mix well. Stuff the mixture into the cavity of the chicken. Close opening with skewers. Roast on a rack in a roasting pan at 350°F. for 2 hours, or until tender and browned. Baste skin with drippings occasionally. Makes 10 servings.

	PROTEIN (grams)	FAT UNSATURATED (grams)	FAT SATURATED (grams)	CARBOHYDRATES (grams)	CALORIES
TOTAL RECIPE	184	23	29	112	1529
EACH SERVING	18	2	3	11	153

ROAST DUCK WITH ORANGE SAUCE

Ducklings are notoriously high in fat. Use them rarely, but when you do, pay particular attention to the techniques of reducing all adhering fat.

1 duckling, about 5 pounds
1 clove garlic, cut in half
¼ teaspoon paprika
2 oranges
3 tablespoons red wine vinegar

1 tablespoon honey
¼ cup Chicken Bouillon
2 tablespoons orange-flavored brandy

Clean and rinse duck thoroughly, then arrange it on a rack in an open roasting pan. Rub skin with cut garlic. Sprinkle skin with paprika. Cut one orange in half. Squeeze juice of half an orange over the duck, then tuck orange rind into the duck's cavity. Roast in a 300°F. oven for 2 hours, then turn heat up to 500°F. for 15 minutes to melt layer of fat under the skin. Pierce duck skin all over with the tines of a fork to permit fat to run off. While duck is at high heat, juice remaining 1½ oranges. Cut rind of oranges into slivers; place in a saucepan, cover with boiling water, and cook for 2 minutes. Add vinegar and honey. Add orange juice, bouillon, and brandy. Bring to a boil, then simmer until mixture is reduced by half. When duck is done, serve with hot orange sauce. Makes 4 servings.

	PROTEIN (grams)	FAT UNSATURATED (grams)	FAT SATURATED (grams)	CARBOHYDRATES (grams)	CALORIES
TOTAL RECIPE	171	19	.27	85	1284
EACH SERVING	43	4.6	6.7	21	321

ROAST TURKEY

Cut calories and roast the turkey without any stuffing. Try the orange brandy trick if you want a shiny surface and a tremendous taste boost.

1 turkey, about 10 pounds
1 teaspoon paprika
½ teaspoon garlic powder

1 cup orange juice
½ cup orange brandy or liqueur

Clean and rinse turkey thoroughly, and arrange it in an open roasting pan. Sprinkle with paprika and garlic powder. Combine orange juice and brandy or liqueur. Roast turkey in a 300°F. oven, 20 minutes to the pound, basting frequently with the orange mixture after the first 30 minutes. Toward the end of roasting time, baste with pan drippings. Makes 16 servings.

	PROTEIN (grams)	FAT UNSATURATED (grams)	FAT SATURATED (grams)	CARBOHYDRATES (grams)	CALORIES
TOTAL RECIPE	430	53	24	28	2682
EACH SERVING	27	3	1.5	2	167

CHICKEN LIVERS AND GRAPEFRUIT

The secret to cooking chicken livers is to simmer them until plump and tender, then serve at once. Chicken livers are rich in iron and worth your menu consideration now and again.

¼ cup grapefruit juice
¼ cup chopped onion
2 tablespoons chopped fresh parsley

1 pound chicken livers, cut in halves
2 cups grapefruit sections

Simmer grapefruit juice and onion in a skillet until onions are tender. Add parsley and chicken livers. Cover and simmer over low heat for 10 minutes, then add grapefruit sections and heat for a moment more. Serve at once. Makes 4 servings.

	PROTEIN (grams)	FAT UNSATURATED (grams)	FAT SATURATED (grams)	CARBOHYDRATES (grams)	CALORIES
TOTAL RECIPE	123	4	4	67	959
EACH SERVING	31	1	1	17	240

POACHED CHICKEN LIVERS OREGANO

Here's a fast iron-rich meal that goes well with a tossed salad. Think of it when you want a low-calorie quick supper. You can serve the livers on hot brown rice or toasted whole-wheat bread points.

1 pound chicken livers
1 onion, sliced thin

1½ cups water
¼ teaspoon dried oregano

Wash and trim chicken livers. Place in a skillet with onion, water, and oregano. Cover tightly and simmer 10 minutes, turning occasionally. Remove with a slotted spoon and serve. Makes 4 servings.

	PROTEIN (grams)	FAT UNSATURATED (grams)	FAT SATURATED (grams)	CARBOHYDRATES (grams)	CALORIES
TOTAL RECIPE	112	4	4	21	780
EACH SERVING	28	1	1	5	195

FISH

The first rule when cooking fish is to be gentle. Poach it at a low simmer rather than boil it, and you'll never eat a tough and tasteless piece of fish. Broil it just until the fish flakes easily and then serve immediately. If you opt for the baking method, be sure that the oven is preheated to at least 325°F. before placing the prepared fish in it.

Naturally, by now, you must have guessed that we do not recommend the usual American method of frying fish. Fish is by nature a lean protein choice. Why add fat when you can cook fish beautifully without it?

The taste of fish depends on its freshness when you purchase it. To tell if a whole fish is really fresh, look at the eyes. If they are bright, clear, and bulging, the fish is fresh. Press the skin if you can—if the pressure leaves no mark of indentation, the fish is fresh. Look at the gills—they should be bright red. Sniff a bit—there should be only a fresh sea odor. Refrigerate fish immediately and use it within a day for best taste results.

You'll need one-third to one-half pound of dressed fish per person. Several recipes in this chapter will show you how to cook a whole fish the Aerobic Nutrition way. There will naturally be some waste when the head, tail, scales, entrails, and fins are removed, but a nicely fleshed three-pound fish should serve six people when cooked.

Here is some information that will help you to cook fish so that you can enjoy it at its peak of tastiness:

HOW TO BAKE.   Place steaks, fillets, or whole fish in a greased baking dish. Bake in a preheated oven at approximately 350°F. or at the temperature suggested in the recipe. Stuff whole fish with an herb and bread stuffing, or marinate fish before baking. For frozen fish, follow package directions.

HOW TO BROIL.   Arrange steaks, fillets, or whole fish on a preheated, well-greased broiler rack. Brush with basting sauce. For steaks and fillets, place rack about 2 inches from heat; for whole or split fish, place rack 3 to 6 inches from heat. Fillets and split fish do not need to be turned. Turn steaks and whole fish once, basting again, to broil second side. Serve immediately.

HOW TO POACH.   Place fish on a flat, greased tray of a poacher or on a strip of greased heavy-duty foil or in cheesecloth. Lower into pan and cover with seasoned liquid or wine. Simmer gently until fish is cooked and remove from liquid. The liquid in which the fish is poached might be a fish stock, court bouillon, or wine that may be used as the base for sauce for the fish.

HOW TO STEAM.   Steaming is like poaching, except that the fish is placed over the liquid. Place fish in a deep pan on a greased perforated rack or tray that will hold it above liquid level. Bring liquid to a boil and cover pan tightly. Cook until done. Season fish after steaming. Liquid used in steaming can be the base for sauce for the fish.

FISH PRIMER

FORM	DEFINITION	PREPARATION	BEST WAYS TO COOK
Whole, fresh	Just as it comes from the water	Have scales and entrails removed. Head, fins, and tail may be removed. Cook whole, or cut into serving-size pieces.	Bake, poach, broil, steam
Drawn, fresh or frozen	Whole fish, eviscerated	Scale. Head, fins, and tail may be removed. Cook whole or in serving-size pieces.	Bake, poach, broil, steam
Dressed, fresh or frozen	Ready to cook	Cut into steaks or fillets.	Bake, poach, broil, steam
Steaks, fresh and frozen	Cross-section cuts of large fish	None	Bake, poach, broil, steam
Fillets, fresh and frozen	Meaty sides of the fish, usually boned	None	Bake, poach, broil, steam
Green, fresh or frozen	Raw, in-shell shrimps	Remove shell and black vein in back, before or after simmering.	Simmer, bake, broil

---

FISH PRIMER (CONT'D)

FORM	DEFINITION	PREPARATION	BEST WAYS TO COOK
Peeled, fresh or frozen	Shrimp from which shell has been removed	Remove black sand vein.	Simmer, bake, broil
Deveined	Peeled shrimp from which the black sand has been removed	None	Simmer, bake, broil
Shucked, fresh or frozen	Removed from shell. Used to describe oysters, clams, and mussels	Wash out sand and bits of shell. If frozen, thaw before cooking.	Steam, bake, sauté
Tail, fresh or frozen	Meat from the tail of the spiny lobster, usually sold in the shell	None	Bake, broil, or simmer

POACHED FISH ROLLS

This fish is rolled up and poached in a milk bath. Tender and terrific.

4 fillets of sole
½ cup low-fat cottage cheese
1 cup skim milk

½ teaspoon dried dillweed
¼ teaspoon paprika

Spread fillets with cottage cheese. Roll up fillets and place in a small skillet. Pour milk over rolls and sprinkle with dillweed and paprika. Cover tightly and cook over very low heat for 15 minutes, or until fish flakes easily. Makes 4 servings.

	PROTEIN (grams)	FAT UNSATURATED (grams)	FAT SATURATED (grams)	CARBOHYDRATES (grams)	CALORIES
TOTAL RECIPE	141	8	8	14	958
EACH SERVING	35	2	2	3.6	240

POACHED SALMON

There is just no comparison between freshly poached salmon and the kind you get out of a can. And did you know how easy it is to do it? Chop some cucumber in a bit of homemade mayonnaise for a fabulous topping.

2 thin center slices fresh salmon
1 quart water
½ cup cider vinegar
1 onion, sliced thin

3 whole cloves
2 sprigs fresh dill
1 bay leaf

Place salmon steak and remaining ingredients in a large saucepan. Bring to a boil, then reduce heat and simmer 15 to 20 minutes, or until salmon is flaky but still whole. Remove from water and serve hot or chilled. Makes 4 servings.

	PROTEIN (grams)	FAT UNSATURATED (grams)	FAT SATURATED (grams)	CARBOHYDRATES (grams)	CALORIES
TOTAL RECIPE	109	8	8	7.4	758
EACH SERVING	27	2	2	1.8	190

POACHED SOLE

Splash a bit of white wine over all and reduce the amount of water if you want to add a bit of extra flavor to this fish. Either way, it's a fast method of serving tender fish.

4 slices fillet of sole
1 cup water
¼ cup lemon juice
1 small bay leaf

1 sprig parsley
¼ cup chopped scallions
2 peppercorns

Place fish slices in a large skillet. Pour water around fish. Pour lemon juice over fish. Add bay leaf, parsley, scallions, and peppercorns around fish. Cover and simmer 5 to 8 minutes, or until fish flakes easily. Serves 4.

	PROTEIN (grams)	FAT UNSATURATED (grams)	FAT SATURATED (grams)	CARBOHYDRATES (grams)	CALORIES
TOTAL RECIPE	136	9	9	8	944
EACH SERVING	34	2.25	2.25	2	236

POACHED SOLE IN CREAM SAUCE

Low-fat yogurt makes an excellent substitute for high-fat cream when you are making a sauce for poached fish. A bit of cornstarch prevents separation of the sauce.

4 small slices fillet of sole
½ cup white wine
1 tablespoon lemon juice

1 sprig fresh dill, cut fine
¼ cup plain low-fat yogurt
1 teaspoon cornstarch

Arrange fillets in a small skillet. Pour wine and lemon juice over fish. Sprinkle with dill. Cover tightly and cook over low heat for 10 minutes, or until fish flakes easily. Combine yogurt and cornstarch; pour over fish and heat for 1 minute more. Makes 4 servings.

	PROTEIN (grams)	FAT UNSATURATED (grams)	FAT SATURATED (grams)	CARBOHYDRATES (grams)	CALORIES
TOTAL RECIPE	136	9	9	5	973
EACH SERVING	34	2.25	2.25	1.25	243

POACHED DILLED SCALLOPS

It doesn't matter whether you buy bay or sea scallops. What does matter is that you cook them fast and just until done to a turn. Serve immediately.

1 pound fresh scallops
½ cup dry white wine
2 tablespoons lemon juice

1 tablespoon chopped fresh dill,
  or 1 teaspoon dried dillweed

Wash scallops and pat dry. Place scallops in a skillet and pour white wine over all. Sprinkle with lemon juice and dill. Cover tightly and cook over low heat for 5 to 8 minutes, or until cooked through. Do not overcook or the scallops will get tough. Makes 3 servings.

	PROTEIN (grams)	FAT UNSATURATED (grams)	FAT SATURATED (grams)	CARBOHYDRATES (grams)	CALORIES
TOTAL RECIPE	105	0	0	19	559
EACH SERVING	35	0	0	6.5	186

BROILED FLOUNDER FILLETS WITH YOGURT CUCUMBER SAUCE

Here's a pretty dish that's certain to win compliments at your house. Tuck some thin lemon slices between the cucumber slices, if desired.

1 pound fillet of flounder, 4 slices
¼ cup plain low-fat yogurt
1 teaspoon cornstarch
1 teaspoon lemon juice
1 teaspoon chopped chives

½ teaspoon chopped fresh parsley
½ teaspoon paprika
¼ teaspoon Worcestershire sauce
½ medium cucumber, peeled

Arrange fillets in a flat baking pan. In a blender, combine yogurt, cornstarch, lemon juice, chives, parsley, paprika, and Worcestershire sauce; blend until smooth. Slice 8 thin slices of cucumber and reserve for garnish; cut up remaining cucumber and add to other ingredients in the blender. Blend until smooth. Spread mixture on fish. Broil in a preheated broiler for 15 minutes, or until fish flakes easily. Garnish with reserved cucumber slices and serve. Makes 4 servings.

	PROTEIN (grams)	FAT UNSATURATED (grams)	FAT SATURATED (grams)	CARBOHYDRATES (grams)	CALORIES
TOTAL RECIPE	137	9	9	8	950
EACH SERVING	34	2	2	2	237

FLOUNDER FLORENTINE

Don't forget the grated carrots. They lift the spinach right out of the mundane.

10-ounce package frozen chopped spinach, thawed
2 carrots, grated
¼ teaspoon ground nutmeg

4 slices fillet of flounder
¼ cup lemon juice
¼ cup white wine
Paprika

Combine spinach, grated carrots, and nutmeg. Spread over fish in a thin layer and roll fish up. Place cut side down in a heavy skillet. Combine lemon juice and wine; pour over and around fish rolls. Dust the tops of fish rolls with paprika. Cover saucepan and cook over low heat for 5 to 7 minutes, or until fish flakes easily. Makes 4 servings.

	PROTEIN (grams)	FAT UNSATURATED (grams)	FAT SATURATED (grams)	CARBOHYDRATES (grams)	CALORIES
TOTAL RECIPE	131	8	8	30	951
EACH SERVING	33	2	2	7.4	238

BROILED FLOUNDER AND BANANAS

This recipe has a Spanish origin and a tantalizing good taste. Whoever thought that a broiled banana could do such wonders for fish?

4 slices fillet of flounder
½ cup lemon-flavored low-fat
 yogurt

1 teaspoon cornstarch
2 ripe bananas
Dash of paprika

Wash and dry fish fillets and arrange flat in a broiling pan. Combine yogurt and cornstarch. Spread half the mixture thinly over fillets. Peel bananas and slice each in half lengthwise. Place cut side down of each half on a fillet. Top with remaining yogurt and sprinkle with paprika. Broil 12 to 15 minutes, or until fish flakes easily. Makes 4 servings.

	PROTEIN (grams)	FAT UNSATURATED (grams)	FAT SATURATED (grams)	CARBOHYDRATES (grams)	CALORIES
TOTAL RECIPE	133	11	11	61	1129
EACH SERVING	33	2.8	2.8	15	282

BROILED DILLED HALIBUT

The thin coating of yogurt will be broiled beyond recognition, but the delicate flavor will remain. Don't forget the bit of dillweed for zest.

4 slices halibut fillets
2 tablespoons lemon juice
½ teaspoon dried dillweed

½ cup plain low-fat yogurt
1 teaspoon cornstarch
½ teaspoon paprika

Arrange fillets in a single layer in a broiling pan. Sprinkle fish with lemon juice and dillweed. Combine yogurt and cornstarch; spread a thin coating over the top of each piece of fish. Sprinkle with paprika. Broil for about 15 minutes, or until the fish flakes easily when tested with a fork. Do not turn fish over during broiling. Makes 4 servings.

	PROTEIN (grams)	FAT UNSATURATED (grams)	FAT SATURATED (grams)	CARBOHYDRATES (grams)	CALORIES
TOTAL RECIPE	114	9	9	5	793
EACH SERVING	28	2.26	2.26	1.17	198

BROILED FISH WITH DILLED LEMON SAUCE

Choose a natural yogurt instead of the kind propped up with fillers. If you can't find the lemon-flavored yogurt, buy plain yogurt and add grated lemon rind to it.

4 slices fillet of flounder
½ teaspoon onion powder
   Dash of pepper
4 teaspoons lemon juice

½ cup lemon-flavored low-fat
   yogurt
2 teaspoons cornstarch
1 teaspoon dried dillweed

Place flounder on a broiling pan. Sprinkle with onion powder and pepper. Drizzle lemon juice over fish. Combine yogurt, cornstarch, and dillweed. Spread mixture in a thin layer over fish. Broil for 8 to 10 minutes, or until fish flakes easily. Makes 4 servings.

	PROTEIN (grams)	FAT UNSATURATED (grams)	FAT SATURATED (grams)	CARBOHYDRATES (grams)	CALORIES
TOTAL RECIPE	124	9	9	12	893
EACH SERVING	31	2.2	2.2	3	223

CASHEW BANANA SOLE

What an unbelievably easy topping for a quick-cooking fish! No need for fish cookery to be boring.

4 large fillets of sole
⅛ teaspoon pepper
   Paprika
1 banana, sliced

2 tablespoons lemon juice
1 tablespoon soft margarine
¼ cup chopped unsalted cashew
   nuts

Arrange fish fillets flat in an oiled baking dish. Sprinkle with pepper and paprika. Cover tightly and bake in a 350°F. oven for 20 minutes. Meanwhile, toss banana slices with lemon juice. Melt margarine in a skillet; add cashews and sliced banana. Cook over low heat for several minutes. Spoon over cooked fish and serve at once. Makes 4 servings.

	PROTEIN (grams)	FAT UNSATURATED (grams)	FAT SATURATED (grams)	CARBOHYDRATES (grams)	CALORIES
TOTAL RECIPE	128	20	11	39	1113
EACH SERVING	32	5	2.7	10	278

LEMON-BROILED FILLET OF SOLE

If you have time to wait, pour the lemon juice over the fish earlier in the day and refrigerate until ready to cook. It will make a plumper fresher-tasting fish.

4 slices fillet of sole
½ cup lemon juice
2 tablespoons grated onion

2 teaspoons chopped fresh parsley
Paprika

Arrange fish slices in a single layer in a large flat baking dish. Pour lemon juice, grated onion, parsley, and paprika over top. Broil 7 minutes, or until fish flakes easily. Makes 4 servings.

	PROTEIN (grams)	FAT UNSATURATED (grams)	FAT SATURATED (grams)	CARBOHYDRATES (grams)	CALORIES
TOTAL RECIPE	121	8	8	12	848
EACH SERVING	30	2	2	3	212

LEMON-HERBED FILLET OF FLOUNDER

The person who claims to be too tired to cook dinner has never mastered the art of cooking fish fast. The dillweed truly enhances the flavor.

4 slices fillet of flounder
½ cup lemon juice
1 tablespoon chopped fresh parsley

½ teaspoon dried dillweed
½ teaspoon onion powder

Soak flounder fillets in lemon juice in refrigerator for at least 1 hour before broiling, turning occasionally. Sprinkle with chopped parsley, dillweed, and onion. Broil 10 minutes, or until fish flakes easily. Makes 4 servings.

	PROTEIN (grams)	FAT UNSATURATED (grams)	FAT SATURATED (grams)	CARBOHYDRATES (grams)	CALORIES
TOTAL RECIPE	121	8	8	10	840
EACH SERVING	30	2	2	2.5	210

MUSHROOM-SAUCED FLOUNDER

Sautéed mushrooms are a plus for steak, but have you ever tried them over broiled fish? Flavor par excellence.

4 slices fillet of flounder
½ cup lemon juice
1 tablespoon grated onion
⅛ teaspoon pepper

1 tablespoon corn oil
¼ pound fresh mushrooms, sliced
¼ teaspoon dried dillweed

Arrange fillets of flounder in one layer in a flat baking dish. Pour lemon juice over and refrigerate, covered, for at least 1 hour. When ready to broil, sprinkle with grated onion and pepper and slip under the broiler for about 10 minutes, or until fish flakes easily. Excess lemon juice will evaporate. Meanwhile, heat oil in a nonstick skillet and sauté mushrooms for several minutes until golden and limp. Add dill. Spoon over broiled fish and serve at once. Makes 4 servings.

	PROTEIN (grams)	FAT UNSATURATED (grams)	FAT SATURATED (grams)	CARBOHYDRATES (grams)	CALORIES
TOTAL RECIPE	123	19	9	18	1002
EACH SERVING	31	4.7	2.3	4.5	250

BAKED COD OREGANO

Baking fish is easy and fast and can help you control your calories. The trick is to start with a preheated oven and to serve the fish immediately.

4 slices cod fillets
1 tablespoon corn oil
½ teaspoon paprika
1 tablespoon butter
1 small onion, diced
1 clove garlic, minced

3 tomatoes, cut up
1 green pepper, seeded and diced
⅛ teaspoon pepper
¼ teaspoon dried oregano
½ cup dry white wine

Preheat oven to 350°F. Paint the cod fillets with corn oil on all sides; arrange in one layer in a baking dish. Sprinkle cod with paprika. Melt butter in a small skillet; sauté onion and garlic, stirring constantly. Add tomatoes, green pepper, pepper, oregano, and wine. Stir and simmer for several minutes. Pour this mixture over the fish. Bake uncovered for about 30 minutes, or until fish flakes easily. Makes 4 servings.

	PROTEIN (grams)	FAT UNSATURATED (grams)	FAT SATURATED (grams)	CARBOHYDRATES (grams)	CALORIES
TOTAL RECIPE	82	20	5	40	844
EACH SERVING	20	5	1.25	10	211

SPANISH BAKED FISH

You may not want to dance the flamenco after this dinner, but you will at least understand why the Spaniards are considered very good cooks.

6 slices codfish
¼ teaspoon dried tarragon
¼ teaspoon black pepper
¼ teaspoon ground nutmeg
1 large onion, thinly sliced
2 tablespoons diced pimiento

6 thick slices tomato
3 tablespoons snipped scallion
   tops
1 cup thinly sliced mushrooms
½ cup dry sherry or white wine
½ cup toasted bread crumbs

Preheat oven to 350°F. Wipe fish with dampened paper toweling. Sprinkle with tarragon, pepper, and nutmeg. Arrange onion slices and pimiento in bottom of 8-by-12-inch baking dish. Top with seasoned fish slices, arranged side by side. Cover each piece of fish with a tomato slice; sprinkle with scallions. Scatter mushrooms over all; add wine and bread crumbs. Bake, uncovered, about 35 to 40 minutes. Makes 6 servings.

	PROTEIN (grams)	FAT UNSATURATED (grams)	FAT SATURATED (grams)	CARBOHYDRATES (grams)	CALORIES
TOTAL RECIPE	123	5.5	4.4	60	966
EACH SERVING	20.5	.9	.7	10	161

BAKED HADDOCK

It takes little effort to make a simple tomato sauce topping for baked fish. Here's the way to do it without additional fat.

4 slices fillet of haddock
1 tablespoon grated onion
½ clove garlic, minced fine
8-ounce can tomato sauce

¼ teaspoon Worcestershire sauce
1 tablespoon lemon juice
¼ teaspoon dried oregano

Arrange fish slices in a greased baking pan. In a small skillet, place onion, garlic, tomato sauce, Worcestershire sauce, lemon juice, and oregano. Simmer 5 minutes. Pour sauce over fish and bake 20 minutes at 400°F. Makes 4 servings.

	PROTEIN (grams)	FAT UNSATURATED (grams)	FAT SATURATED (grams)	CARBOHYDRATES (grams)	CALORIES
TOTAL RECIPE	90	9	13	48	822
EACH SERVING	23	2.3	3.3	12	206

BAKED RED SNAPPER AU VIN

If you are squeamish, have the fishman cut off the head and tail. Otherwise, cook the fish cleaned and whole. Bass or other whole fish may be substituted for red snapper, and tomato juice may be substituted for wine.

¼ cup diced green pepper
¼ cup diced onion
2 tablespoons chopped fresh parsley
1 teaspoon dried tarragon

½ cup Burgundy or other dry red wine
2 cups chopped tomatoes
1 red snapper, about 5 pounds, cleaned

Combine green pepper, onion, parsley, tarragon, wine, and tomatoes. Place fish in a greased baking dish. Pour liquid mixture over the fish and bake in a 350°F. oven for 40 minutes. Baste occasionally with the sauce. Serves 6.

	PROTEIN (grams)	FAT UNSATURATED (grams)	FAT SATURATED (grams)	CARBOHYDRATES (grams)	CALORIES
TOTAL RECIPE	195	15	15	28	1412
EACH SERVING	32.5	2.5	2.5	5	235

RED SNAPPER CREOLE

Start with a hot oven and you can't miss when baking fish. This Creole sauce is especially good.

1 red snapper, about 3 pounds, cleaned
1 onion, diced
1 small green pepper, diced
2 stalks celery, diced
1 tablespoon chopped fresh parsley

3 tomatoes, chopped fine
½ cup dry red wine
1 bay leaf
¼ teaspoon dried oregano

Wash fish thoroughly, removing head if desired. Combine onion, green pepper, celery, parsley, chopped tomatoes, wine, bay leaf, and oregano in a small saucepan. Cover and simmer for 10 minutes. Meanwhile, arrange fish in a baking dish. Pour sauce over fish. Bake in a 350°F. oven for 30 minutes, or until fish flakes easily. Add a small amount of water, if needed. Makes 6 servings.

	PROTEIN (grams)	FAT UNSATURATED (grams)	FAT SATURATED (grams)	CARBOHYDRATES (grams)	CALORIES
TOTAL RECIPE	198	15	15	40	1468
EACH SERVING	33	2.5	2.5	6.7	245

BAKED STUFFED RED SNAPPER

Be sure to use whole-grain bread for the stuffing, rather than the refined kind. It has extra nutrition and extra good taste.

1 dressed red snapper, about 3 pounds
½ cup diced celery
¼ cup diced onion
¼ cup water

2 cups whole-grain dry bread cubes
1 egg, beaten
¼ teaspoon dried thyme

Clean, wash, and dry fish. In a skillet, cook celery and onion in water. Add bread cubes, beaten egg, and thyme. If too dry, add a small amount of water to moisten through. Stuff fish loosely and close with skewers. Place fish in a nonstick-surfaced baking dish. Bake in a 350°F. preheated oven for 45 to 60 minutes, or until fish flakes easily. Makes 6 servings.

	PROTEIN (grams)	FAT UNSATURATED (grams)	FAT SATURATED (grams)	CARBOHYDRATES (grams)	CALORIES
TOTAL RECIPE	134	18	18	62	1276
EACH SERVING	22	3	3	11	212

BAKED SEA BASS

To keep fish moist and tender, don't overcook it. Bake only until the fish flakes easily.

1 sea bass, about 3 pounds
1 small onion, sliced thin
¼ cup finely chopped green pepper
1 cup chopped tomatoes

½ teaspoon dried oregano
¼ teaspoon pepper
½ cup water
½ cup dry red wine

Arrange fish in a baking dish. Top with onion slices, green pepper, tomatoes, oregano, and pepper. Pour water and wine around fish. Bake in a 350°F. preheated oven for 45 to 60 minutes, or until fish flakes easily. Baste several times, adding more water if necessary. Makes 6 servings.

	PROTEIN (grams)	FAT UNSATURATED (grams)	FAT SATURATED (grams)	CARBOHYDRATES (grams)	CALORIES
TOTAL RECIPE	134	18	18	62	1276
EACH SERVING	22	3	3	10	213

BOILED CARP

Actually this should be called poached carp, because you must turn the heat down low after the water comes to a boil. You may substitute cod for carp in this recipe.

4 slices fresh carp
1 onion, sliced thin
½ teaspoon dried thyme
1 teaspoon sugar

2 peppercorns
1 bay leaf
1 whole clove

Arrange fish slices in the bottom of a heavy skillet. Add onion slices, thyme, sugar, peppercorns, bay leaf, and clove. Cover with boiling water. Cover skillet and simmer for 30 minutes, or until fish flakes easily. Serve hot or cold. Makes 4 servings.

	PROTEIN (grams)	FAT UNSATURATED (grams)	FAT SATURATED (grams)	CARBOHYDRATES (grams)	CALORIES
TOTAL RECIPE	75	2.6	2.6	7	472
EACH SERVING	19	.65	.65	1.8	118

BOILED FISH

This is a lovely dish to serve hot or cold. Use it as the base for a fish salad if desired.

4 cod or halibut steaks
1 small onion, diced
1 carrot, peeled and diced
1 sprig parsley
2 quarts water

½ cup tarragon vinegar
1 teaspoon sugar
1 bay leaf
2 whole cloves

Arrange fish steaks on the bottom of a heavy saucepan, preferably on a rack. Add onion, carrot, and parsley. Cover with water and vinegar; add sugar, bay leaf, and cloves. Bring quickly to the boiling point; lower heat to keep liquid just below the boiling point. Simmer for 10 to 15 minutes, or until fish flakes easily. Makes 4 servings.

	PROTEIN (grams)	FAT UNSATURATED (grams)	FAT SATURATED (grams)	CARBOHYDRATES (grams)	CALORIES
TOTAL RECIPE	76	2.6	2.6	18	517
EACH SERVING	19	.65	.65	4.5	129

BOILED SHRIMP

The bay leaves and whole cloves will give a wonderful flavor and mask any fishy taste. When you rinse shrimp under cold water the shells will slip off with ease.

1 pound shrimp with shells	2 peppercorns
3 cups water	2 whole cloves
2 bay leaves	¼ cup lemon juice

Wash shrimp. In a large saucepan, bring to a boil the water, bay leaves, peppercorns, cloves, and lemon juice. Add shrimp and cook over low heat for 5 minutes, or until shells turn pink. Drain. Rinse shrimp to cool down. Remove shells and black veins. Chill until ready to serve. Makes 4 servings.

	PROTEIN (grams)	FAT UNSATURATED (grams)	FAT SATURATED (grams)	CARBOHYDRATES (grams)	CALORIES
TOTAL RECIPE	110	0	0	8	541
EACH SERVING	28	0	0	2	135

BROILED BUTTERFLY SHRIMP

Once you discover how easy it is to butterfly shrimp, you'll be showing off all the time. The natural indentation in the back of the shrimp shows you where to start cutting.

1 pound large shrimp	1 teaspoon finely chopped fresh
1 teaspoon corn oil	parsley
1 clove garlic, peeled and minced fine	Lemon wedges

Peel shrimp, leaving the tails intact. Cut down the backs to the tails; clean and flatten into a butterfly shape. Combine oil, garlic, and parsley. Arrange shrimp on a broiling pan; brush lightly with garlic mixture. Broil 2 to 3 minutes on each side. Serve with lemon wedges. Makes 4 servings.

	PROTEIN (grams)	FAT UNSATURATED (grams)	FAT SATURATED (grams)	CARBOHYDRATES (grams)	CALORIES
TOTAL RECIPE	111	4	.45	13	598
EACH SERVING	28	1	.11	3	149

SHRIMP PILAF

Add the pinch of saffron if you can find it in your local store. It will turn the rice pale yellow and add a touch of class.

1 tablespoon corn oil
1 onion, chopped
2 cups chopped tomatoes
1 cup diced celery
¼ teaspoon paprika

⅛ teaspoon pepper
½ cup chicken broth
  Pinch of saffron (optional)
2 cups cooked rice
1 cup cooked peeled shrimp

Heat oil in a heavy saucepan; sauté onion until golden. Add tomatoes, celery, paprika, pepper, chicken broth, and saffron; stir well. Cook over low heat for 10 minutes. Add cooked rice and shrimp; mix thoroughly. Spoon into a greased casserole. Cover. Bake in a 325°F. oven for 25 minutes. Makes 4 servings.

	PROTEIN (grams)	FAT UNSATURATED (grams)	FAT SATURATED (grams)	CARBOHYDRATES (grams)	CALORIES
TOTAL RECIPE	24	11	1	137	775
EACH SERVING	6	3	.25	34	194

SHRIMP CREOLE

This dish is fine for the smaller, less expensive shrimp. Use it for a buffet supper, ringed with hot cooked rice, or serve it over cooked brown rice.

2 onions, sliced
1 clove garlic, crushed
3 tomatoes, chopped fine
1 green pepper, seeded and chopped fine
1 cup water

10-ounce package frozen peas, or 1½ cups shelled fresh peas
1 tablespoon chili powder
1 tablespoon cornstarch
1 tablespoon vinegar
2 cups cooked peeled shrimp

Place onions, garlic, tomatoes, green pepper, water, and peas into a heavy saucepan. Cover and cook over low heat until vegetables are tender, about 15 minutes. Combine chili powder, cornstarch, vinegar, and just enough additional water to make a thin paste; stir some of the hot liquid into the paste and stir smooth. Pour all back into the vegetables, stir constantly, and simmer until thickened. Add cooked shrimp and heat through. Makes 4 servings.

	PROTEIN (grams)	FAT UNSATURATED (grams)	FAT SATURATED (grams)	CARBOHYDRATES (grams)	CALORIES
TOTAL RECIPE	71	16	4	111	951
EACH SERVING	17	4	1	28	238

STEAMED CLAMS

If you find any sand in your broth, just let it settle to the bottom of the bowl and sip off the steaming goodness with nary a care.

2 dozen small steamer clams with tightly closed shells
2 cups water

2 tablespoons lemon juice
1 large sprig parsley

Scrub *live* clams thoroughly to remove sand from shells. Do this just before cooking, chemicals from water may kill clams. Place clams into a large heavy saucepan. Add water, lemon juice, and parsley. Bring to a boil, then reduce heat and simmer for 10 minutes, or until shells are open. Discard any shells that do not open naturally. Discard parsley. Pour broth into bowls; divide clams still in the shells among the bowls. Makes 4 servings.

	PROTEIN (grams)	FAT UNSATURATED (grams)	FAT SATURATED (grams)	CARBOHYDRATES (grams)	CALORIES
TOTAL RECIPE	32	0	0	5	196
EACH SERVING	8	0	0	1.25	49

CIOPPINO

When is a soup really a seafood entrée? When it is cioppino—served in a bowl as a main course, of course.

3 cups chopped tomatoes
1 clove garlic, minced
1 small onion, diced fine
2 tablespoons chopped fresh
parsley
1 small bay leaf

½ teaspoon dried oregano
¼ cup dry red wine
12 large shrimp, unshelled, heads removed
2 cod fillets, cut in 1½-inch squares

Combine tomatoes, garlic, onion, parsley, bay leaf, oregano, and wine in saucepan; simmer about 15 minutes. Add the uncooked seafood. Cover, bring to a boil, reduce heat, and simmer 15 minutes. Serves 4.

	PROTEIN (grams)	FAT UNSATURATED (grams)	FAT SATURATED (grams)	CARBOHYDRATES (grams)	CALORIES
TOTAL RECIPE	81	4	4	52	689
EACH SERVING	20	1	1	13	172

JAMBALAYA

Filé powder is made from the sassafras root and is very popular in Louisiana. You may have to go to a gourmet shop to find it elsewhere.

1 small onion, finely chopped
1 medium green pepper, finely chopped
2 cloves garlic, minced
2 tablespoons vegetable oil
1 cup chopped tomatoes
½ cup sliced mushrooms
½ teaspoon filé powder
¼ teaspoon pepper
2 tablespoons sherry
2 dozen cooked peeled shrimp
2 cups cooked brown rice

In a heavy saucepan, sauté onion, green pepper, and garlic in oil. Stir in tomatoes, mushrooms, filé powder, and pepper. Stir in sherry. Bring to a boil. Add shrimp. Serve over cooked rice. Serves 4.

	PROTEIN (grams)	FAT UNSATURATED (grams)	FAT SATURATED (grams)	CARBOHYDRATES (grams)	CALORIES
TOTAL RECIPE	34	22	2.7	127	950
EACH SERVING	8	5	7	32	237

HALIBUT LOAF

Whether you are working with cooked leftover fish or poaching fish just for this dish, you'll enjoy the change of pace with a loaf as light as a mousse.

3 eggs
2½ cups flaked, cooked halibut
½ cup whole-grain bread crumbs
⅛ teaspoon pepper
1 tablespoon minced fresh parsley
1 tablespoon dried dillweed

Separate the eggs. Beat the yolks until lemon-colored and the whites until stiff. Flake the fish and add it with the remaining ingredients to the egg yolks. Fold in the egg whites. Bake in a nonstick-surfaced loaf pan at 350°F. for 40 to 45 minutes. Serves 6.

	PROTEIN (grams)	FAT UNSATURATED (grams)	FAT SATURATED (grams)	CARBOHYDRATES (grams)	CALORIES
TOTAL RECIPE	140	19	15	38	1220
EACH SERVING	23	3	2.5	6	203

SALMON BROCCOLI LOAF

Use fresh poached salmon if you can get it, along with a quarter cup of the poaching liquid, instead of the canned variety. This is a perfect Sunday-night supper dish.

2 large lemons
16-ounce can salmon, including liquid from can
2 cups toasted whole-wheat bread crumbs

10-ounce package frozen chopped broccoli, thawed
3 eggs, beaten
¼ teaspoon pepper
1 teaspoon dried dillweed

Squeeze juice from lemons and pare the yellow rind from lemons; cut rind into slivers. Flake the salmon into a bowl; add liquid from can, lemon rind slivers, and the juice of the lemons. Stir in bread crumbs, broccoli, eggs, pepper, and dillweed. Mix well. Spoon mixture into a loaf pan. Bake in a 350°F. oven for 30 minutes. Serve hot or cold. Makes 8 servings.

	PROTEIN (grams)	FAT UNSATURATED (grams)	FAT SATURATED (grams)	CARBOHYDRATES (grams)	CALORIES
TOTAL RECIPE	148	29	21	177	1936
EACH SERVING	18.5	3.5	2.6	22	242

SKILLET FISH COMBO

Although fresh fish is the very best choice, here's a combination that can make use of frozen fish and vegetables for a last-minute supper. Serve on cooked rice for a nutritious meal.

10-ounce package frozen mixed vegetables
1 cup water
4 fillets of flounder or other fish

2 tablespoons lemon juice
½ teaspoon dried dillweed
⅛ teaspoon paprika

Place frozen mixed vegetables and water in a skillet, cover, and cook for 4 minutes, or until vegetables are hot. Arrange fish over bed of vegetables. Add additional water if mixture seems dry. Sprinkle fish with lemon juice, dill, and paprika. Cover and simmer for 8 minutes, or until fish is cooked through and flakes easily. Makes 4 servings.

	PROTEIN (grams)	FAT UNSATURATED (grams)	FAT SATURATED (grams)	CARBOHYDRATES (grams)	CALORIES
TOTAL RECIPE	130	8	8	41	1001
EACH SERVING	32.4	2	2	10.3	250

VEGETABLES

Meat-and-potatoes people are missing a lot of good nutrients from vegetables, as well as a lot of good-tasting food. A large variety of light and dark green and yellow vegetables in your menu gives you large quantities of vitamins A and C, along with many trace minerals that are important to optimum health.

There are only a few important rules to remember about vegetables in your diet. When peeling vegetables, try to cut thin so you don't throw away valuable minerals. When possible, eat them raw. When cooking, preserve nutrients by using the least amount of liquid possible and heating only until tender. Vegetables should be steamed if possible. The Southern style of cooking vegetables for several hours in a bath that contains plenty of salt pork is just not compatible with the Aerobic Nutrition plan for better health.

To keep the colors fresh, the French "blanch" their green vegetables (dip in boiling water for a moment and then into iced water to stop the cooking action), and then cook them just before serving. Another way to preserve color in vegetables is to add lemon juice. This prevents white vegetables from turning light tan, red vegetables from turning brown, and green vegetables from paling too much. Yellow vegetables such as carrots and sweet potatoes do not need any additives to preserve their color, and are cooked covered.

Cook frozen vegetables as directed on the package, using as little water as possible. A good technique for heating canned low-sodium packed vegetables is to drain off the liquid into a saucepan and cook the liquid until it reduces to half the amount. Then add the vegetables and heat in this double-strength juice. Since canned vegetables are already cooked, only a few moments are required to bring them to serving temperature.

Always keep color and variety in mind, both for eye appeal and for balanced nutrition, as you plan to use nature's valuable accessories to enhance your meals. Buy only the amount that you will use within a short period of time, as vegetables are highly perishable. Sort the vegetables before storing, and discard any that are bruised, soft, or decayed. Here is a list that will help you get the most food return for your money, with additional advice on how to store each kind of vegetable:

ABOUT VEGETABLES

ARTICHOKES.   Select those that feel compact and heavy. Leaves should be large and fleshy, tightly closed, and of good color, although a few dark spots are all right. The size will not affect flavor or quality.

ASPARAGUS.   Stalks should be mostly green with compact tips. Remove tough white parts of stalks. Store in refrigerator crisper in a plastic bag. Use within one or two days.

BEANS, LIMA.   Select well-filled pods that are clean, fresh, and of good color. Old and tough beans will have shriveled, spotted, or flabby pods. Shelled lima beans should be plump and of good green or green-white color. Refrigerate and use within one or two days.

BEANS, SNAP.   Select pods with small seeds; overmature pods may be tough. Avoid dry-looking or wilted pods. Refrigerate and use within one or two days.

BEETS.   Select smooth and firm beets. Soft or shriveled beets may be tough. Store beets, covered, in the refrigerator, and use within one or two weeks.

BROCCOLI.   Select stalks that are clean with compact green clusters. Avoid those with yellow flower clusters. The stalks should be dark green, tender, and firm. Dirty spots may indicate insects. Store in refrigerator in a plastic bag and use within one or two days.

BRUSSELS SPROUTS.   Select firm sprouts of good green color. Avoid those that have worm-eaten or wilted leaves, or a dirty appearance. Store in the refrigerator in a plastic bag and use within one or two days.

CABBAGE.   Select crisp, firm heads that feel heavy for their size. Avoid those that are discolored, soft, or have wormholes. Store in a plastic bag in the refrigerator and use within one or two weeks.

CARROTS.   Select those of good color that are smooth and firm. Avoid wilted or shriveled carrots, and large ones that may have a pithy core, and those that are cracked. Remove tips and tops and store in a plastic bag in the refrigerator for one to two weeks.

CAULIFLOWER.   Select a white, clean, firm, and compact head with fresh green leaves. Avoid spotted or bruised heads. Store, covered, in the refrigerator and use within three to five days.

CELERY.   Select crisp, clean celery with branches that will snap easily. Avoid soft, pithy, or stringy stalks. Wrap in plastic bag and store in crisper of refrigerator. Use within one or two weeks.

CORN.   Select ears with plump kernels and fresh green husks. Avoid dry or yellowed husks. Cook as soon after purchase as possible.

CUCUMBERS.   Select firm, green, well-shaped cucumbers. Avoid those that are withered or overmature, and those that have decay spots. Store in refrigerator crisper and use within three to five days.

EGGPLANT.   Select firm, dark-purple, heavy eggplant. Avoid those that are soft or scarred. Decay appears as brown spots on the surface. Store in a cool place (60°F.) or store in refrigerator in a plastic bag.

LETTUCE.   Select crisp, clean heads that are firm and heavy for their size. Avoid those that have rust spots and those with an excess of outer leaves. Wash and dry before storing; wrap in paper toweling and store in crisper of refrigerator. Use within one or two days.

MUSHROOMS.   Select clean, white, firm mushrooms with light-colored gills on the underside. Avoid dark and discolored mushrooms. Store in a plastic bag in the refrigerator and use within one or two days.

ONIONS.   Select clean, hard onions with dry skins; avoid those with developing seed-stem and those that feel moist at the neck, which is an indication of decay inside. Store in a cool place at 60°F. and they will keep for a month or so.

PARSLEY.   Select bright-green, crisp-appearing leaves; avoid yellowing wilted-looking leaves. Wash thoroughly, shake dry, and place in a tightly covered jar in the refrigerator. Use within one or two weeks.

PEAS.   Select light-green, firm, and well-filled pods; avoid flat, wilted, or yellowing pods. Store in pods in refrigerator until wanted. Use within one or two days.

PEPPERS.   Select firm, fresh-colored peppers; avoid shriveled, spotted, or dull-appearing ones. Wash and dry. Store in crisper in the refrigerator and use within three to five days.

POTATOES.   Select firm, smooth, well-shaped potatoes; avoid sprouting, wilted, leathery, or discolored ones. Keep at room temperature and in a dark place for three to four weeks. When they are exposed to light, the exposed portion turns green and may taste bitter.

RADISHES.   Select smooth, firm, crisp radishes of good color; avoid wilted, decayed, and pithy ones. Remove tops and store in a plastic bag in the crisper of the refrigerator. Use within one to two weeks.

SPINACH.   Select leaves that are clean, crisp, and fresh-green in color; avoid wilted, bruised, and yellowed leaves. Decay appears as a slimy spot. Wash and dry. Wrap in paper toweling and store in the crisper of the refrigerator. Use within one or two days.

TOMATOES.   Select well-formed plump and uniformly red ones; avoid those that have bruise marks or are soft or discolored. Store uncovered in the refrigerator crisper. Keep unripened tomatoes at room temperature, away from direct sunlight until ripe, and then refrigerate. Use within three to five days.

ZUCCHINI. Select crisp, dark-green zucchini; avoid soft spots, mold growth, and wilted appearance. Wash, dry, and wrap in plastic. Store in refrigerator. Use within three to five days.

GLOBE ARTICHOKES

Serve this as a salad, vegetable, or first-course appetizer. Make a few extras to serve cold the next day.

6 globe artichokes of uniform size
2 tablespoons lemon juice
2 bay leaves
2 cloves

2 peppercorns
1 clove garlic, minced
3 teaspoons vegetable oil

Wash artichokes and drain upside down. Remove the thick, loose leaves around base and clip off tip of each leaf. Bang each artichoke upside down on a hard surface to force leaves to open slightly. Place artichokes in skillet. Add water to cover bottom of skillet by 1 inch. Add remaining ingredients except oil to water. Drizzle ½ teaspoon oil into leaves of each artichoke. Cover and cook 25 to 35 minutes, or until leaf pulls out easily and is tender. Drain.

To eat artichokes, pull off each leaf and hold it by the tip. Remove the fleshy part of the base of the leaf with the teeth and discard the remainder of the leaf. When all the leaves are removed, discard the choke (the "hairy" part above the heart). Eat the heart with a knife and a fork. Serves 6.

	PROTEIN (grams)	FAT UNSATURATED (grams)	FAT SATURATED (grams)	CARBOHYDRATES (grams)	CALORIES
TOTAL RECIPE	20	33	4	75	558
EACH SERVING	3	5.5	.68	12	93

STEAMED ASPARAGUS WITH LEMON PARSLEY SAUCE

Use only when dainty asparagus is fresh on the market. If you don't have a double boiler to invert as suggested, cook flat in a skillet and enjoy anyway.

1 pound asparagus, trimmed and scaled
¼ cup lemon juice

2 tablespoons chopped fresh parsley

Tie asparagus into a stack, using white kitchen cord. Place upright, stems down, in the bottom half of a double boiler. Fill with 3 inches of water. Invert top half of double boiler and place over asparagus tops. (This forms a high cooking unit in which the tougher stems can simmer while the tender tops can steam.) Cook for 10 minutes, or until asparagus stems are tender. Combine lemon juice and chopped parsley; pour over cooked asparagus that has been untied and arranged in a serving dish. Makes 4 servings.

	PROTEIN (grams)	FAT UNSATURATED (grams)	FAT SATURATED (grams)	CARBOHYDRATES (grams)	CALORIES
TOTAL RECIPE	12	0	0	6	137
EACH SERVING	3	0	0	1.5	34

GREEN BEANS OREGANO

Green beans and tomatoes are compatible in the garden and at the table too. Oregano gives the dish just the herbal lift to make it special.

1 pound fresh green beans, trimmed and sliced
3 tomatoes, cut in small wedges
1 small onion, sliced
½ teaspoon dried basil
⅛ teaspoon white pepper
¼ teaspoon dried oregano

Place green beans in a heavy saucepan. Add 1 inch of water. Add tomato wedges, onion, basil, pepper, and oregano. Cook uncovered until beans are tender, about 15 minutes. Drain and serve. Makes 6 servings.

	PROTEIN (grams)	FAT UNSATURATED (grams)	FAT SATURATED (grams)	CARBOHYDRATES (grams)	CALORIES
TOTAL RECIPE	13	0	0	52	238
EACH SERVING	2	0	0	8.7	40

GREEN BEANS PARMESAN

When you are tired of green beans, perk them up this way and watch the calls for seconds.

10-ounce package frozen green beans, or fresh and trimmed
2 tomatoes, cut in small wedges
1 tablespoon chopped onion

1 teaspoon lemon juice
½ teaspoon dried basil
1 teaspoon grated Parmesan cheese

Place green beans in a heavy saucepan; add ½ inch of water to saucepan. Add tomatoes, onion, lemon juice, and basil. Cook, covered, until beans are just tender and most of the water has evaporated. Sprinkle with cheese and toss. Makes 4 servings.

	PROTEIN (grams)	FAT UNSATURATED (grams)	FAT SATURATED (grams)	CARBOHYDRATES (grams)	CALORIES
TOTAL RECIPE	9	.1	.2	35	165
EACH SERVING	2.3	.02	.05	8.8	41

CREOLE GREEN BEANS

Do try to add the okra pod to keep the Creole flavor authentic—it gives the green beans a titillating taste.

1 pound green beans, trimmed
2 tomatoes, chopped
½ green pepper, diced
½ small onion, diced

1 okra pod, sliced thin (optional)
¼ cup water
⅛ teaspoon pepper

In a medium saucepan combine all ingredients. Cover and cook over low heat until beans are tender, about 10 to 15 minutes. Serves 6.

	PROTEIN (grams)	FAT UNSATURATED (grams)	FAT SATURATED (grams)	CARBOHYDRATES (grams)	CALORIES
TOTAL RECIPE	14	0	0	56	258
EACH SERVING	2.3	0	0	9	43

WAX BEANS AMANDINE

Marjoram should be a staple on your spice rack. The crunch of slivered almonds gives this dish a gourmet touch.

1 pound wax beans
1 tablespoon soft margarine
¼ cup sliced blanched unsalted almonds

½ teaspoon dried marjoram
⅛ teaspoon pepper

Trim ends of wax beans and place in a large saucepan; cover with water and cook uncovered over low heat until tender. Drain. Meanwhile, in a small saucepan, melt margarine. Add almonds and heat over medium heat, stirring occasionally until almonds are light brown. Add marjoram and pepper. Cook a minute more and pour over drained cooked beans. Serve at once. Makes 6 servings.

	PROTEIN (grams)	FAT UNSATURATED (grams)	FAT SATURATED (grams)	CARBOHYDRATES (grams)	CALORIES
TOTAL RECIPE	13	20	3	33	362
EACH SERVING	2.1	3.3	.5	5.5	60

CREOLE LENTILS

Here's a way to get complete protein with a vegetarian combination of a legume and a grain. Increase the serving portions if meat, poultry, or fish will not be served.

½ cup dried lentils
1 tablespoon salad oil
1 green pepper, chopped fine
1 small onion, chopped fine
1 cup chopped tomatoes

½ teaspoon dried thyme
⅛ teaspoon pepper
⅛ teaspoon filé powder (optional)
2 cups cooked whole-grain rice

Cover lentils with water and soak overnight. Drain, cover with fresh water, and simmer for 50 minutes or until tender. Heat oil in a skillet; sauté green pepper and onions until limp. Add tomatoes, thyme, pepper, and filé powder. Drain lentils and add to skillet; simmer until heated through. Pour over cooked rice and serve hot. Makes 6 servings.

	PROTEIN (grams)	FAT UNSATURATED (grams)	FAT SATURATED (grams)	CARBOHYDRATES (grams)	CALORIES
TOTAL RECIPE	39	11	1.4	186	1040
EACH SERVING	6.5	1.8	.2	31	173

BAKED LIMA BEANS

This casserole dish is fit to bring to a pot-luck supper, and it's full of subtle flavors and good vitamins.

2 cups dried lima beans
2 tablespoons soft margarine
2 onions, sliced thin
2 carrots, diced
1 cup chopped tomatoes

1 clove garlic, finely minced
½ teaspoon dried basil
⅛ teaspoon pepper
1 cup tomato juice

Soak lima beans for several hours or overnight. Discard soaking water. Heat margarine in a skillet, add onions, and sauté until limp. Place lima beans in a greased casserole; add onions and whatever fat remains. Add carrots, tomatoes, garlic, basil, and pepper. Mix well. Pour tomato juice over all. Bake in a 350°F. oven for 2 hours, or until beans are tender. Keep casserole tightly covered with a lid or with foil. Makes 6 servings.

	PROTEIN (grams)	FAT UNSATURATED (grams)	FAT SATURATED (grams)	CARBOHYDRATES (grams)	CALORIES
TOTAL RECIPE	35	12	3	117	733
EACH SERVING	6	2	.50	19	122

MINTED GREEN PEAS

No need for butter when you find another way to flavor peas. Here's a refreshing use for mint.

4 cups shelled green peas
¼ cup chopped fresh mint

⅛ teaspoon pepper
½ cup water

Combine peas with remaining ingredients, cover, and cook for 5 minutes, or until peas are just tender. (An alternate method is to place ingredients in a steam unit over boiling water.) Serves 8.

	PROTEIN (grams)	FAT UNSATURATED (grams)	FAT SATURATED (grams)	CARBOHYDRATES (grams)	CALORIES
TOTAL RECIPE	36	0	0	84	488
EACH SERVING	4.5	0	0	10.5	61

BOILED BEETS À L'ORANGE

Don't throw the beet tops out. Cook them as you would spinach and have a green vegetable for another meal.

1 bunch small beets (about 1 pound), tops removed, washed
1 cup water
1 teaspoon grated orange peel

¼ teaspoon dried dillweed
2 tablespoons frozen orange juice concentrate

Place beets and water in a heavy saucepan. Cover and boil until beets are tender, about 15 minutes. Remove beets and scrape off skins. Slice beets. Pour off all but ½ cup of the cooking liquid. Add orange peel, dillweed, and orange juice concentrate. Bring liquid to a boil and reduce to half. Add beets and heat through. Makes 4 servings.

	PROTEIN (grams)	FAT UNSATURATED (grams)	FAT SATURATED (grams)	CARBOHYDRATES (grams)	CALORIES
TOTAL RECIPE	8	0	0	58	250
EACH SERVING	2	0	0	15	62

BROCCOLI WITH PARSLEY SAUCE

Be sure to soak the fresh broccoli in deep water to be rid of any mites or cabbage worms. The simple parsley butter makes an appetizing sauce.

1 pound fresh broccoli, or two
   10-ounce packages frozen
2 tablespoons soft margarine

1 tablespoon chopped fresh
   parsley, or 1 teaspoon dried
1 lemon, cut in wedges

Trim fresh broccoli and wash well. Cut lengthwise if stems are thick. Steam or cook in a small amount of water until just tender, 10 to 15 minutes. Melt margarine and stir in parsley. Place cooked broccoli on a warm platter, pour parsley butter over all, and serve with lemon wedges. Makes 6 servings.

	PROTEIN (grams)	FAT UNSATURATED (grams)	FAT SATURATED (grams)	CARBOHYDRATES (grams)	CALORIES
TOTAL RECIPE	17	12	3	34	307
EACH SERVING	3	2	.50	6	51

SKILLET BROCCOLI

If you have stored some chicken broth as ice cubes in your freezer, you'll have merely to thaw two of them for the broth needed here. It's the way to make a freezer bank pay off.

2 large stalks fresh broccoli, cut
   in chunks
1 onion, sliced thin

½ cup chicken broth
⅛ teaspoon powdered ginger
⅛ teaspoon pepper

Place all ingredients in a skillet. Cover and simmer over low heat just until broccoli is tender. Serve at once. Makes 4 servings.

	PROTEIN (grams)	FAT UNSATURATED (grams)	FAT SATURATED (grams)	CARBOHYDRATES (grams)	CALORIES
TOTAL RECIPE	12	0	0	16.7	116
EACH SERVING	3	0	0	4.2	29

SWEET-AND-SOUR RED CABBAGE

This recipe keeps well in the refrigerator for several days. Indeed, it seems to get better with age.

1 medium head red cabbage, shredded
1½ cups water
2 tablespoons frozen apple juice concentrate

2 tablespoons lemon juice
1 tablespoon wine vinegar
2 whole cloves
½ teaspoon powdered ginger

Place shredded cabbage in a deep saucepan. Add remaining ingredients. Cover and simmer 35 minutes, stirring occasionally, or until cabbage is tender. Makes 8 servings.

	PROTEIN (grams)	FAT UNSATURATED (grams)	FAT SATURATED (grams)	CARBOHYDRATES (grams)	CALORIES
TOTAL RECIPE	14	0	0	64	278
EACH SERVING	1.75	0	0	8	35

DILLED CARROT RING

This hostess conversation-piece recipe is not difficult to make. Use the same formula for two cups of any compatible vegetable, and fill the unmolded ring with peas or any vegetable of contrasting color.

2 cups diced cooked carrots
½ teaspoon grated onion
1 teaspoon dried dillweed

⅛ teaspoon pepper
3 eggs, well beaten
1 cup skim milk

Combine all ingredients. Pour into an oiled ring mold and bake in a 350°F. oven for 40 minutes. Unmold and serve. Serves 6.

	PROTEIN (grams)	FAT UNSATURATED (grams)	FAT SATURATED (grams)	CARBOHYDRATES (grams)	CALORIES
TOTAL RECIPE	31	9	5.5	35	424
EACH SERVING	5	1.5	1	6	71

HERBED CARROTS

Why serve plain old carrots when with a little kitchen wizardry you can avoid the humdrum? Use the food processor to make fast even slices and lighten the chore.

4 large carrots, scraped and
   sliced thin
2 tablespoons finely chopped
   onion

½ cup orange juice
¼ teaspoon dried rosemary
½ teaspoon chopped fresh parsley

Place carrots in a heavy saucepan; add onion, orange juice, rosemary, and parsley. Cover and cook over low heat until carrots are just tender. Add more orange juice, if needed. Makes 4 servings.

	PROTEIN (grams)	FAT UNSATURATED (grams)	FAT SATURATED (grams)	CARBOHYDRATES (grams)	CALORIES
TOTAL RECIPE	4	0	0	42	181
EACH SERVING	1	0	0	10	45

FRESH CARROTS AND MUSHROOMS TARRAGON

Zip these carrots through the food processor or an electric slicing machine for quick preparation.

8–10 medium carrots (1 pound)
   1 cup water
   1 teaspoon dried tarragon
   1 tablespoon corn oil
     margarine

¼ pound fresh mushrooms,
   sliced

Pare carrots and cut into ¼-inch crosswise slices. Place in medium saucepan; add water and tarragon. Cover and cook over medium heat 20 to 30 minutes, until tender. While carrots are cooking, heat margarine in a small skillet; add mushrooms and cook until tender. If there is much water left in the pan with the carrots, drain the carrots. Add mushrooms to carrots and mix lightly. Makes 8 servings.

	PROTEIN (grams)	FAT UNSATURATED (grams)	FAT SATURATED (grams)	CARBOHYDRATES (grams)	CALORIES
TOTAL RECIPE	9	22	2.7	61	511
EACH SERVING	1.1	2.7	.33	7.6	64

CELERY AMANDINE

Celery is so low in calories that they are almost negligible. You can afford to have the luxury of a few slivered almonds in the sauce.

1 medium bunch celery, cut into 1-inch pieces
1 cup Chicken Bouillon or water

2 tablespoons chopped fresh parsley
2 tablespoons slivered almonds
1 tablespoon soft margarine

Place celery, chicken bouillon or water, and parsley in a saucepan. Cover and cook until just tender. Remove celery to a serving plate. Cook liquid until it almost evaporates, leaving about 3 tablespoons of liquid in the saucepan. Add almonds and margarine, stirring until margarine melts. Pour over celery. Makes 6 servings.

	PROTEIN (grams)	FAT UNSATURATED (grams)	FAT SATURATED (grams)	CARBOHYDRATES (grams)	CALORIES
TOTAL RECIPE	10	16	2.8	35	339
EACH SERVING	1.6	2.6	.47	6	56

CARROT AND CELERY SOUFFLÉ

Cut this soufflé into pie-shaped pieces and serve as a vegetable, or use it as a meatless main course for four.

1 cup dry bread crumbs
¼ cup skim milk
1¼ cups mashed cooked carrots
½ cup chopped celery
2 tablespoons chopped onion

2 eggs, separated
1 teaspoon chopped fresh parsley
⅛ teaspoon pepper

Mix bread crumbs with milk to moisten. Add carrots, celery, onion, and beaten egg yolks. Beat egg whites until stiff and fold into mixture. Add parsley and pepper. Pour into greased baking dish and bake in a 350°F. oven for 30 to 40 minutes. Serves 8.

	PROTEIN (grams)	FAT UNSATURATED (grams)	FAT SATURATED (grams)	CARBOHYDRATES (grams)	CALORIES
TOTAL RECIPE	30	9	5	95	652
EACH SERVING	4	1	.6	12	82

BRUSSELS SPROUTS/TOMATO COMBO

For a change of flavor and a diverting taste, try this method of cooking young sprouts with tomatoes and seasonings. Very good with beef.

1 pint fresh Brussels sprouts
2 tomatoes
½ cup water
½ teaspoon dried tarragon

⅛ teaspoon pepper
1 teaspoon lemon juice
1 teaspoon chopped fresh parsley

Wash Brussels sprouts thoroughly and cut in half lengthwise; place in a saucepan. Cut tomatoes into thin wedges and add to saucepan. Add remaining ingredients. Cover tightly and cook 10 to 15 minutes, until tender but not mushy. Makes 4 servings.

	PROTEIN (grams)	FAT UNSATURATED (grams)	FAT SATURATED (grams)	CARBOHYDRATES (grams)	CALORIES
TOTAL RECIPE	17	0	0	37	194
EACH SERVING	4.25	0	0	9	48

BAKED CHINESE CABBAGE AND TOMATOES

This same recipe works fine with regular cabbage too. Either way, it's an agreeable dish.

4 cups shredded Chinese cabbage
1 small onion, chopped
⅛ teaspoon paprika

2 eggs, beaten
2 cups chopped tomatoes

Arrange cabbage and onion in greased baking dish and season with paprika. Combine eggs and tomatoes, and pour over cabbage. Place dish in pan of hot water. Bake in 350°F. oven for 40 minutes or until firm. Serves 8.

	PROTEIN (grams)	FAT UNSATURATED (grams)	FAT SATURATED (grams)	CARBOHYDRATES (grams)	CALORIES
TOTAL RECIPE	23	6	4	39	336
EACH SERVING	3	.75	.50	5	42

BAKED CAULIFLOWER

There are those who do not like the flavor of plain steamed cauliflower. With added seasonings, however, cauliflower can become a gratifying vegetable.

1 large head cauliflower
1 onion, diced
2 tablespoons chopped fresh parsley
1 clove garlic, minced

2 cups chopped tomatoes
½ teaspoon paprika
¼ teaspoon pepper
¼ cup grated Parmesan cheese

Preheat oven to 350°F. Wash cauliflower and break into small flowerets. In a covered casserole, combine onion, parsley, garlic, and tomatoes; add paprika, pepper, and grated cheese. Add cauliflowerets and mix thoroughly. Cover and bake 40 minutes, or until cauliflower is tender. Makes 6 servings.

	PROTEIN (grams)	FAT UNSATURATED (grams)	FAT SATURATED (grams)	CARBOHYDRATES (grams)	CALORIES
TOTAL RECIPE	39	2	3.5	76	470
EACH SERVING	6.5	.33	.58	13	78

BROILED STUFFED MUSHROOMS

Serve these stuffed mushrooms with a meat or poultry dish, or use them as an appetizer at a cocktail party.

6 giant mushrooms
2 tablespoons wheat germ
1 tablespoon chopped fresh
   parsley

½ teaspoon garlic powder
¼ teaspoon dried oregano

Remove stems from mushrooms and chop fine. Add wheat germ, parsley, garlic powder, and oregano; mix well. Spoon into cavities of mushroom caps. Broil for 5 minutes, or until mushrooms are tender. Makes 6 servings.

	PROTEIN (grams)	FAT UNSATURATED (grams)	FAT SATURATED (grams)	CARBOHYDRATES (grams)	CALORIES
TOTAL RECIPE	7	.92	.20	11	80
EACH SERVING	1.16	.15	.03	2	13

BROILED TOMATOES

The secret of success with broiled tomatoes is not to cook them too long. Soft on the inside and firm on the outside is the culinary goal.

2 large tomatoes, cut in half
   through the wide middle
2 tablespoons wheat germ
1 tablespoon grated onion

1 tablespoon chopped fresh
   parsley
⅛ teaspoon pepper

Arrange tomatoes, cut sides up, on a broiling pan. Combine wheat germ, onion, parsley, and pepper; spoon mixture over the cut side of tomatoes. Broil for 5 minutes, or until tomatoes are softened and topping is lightly browned. Serve at once. Makes 4 servings.

	PROTEIN (grams)	FAT UNSATURATED (grams)	FAT SATURATED (grams)	CARBOHYDRATES (grams)	CALORIES
TOTAL RECIPE	8	.92	.20	24	132
EACH SERVING	2	.23	.05	6	33

EGGPLANT PARMESAN

Here's another meatless dish that can double as a main course. The mozzarella is an excellent source of protein, but be sure that it is the less fatty variety.

1-pound can tomatoes
2 tablespoons tomato paste
1 teaspoon dried oregano
1 eggplant, peeled and sliced thin

1 pound sliced mozzarella (part skim milk) cheese
¼ cup grated Parmesan cheese

Preheat oven to 350°F. Combine tomatoes, tomato paste, and oregano; blend in an electric blender. Spoon some of the tomato mixture into a thin layer in a large flat baking dish; cover with slices of eggplant and top with a layer of sliced mozzarella cheese. Sprinkle with grated Parmesan cheese. Repeat layers of sauce, eggplant, and cheese, using all ingredients and ending with sauce. Sprinkle Parmesan cheese over the top. Bake 35 minutes, or until eggplant is fork tender. Makes 6 servings.

	PROTEIN (grams)	FAT UNSATURATED (grams)	FAT SATURATED (grams)	CARBOHYDRATES (grams)	CALORIES
TOTAL RECIPE	96	2	3.5	57	696
EACH SERVING	16	.33	.58	10	116

STUFFED EGGPLANTS

Use this recipe when the rest of the meal seems to be lightweight, or serve by itself as a main course for lunch.

2 medium eggplants
1 onion, diced
4 stalks celery, diced
1 cup tomato juice
½ teaspoon dried thyme

½ teaspoon dried oregano
1 egg
½ cup cornflake crumbs
¼ cup grated Parmesan cheese

Cut eggplants in half and scoop out flesh carefully, leaving unbroken shells. Dice scooped-out eggplant flesh; place in a saucepan with onion, celery, tomato juice, thyme, and oregano. Simmer until vegetables are tender. Remove from heat. Preheat oven to 350°F. Add egg and cornflake crumbs to mixture in saucepan and stir in half the cheese. Fill eggplant shells with this mixture; sprinkle with remaining cheese. Bake for 20 minutes. Makes 4 servings.

	PROTEIN (grams)	FAT UNSATURATED (grams)	FAT SATURATED (grams)	CARBOHYDRATES (grams)	CALORIES
TOTAL RECIPE	33	5.2	5.4	99	623
EACH SERVING	8.2	1.2	1.3	24.7	156

RATATOUILLE

The French have a way with food, and this is one way they cook a vegetable stew. Great hot, and pretty good cold the next day for refrigerator raiders.

1 eggplant, peeled and diced into
   ½-inch cubes
1 zucchini, cut into ¼-inch slices
3 tomatoes, chopped
1 large onion, sliced
2 green peppers, seeded and
   diced

1 clove garlic, minced fine
2 tablespoons tomato paste
¼ cup water
¼ cup dry sherry wine
½ teaspoon dried oregano
¼ teaspoon pepper

Combine all ingredients in a heavy saucepan. Cover and cook over low heat for 20 minutes, or until all vegetables are tender. Stir occasionally. Remove cover and let juices evaporate to half. Makes 6 servings.

	PROTEIN (grams)	FAT UNSATURATED (grams)	FAT SATURATED (grams)	CARBOHYDRATES (grams)	CALORIES
TOTAL RECIPE	15	0	0	67	323
EACH SERVING	2.5	0	0	11	54

SPINACH CHEESE SOUFFLÉ

There are no egg yolks in this dish, which can be a main course for luncheon. It's a low-fat, high-protein delight.

10-ounce package frozen chopped spinach	¼ teaspoon garlic powder
½ cup low-fat cottage cheese	¼ teaspoon ground nutmeg
	2 egg whites

Cook spinach in a small amount of water and drain well. Add cottage cheese, garlic, and nutmeg. Beat egg whites until stiff peaks form; fold through spinach mixture. Pour into a greased baking dish. Bake in a 350°F. oven for 20 minutes, or until firm. Makes 4 servings.

	PROTEIN (grams)	FAT UNSATURATED (grams)	FAT SATURATED (grams)	CARBOHYDRATES (grams)	CALORIES
TOTAL RECIPE	33	0	0	14	188
EACH SERVING	8	0	0	3.5	47

SPINACH COTTAGE CHEESE BAKE

If you want to skip the egg white, here's a shortcut to get approximately the same dish as the previous recipe. Good for an appetizer course or as a nutritious hot lunch.

10-ounce package frozen chopped spinach, cooked and drained	1 cup low-fat cottage cheese
	¼ teaspoon ground nutmeg

Preheat oven to 350°F. Spoon spinach into a lightly buttered baking dish. Top with cottage cheese and sprinkle with nutmeg. Bake 15 minutes and serve at once. Makes 3 servings.

	PROTEIN (grams)	FAT UNSATURATED (grams)	FAT SATURATED (grams)	CARBOHYDRATES (grams)	CALORIES
TOTAL RECIPE	43	0	0	16	240
EACH SERVING	14	0	0	5	80

SPINACH SOUFFLÉ

Double this recipe and bake it in a small ring mold set in a pan of water. Very nice as a vegetable for a special dinner.

10-ounce package frozen chopped spinach	½ teaspoon onion powder
	2 egg whites

Preheat oven to 350°F. Cook frozen spinach and drain very well. Add onion powder. Beat egg whites until stiff peaks form. Fold cooked and drained spinach through beaten whites. Spoon into a buttered baking dish. Bake for 20 minutes, or until firm. Cut into serving portions. Makes 3 servings.

	PROTEIN (grams)	FAT UNSATURATED (grams)	FAT SATURATED (grams)	CARBOHYDRATES (grams)	CALORIES
TOTAL RECIPE	16	0	0	43	102
EACH SERVING	5	0	0	14	34

SPINACH WITH ORANGE SAUCE

What a way to pep up Popeye's favorite food, combining high calcium with a source of vitamin C. A simple proof that nutritious can also be delicious.

10-ounce package frozen chopped spinach	½ teaspoon onion powder
2 tablespoons frozen orange juice concentrate	⅛ teaspoon ground nutmeg

Cook spinach in a small amount of water; drain. Combine orange juice concentrate, onion powder, and nutmeg in a small saucepan; heat. Pour over cooked spinach and mix well. Makes 3 servings.

	PROTEIN (grams)	FAT UNSATURATED (grams)	FAT SATURATED (grams)	CARBOHYDRATES (grams)	CALORIES
TOTAL RECIPE	10	0	0	40	188
EACH SERVING	3.3	0	0	13	63

STEWED TOMATOES AND SPROUTS

When you are raising soybean sprouts and want to find a new way to use them, think of this recipe that will give you high-quality mouthfuls.

3 cups soybean sprouts
2 cups boiling water
2 tablespoons chopped onion
2 tablespoons chopped green pepper

1 stalk celery, thinly sliced
2 cups diced tomatoes
1 bay leaf
¼ teaspoon dried basil

Drop bean sprouts into boiling water and cook for 10 minutes; drain, reserving liquid. Place onion, green pepper, celery, tomatoes, bay leaf, and basil in a saucepan. Add ¼ cup of the drained soybean water and cover and cook over low heat for 10 minutes. Remove bay leaf. Add drained sprouts and cook 5 minutes more. Makes 6 servings.

	PROTEIN (grams)	FAT UNSATURATED (grams)	FAT SATURATED (grams)	CARBOHYDRATES (grams)	CALORIES
TOTAL RECIPE	25	0	0	42	261
EACH SERVING	4	0	0	7	43

CROOKNECK SQUASH WITH LEMON DILL SAUCE

There are so few pleasant yellow vegetables that this is sure to become a favorite. Just a hint of lemon sets it off.

2 large yellow crookneck squash, sliced
1 cup water

1 small onion, sliced thin
¼ cup lemon juice
1 teaspoon dried dillweed

Place sliced squash and water into a saucepan; add onion. Cover and simmer for 5 minutes, or until tender. Pour off liquid. Combine lemon juice and dillweed; pour over squash and toss to coat well. Makes 6 servings.

	PROTEIN (grams)	FAT UNSATURATED (grams)	FAT SATURATED (grams)	CARBOHYDRATES (grams)	CALORIES
TOTAL RECIPE	7	0	0	32	138
EACH SERVING	1	0	0	5	23

ZUCCHINI CHEDDAR BAKE

When the garden is coming up zucchini, or when you just strike a lucky market price, here's a way to turn that vegetable into something incredible.

4 cups sliced zucchini, cut ¼
   inch thick
2 tomatoes, chopped
¼ cup chopped onion

¼ cup chopped green pepper
¼ teaspoon dried oregano
¼ cup water
½ cup shredded Cheddar cheese

In a nonstick skillet, place zucchini, tomatoes, onion, green pepper, and oregano. Add water. Cover and cook over low heat about 15 minutes, or until zucchini is tender. Fold in cheese, stirring until it is melted. Makes 6 servings.

	PROTEIN (grams)	FAT UNSATURATED (grams)	FAT SATURATED (grams)	CARBOHYDRATES (grams)	CALORIES
TOTAL RECIPE	25	6	10	43	417
EACH SERVING	4	1	1.66	7	69

ZUCCHINI ITALIENNE

Don't cook zucchini until it's limp. Leave it a little crisp and you'll marvel at the difference.

2 medium zucchini, sliced thin
3 tomatoes, chopped
1 onion, sliced thin
1 clove garlic, minced fine
2 tablespoons tomato paste

½ teaspoon dried oregano
½ teaspoon dried thyme
⅛ teaspoon pepper
½ cup red wine

Place zucchini, tomatoes, onion, and garlic in a large skillet. Add tomato paste, oregano, thyme, and pepper. Mix well. Add dry red wine. Cover and cook until vegetables are tender, about 15 minutes. Makes 4 servings.

	PROTEIN (grams)	FAT UNSATURATED (grams)	FAT SATURATED (grams)	CARBOHYDRATES (grams)	CALORIES
TOTAL RECIPE	12	0	0	53	297
EACH SERVING	3	0	0	13	74

BAKED HONEYED ACORN SQUASH

When you crave a sweet-tasting accompaniment to a poultry or meat meal, try baking squash with margarine and honey. It should gladden all the sweet tooths at the table.

2 acorn squash
2 teaspoons soft margarine

2 teaspoons honey
¼ teaspoon ground cinnamon

Preheat oven to 350°F. Cut acorn squash in half lengthwise. Scoop out and discard seeds. Place squash, cut side up, in a baking pan. Fill cavities with dots of margarine and honey. Sprinkle with cinnamon. Bake for 25 to 30 minutes, or until fork tender. Makes 4 servings.

	PROTEIN (grams)	FAT UNSATURATED (grams)	FAT SATURATED (grams)	CARBOHYDRATES (grams)	CALORIES
TOTAL RECIPE	12	6	1.4	99	455
EACH SERVING	3	1.5	.35	25	114

BAKED STUFFED POTATOES PARMESAN

This is the way to escape the buttered baked potato routine and still enjoy some extra gusto. Potatoes may be prepared ahead of time and refrigerated. Bake just before serving. They also freeze extremely well, so bake up a bunch and stuff them for another day.

4 large baking potatoes
¼ cup skim milk
1 egg, slightly beaten

½ small onion, grated
4 teaspoons grated Parmesan cheese

Bake potatoes in a 350°F. oven for 1 hour, or until tender. Remove from oven. Cut each potato in half horizontally. Scoop out potato and reserve the shells.

Mash potatoes; add skim milk, beaten egg, and grated onion. Beat potatoes until fluffy. Spoon back into the shells. Top with a sprinkling of grated Parmesan cheese. Return to oven for 15 minutes, or until heated through. Makes 8 servings.

	PROTEIN (grams)	FAT UNSATURATED (grams)	FAT SATURATED (grams)	CARBOHYDRATES (grams)	CALORIES
TOTAL RECIPE	27	3.5	3	136	714
EACH SERVING	3	.45	.38	17	89

MASHED POTATOES

No need for butter and cream in your mashed potatoes when you can use low-fat yogurt for the same purpose. Adding an egg to the potato casserole puffs it up during the extra baking time.

6 medium potatoes, peeled and
  quartered
2 cups water
1 sliced onion

½ cup plain low-fat yogurt
1 tablespoon chopped chives
1 egg, beaten slightly

Place potatoes, water, and onion into a saucepan. Cook about 20 minutes, or until tender. Drain. Whip with a whisk or electric beater. Add yogurt, chopped chives, and beaten egg. Beat until fluffy. Spoon into a greased casserole. Bake in a 350°F. oven for 20 minutes. Makes 8 servings.

	PROTEIN (grams)	FAT UNSATURATED (grams)	FAT SATURATED (grams)	CARBOHYDRATES (grams)	CALORIES
TOTAL RECIPE	35	3.6	3	207	1027
EACH SERVING	4.4	.45	.37	26	128

MASHED SWEET POTATO CASSEROLE

Here's the way to stretch four sweet potatoes to feed six people happily. Such a nice addition to a poultry or lamb meal.

4 large sweet potatoes
1 cup water
¼ cup pineapple juice

1 egg, beaten
¼ teaspoon ground nutmeg
⅛ teaspoon pepper

Peel sweet potatoes and cut into quarters. Place in a saucepan with water. Cover and cook over low heat until tender. Drain. Mash with pineapple juice. Add beaten egg, nutmeg, and pepper; beat until fluffy. Spoon into a greased casserole. Bake in a 350°F. oven for 30 minutes. Makes 6 servings.

	PROTEIN (grams)	FAT UNSATURATED (grams)	FAT SATURATED (grams)	CARBOHYDRATES (grams)	CALORIES
TOTAL RECIPE	18	3	1.85	179	856
EACH SERVING	3	.50	.30	30	143

PASTA AND RICE

Pasta and grains are the "good guys" of complex carbohydrates. It's a mistake to lump all carbohydrates together as "bad guys" along with the simple carbohydrates of sugar in the diet. Remember that the Aerobic Nutrition goal is to increase your intake of complex carbohydrates to 63 percent of the calories in your diet, while reducing your sugar intake to a mere 5 percent.

Try to use pasta made from unbleached flour and to use rice that is brown or in its least polished form to benefit from the nutrients that are otherwise refined out of your food.

You can make your own pasta rather quickly if you have a pasta machine in your kitchen. The process can be fun, as family members take turns rolling the dough through and draping it over surfaces to dry.

If this is not your idea of fun, then take a walk down the aisles of your supermarket and study the many types of pasta that are available to you. What is readily available in local grocery stores in foreign countries somehow has become rarefied food in America, all too often available only in health food stores. Your health food store will have less refined wheat products and may be the only place nearby to purchase brown rice. Why don't all food stores offer a healthy assortment of choices?

You will find many pasta dishes in this chapter that can be used as side dishes or that can serve as a main meatless entrée. There are also several combinations of legumes and rice that give the complete protein of meat but none of the fat. Consider these when you plan your menus so that several times a week you can eliminate animal protein altogether, with no damage to your nutritional intake.

Notice, also, how nicely vegetables (which are also a complex carbohydrate) can be combined with pasta dishes, particularly in the noodle and lasagna categories. Be sure to use low-fat cottage cheese and low-fat yogurt when making noodle-cheese puddings. These can be served as a main course or cut into small servings as a meat accompaniment.

The recipes in this chapter have been nearly stripped of fat, but they are so flavorful and filling that you'll barely know the difference. Get on with good health and think of pasta and rice for many meals throughout the week.

HOMEMADE PASTA

For total control of ingredients and total freshness, don't hesitate to make your own pasta. This dough can be turned into broad lasagna noodles, narrower noodles for soups and baked puddings, and slender flat noodles known as fettucine. There are no preservatives, so cook within the time directed.

2 cups unbleached flour	¼ teaspoon salt
3 eggs	3 tablespoons cold water

Sift flour into a pile in a large bowl. Make a well in the center. Drop in the eggs, salt, and 1 tablespoon of the water. Mix and add the rest of the water, working it into the dough. Flour your hands and knead the dough on a floured board until you can work it into a smooth ball that no longer sticks to your hands. Cover the ball of dough and let it stand for 1 hour. Then process the dough through a pasta machine or roll segments of the dough on a floured board until very thin. Roll each segment up and slice into noodles. Arrange noodles over a clean cloth to dry for 15 minutes. Then drop into a pot of boiling water and cook for 6 to 8 minutes. Drain well before serving. Makes 8 servings.

	PROTEIN (grams)	FAT UNSATURATED (grams)	FAT SATURATED (grams)	CARBOHYDRATES (grams)	CALORIES
TOTAL RECIPE	46	8.7	5.4	192	1156
EACH SERVING	5.6	2	6.6	24	144

CLAM SAUCE

For a simple main dish when served over pasta and rice, or as a side dish for a fish dinner, this sauce has piquant appeal. Be sure to add the natural clam juice to the simmering sauce.

1 clove garlic, minced	½ teaspoon dried oregano
1 onion, diced fine	½ teaspoon dried thyme
½ green pepper, diced fine	½ teaspoon pepper
3 cups chopped tomatoes	1 cup chopped clams
½ cup water	

In a large saucepan, combine garlic, onion, green pepper, tomatoes, water, oregano, thyme, and pepper. Cover and simmer over low heat for 30 minutes. Add chopped clams. Simmer uncovered 5 minutes more. Serves 4.

	PROTEIN (grams)	FAT UNSATURATED (grams)	FAT SATURATED (grams)	CARBOHYDRATES (grams)	CALORIES
TOTAL RECIPE	37	0	0	66	426
EACH SERVING	9	0	0	17	107

MEAT SAUCE

There's no need to cook meat sauce for hours when you use this method. A crisp salad rounds out the pasta or rice offering.

1 tablespoon corn oil	½ teaspoon dried oregano
1 onion, sliced thin	4 tomatoes, chopped fine
2 large cloves garlic, mashed	1 green pepper, chopped fine
½ pound lean ground beef	2 tablespoons tomato paste
½ teaspoon pepper	

Heat oil in a skillet. Sauté onion and garlic for several minutes. Add ground beef and cook while breaking apart into particles. Add pepper and oregano.

Stir well. Add tomatoes, green pepper, and tomato paste; mix well. Cover and simmer over low heat for 20 minutes. Makes 4 servings.

	PROTEIN (grams)	FAT UNSATURATED (grams)	FAT SATURATED (grams)	CARBOHYDRATES (grams)	CALORIES
TOTAL RECIPE	58	21	12	53	769
EACH SERVING	15	5	3	13	192

SPAGHETTI MILANESE

Just a few chicken livers can turn a simple spaghetti sauce into a gallant Italian treat. It's a meal-in-one that requires only a vegetable or salad to give balanced and good nutrition.

1 tablespoon corn oil
1 large onion, finely diced
1 cup sliced fresh mushrooms
2 cloves garlic, minced
8 chicken livers
1 teaspoon dried oregano
½ teaspoon pepper

½ teaspoon dried basil
4 large tomatoes, chopped fine
½ cup tomato juice
¼ cup dry red wine
1 pound spaghetti, cooked and drained

Heat oil in a skillet. Add onion, mushrooms, and garlic; sauté until onions are golden. Cut livers into small chunks; add to skillet and brown on all sides. Stir constantly to prevent sticking. Add oregano, pepper, and basil. Add tomatoes, tomato juice, and wine. Simmer for 15 minutes over low heat. Serve over spaghetti. Makes 8 servings.

	PROTEIN (grams)	FAT UNSATURATED (grams)	FAT SATURATED (grams)	CARBOHYDRATES (grams)	CALORIES
TOTAL RECIPE	124	24	10	386	2473
EACH SERVING	16	3	1.2	48	310

SPINACH LASAGNA

Take this to a potluck supper or savor it at home. Makes a great luncheon or side dish for a company meal.

8-ounce package lasagna
noodles, cooked and drained
2 cups low-fat ricotta cheese
1 egg, beaten
10-ounce package frozen
chopped spinach, thawed and
drained
¼ cup sliced scallions, including
tops

2 cups tomato sauce
½ teaspoon dried oregano
1 cup shredded low-fat
mozzarella cheese
2 tablespoons grated Parmesan
cheese

Rinse cooked noodles to prevent sticking. Combine ricotta cheese, egg, spinach, and scallions. Combine tomato sauce and oregano. Spoon a third of the sauce over the bottom of an 8-by-12-inch baking dish. Arrange a layer of noodles side by side over the sauce. Spread half the ricotta cheese mixture over noodles. Top with another layer of noodles. Spoon a thin layer of sauce over noodles. Spread remaining ricotta cheese mixture over all. Top with final layer of noodles. Pour remaining sauce over top. Sprinkle with mozzarella cheese and Parmesan cheese. Bake in a 350°F. oven for 40 minutes, or until top is browned and cheese is melted. Makes 8 servings.

	PROTEIN (grams)	FAT UNSATURATED (grams)	FAT SATURATED (grams)	CARBOHYDRATES (grams)	CALORIES
TOTAL RECIPE	158	9	6	235	1780
EACH SERVING	20	1.1	.75	30	222

ZUCCHINI LASAGNA

When the garden is producing more zucchini than the family can possibly eat, bury it in pasta strips and cheese for an enticing meal-in-one.

1-pound can tomatoes
½ cup chopped onion
1 teaspoon dried oregano
8 lasagna noodles, cooked and
drained

4 cups zucchini slices
1 pound sliced mozzarella (part
skim milk) cheese
¼ cup grated Parmesan cheese

Simmer tomatoes, onion, and oregano, covered. Cook over low heat 20 minutes, stirring occasionally. Layer half the cooked lasagna noodles in a buttered baking dish. Top with half the zucchini slices, one-third of the tomato sauce, and half the mozzarella cheese. Repeat layers of noodles, zucchini, sauce, and mozzarella cheese. Top with remaining sauce. Sprinkle Parmesan cheese over top. Bake in a preheated 375°F. oven for 35 minutes, or until zucchini is tender. Makes 6 servings.

	PROTEIN (grams)	FAT UNSATURATED (grams)	FAT SATURATED (grams)	CARBOHYDRATES (grams)	CALORIES
TOTAL RECIPE	127	7	7	222	1584
EACH SERVING	21	1	1	37	264

CABBAGE-APPLE-NOODLE BAKE

Here's another dish that can double as a main course or a side course with meat. However you serve it, it's a winner.

6 cups shredded cabbage
2 cups peeled, thinly sliced
  cooking apples
2 tablespoons soft margarine
  8-ounce package wide noodles,
  cooked and drained

2 cups low-fat cottage cheese
1 egg, beaten
½ teaspoon ground cinnamon
¼ teaspoon ground nutmeg
½ teaspoon ground allspice
⅛ teaspoon pepper

Using a large skillet, sauté cabbage and apples in margarine until tender, about 15 to 20 minutes. Add cooked noodles and toss through. Combine cottage cheese, egg, cinnamon, nutmeg, allspice, and pepper; add to cabbage mixture and toss through. Pour into a greased casserole. Top with additional cinnamon and nutmeg, if desired. Bake in a 350°F. oven for 30 minutes, or until top is lightly browned. Makes 8 servings.

	PROTEIN (grams)	FAT UNSATURATED (grams)	FAT SATURATED (grams)	CARBOHYDRATES (grams)	CALORIES
TOTAL RECIPE	110	20	8	259	1791
EACH SERVING	14	2.5	1	32	224

BROCCOLI NOODLE CASSEROLE

Use this either as a combined vegetable/pasta part of the meal or as a meatless dish. Ricotta cheese provides a good part of the protein.

8-ounce package wide noodles,
cooked and drained
1 pound broccoli, cooked and
chopped into small pieces
1 cup low-fat ricotta cheese

1 egg, beaten
4 tablespoons grated Parmesan
cheese
½ teaspoon dried oregano
⅛ teaspoon pepper

Combine the cooked noodles and broccoli. Combine ricotta cheese, egg, 2 tablespoons of the Parmesan cheese, oregano, and pepper. Add the noodle-broccoli mixture and toss lightly to mix through. Pour all into a greased casserole. Top with remaining Parmesan cheese. Bake in a 350°F. oven for 30 minutes, or until top is lightly browned. Makes 8 servings.

	PROTEIN (grams)	FAT UNSATURATED (grams)	FAT SATURATED (grams)	CARBOHYDRATES (grams)	CALORIES
TOTAL RECIPE	93	10	8	196	1360
EACH SERVING	12	1.2	1	24.5	170

CAULIFLOWER NOODLE PUDDING

Here's a way to serve cauliflower without anyone being the wiser. There's a faint cabbagey flavor that only the most discerning will detect.

8-ounce package whole-wheat
noodles, cooked and drained
2 cups chopped cooked
cauliflower
2 cups skim-milk ricotta cheese

1 egg
1 tablespoon chopped fresh
parsley
2 tablespoons grated Parmesan
cheese

Combine noodles and cauliflower. Combine ricotta cheese, egg, and parsley; add to noodles. Pour into a greased 8-by-12-inch baking pan or casserole. Top with grated Parmesan cheese. Bake in a 350°F. oven for 30 minutes, or until top is lightly browned. Makes 8 servings.

	PROTEIN (grams)	FAT UNSATURATED (grams)	FAT SATURATED (grams)	CARBOHYDRATES (grams)	CALORIES
TOTAL RECIPE	114	9	6.6	187	1411
EACH SERVING	14	1	.8	23	176

COTTAGE CHEESE NOODLE PUDDING

Serve this as a main course, a side dish, or even an interesting dessert. Honey and raisins make it a versatile taste treat.

8 ounces broad noodles
1 cup low-fat cottage cheese
1 cup plain low-fat yogurt
2 tablespoons lemon juice

1 teaspoon vanilla extract
1 tablespoon honey
½ teaspoon ground cinnamon
½ cup seedless raisins

Boil noodles as directed on the package, eliminating salt in the cooking water. Mix together cottage cheese, yogurt, lemon juice, vanilla, honey, cinnamon, and raisins; toss mixture through noodles. Spoon into a well-greased baking dish. Bake in a 350°F. oven for 1 hour, or until lightly browned. Makes 8 servings.

	PROTEIN (grams)	FAT UNSATURATED (grams)	FAT SATURATED (grams)	CARBOHYDRATES (grams)	CALORIES
TOTAL RECIPE	65	5	3	245	1334
EACH SERVING	8	.6	.37	31	167

MEATLESS LASAGNA

It's not necessary to add meat to this dish, but if you want to, just brown a half pound of lean ground beef in the sauce and proceed as directed.

8-ounce package lasagna
  noodles
¼ cup water
1 onion, chopped fine
1 green pepper, chopped fine
3 cups chopped tomatoes

¼ teaspoon pepper
½ teaspoon dried oregano
¼ teaspoon garlic powder
1 pint low-fat ricotta cheese
1 egg
½ cup grated Parmesan cheese

Cook lasagna noodles until soft and pliable but still firm; rinse under cold water and drain well. Meanwhile, heat water in a skillet. Add onion, green pepper, tomatoes, pepper, oregano, and garlic powder. Cover and simmer for 10 minutes. Spread a thin layer of this sauce over the bottom of a rectangular baking dish. Arrange a layer of cooked lasagna noodles side by side. Beat ricotta cheese and egg together; spread a layer of this mixture over the noodles. Sprinkle lightly with some of the grated Parmesan cheese. Arrange another layer of noodles over this; top with remaining cheese mixture and sprinkle with Parmesan cheese. Arrange remaining noodles over top; spoon tomato sauce over all. Sprinkle with remaining Parmesan cheese. Bake in a 350°F. oven for 30 minutes. Makes 6 servings.

	PROTEIN (grams)	FAT UNSATURATED (grams)	FAT SATURATED (grams)	CARBOHYDRATES (grams)	CALORIES
TOTAL RECIPE	115	7	5	222	1528
EACH SERVING	19	1.2	.83	37	254

NOODLE BOWS AND CHEESE

It's fun to experiment with all the shapes and sizes of pasta that are available. Here are the most attractive pasta bows combined with cheese for lunch or dinner.

1-pound package noodle bows
1 cup freshly grated Parmesan cheese
1 cup diced Swiss cheese
1 cup diced low-fat mozzarella cheese

3 tablespoons cornstarch
3 cups skim milk
¼ teaspoon pepper
⅛ teaspoon ground nutmeg

Cook noodle bows in boiling water according to package directions. Drain in colander. Add ¾ cup Parmesan cheese, Swiss cheese, and mozzarella cheese, and mix well. In a saucepan combine cornstarch and milk; cook, stirring constantly, until sauce thickens. Add pepper and nutmeg. Turn half the noodle-cheese mixture into an oiled baking dish; top with half of the sauce. Repeat layers. Sprinkle remaining ¼ cup grated Parmesan cheese on top. Bake in a 350°F. oven for 25 minutes. Makes 12 servings.

	PROTEIN (grams)	FAT UNSATURATED (grams)	FAT SATURATED (grams)	CARBOHYDRATES (grams)	CALORIES
TOTAL RECIPE	184	31	38	395	3078
EACH SERVING	15	2.6	3.2	33	256

PINEAPPLE NOODLE PUDDING

Are you at a loss for something to serve for luncheon or as a side course with dinner? Try this delectable pineapple concoction for gustatorial pleasure.

8-ounce package broad noodles	8-ounce can unsweetened
3 eggs	pineapple tidbits, drained
½ pound low-fat cottage cheese	¼ cup bread crumbs
1 cup plain low-fat yogurt	

Preheat oven to 350°F. Cook noodles according to package directions, or boil in water for about 8 minutes until tender. Drain. Beat eggs; add cottage cheese, yogurt, and pineapple tidbits. Fold noodles into this mixture. Pour noodle mixture into lightly greased 8-by-12-inch baking dish. Top with bread crumbs. Bake for 1 hour. Makes 8 servings.

	PROTEIN (grams)	FAT UNSATURATED (grams)	FAT SATURATED (grams)	CARBOHYDRATES (grams)	CALORIES
TOTAL RECIPE	70	16	11	207	1422
EACH SERVING	9	2	1.3	26	178

STUFFED BAKED MANICOTTI

This high-protein dairy dish is suitable for luncheon or dinner. Add a vegetable or salad and enjoy a low-budget offering.

1-pound package manicotti pasta	2 tablespoons tomato paste
1 pound low-fat ricotta cheese	1 teaspoon dried oregano
3 tablespoons Parmesan cheese	¼ cup Italian-seasoned bread crumbs
16-ounce can tomatoes	

Cook manicotti according to package directions; remove from water as soon as pasta is pliable. Combine ricotta cheese and Parmesan cheese; stuff noodle tubes with the mixture and place side by side in a greased flat casserole. Blend tomatoes, tomato paste, and oregano in an electric blender; spoon over stuffed manicotti and top with bread crumbs. Bake for 30 minutes in a 350°F. oven, or until manicotti is fork tender. Makes 8 servings.

	PROTEIN (grams)	FAT UNSATURATED (grams)	FAT SATURATED (grams)	CARBOHYDRATES (grams)	CALORIES
TOTAL RECIPE	149	13	9	383	2430
EACH SERVING	18.6	1.6	1.1	48	304

LENTIL AND RICE CASSEROLE

Here is one more legume-and-grain dish that gives the complete protein that vegetarians need for meatless dining. All others may use it as a side dish that is well worth the effort to prepare.

⅔ cup dried lentils
1 cup rice
1 onion, diced
1 clove garlic, minced fine
5 stalks celery, diced fine
2½ cups cooked tomatoes

1 teaspoon dried thyme
¼ teaspoon white pepper
1 teaspoon dried dillweed
¼ cup whole-wheat bread crumbs

Soak lentils in water overnight. Simmer slowly in the same water until lentils are tender, about 2 hours. Place rice and 3 cups water in a saucepan; bring to a boil, then cover and simmer for 20 minutes, fluffing once with a fork during cooking. In the meantime, cook onion, garlic, and celery in ¼ cup water until soft, about 7 minutes. Add tomatoes, drained lentils with ½ cup of the lentil cooking water, rice, thyme, pepper, and dillweed. Mix well. Pour into a 2-quart nonstick-surface baking pan. Pour lentil-rice mixture into baking dish. Sprinkle crumbs over the top. Bake in a 350°F. oven for 30 minutes. Makes 6 servings.

	PROTEIN (grams)	FAT UNSATURATED (grams)	FAT SATURATED (grams)	CARBOHYDRATES (grams)	CALORIES
TOTAL RECIPE	56	.82	.26	290	1411
EACH SERVING	9	.14	.04	48	235

BLACK BEANS AND RICE

This is a native Brazilian dish that combines a legume with a grain for complete protein without meat.

½ cup black beans
1 cup chopped onions
1 green pepper, diced fine
1 clove garlic, minced fine

1 tablespoon corn oil
½ teaspoon pepper
2 cups cooked rice

Wash black beans. Place in a deep pot and cover with about 4 cups water. Bring to a boil. Meanwhile, in a large skillet, sauté onions, green pepper, and garlic in hot corn oil; when onions are limp and translucent, pour all into the bean pot. Add pepper. Cook beans until soft, adding more water if necessary. Serve on mounds of cooked hot rice. Makes 6 servings.

	PROTEIN (grams)	FAT UNSATURATED (grams)	FAT SATURATED (grams)	CARBOHYDRATES (grams)	CALORIES
TOTAL RECIPE	34	11	1.4	179	986
EACH SERVING	5.6	1.8	.2	30	164

BROWN RICE MUSHROOM RING

This makes a pretty setting for a vegetable filling. Brown rice makes it a healthier and crunchier choice.

1 cup brown rice
2½ cups water
½ pound mushrooms, trimmed and sliced

1 tablespoon grated onion
3 tablespoons chopped fresh parsley

Wash rice well, and cook in boiling water for 25 minutes, covered. Stir occasionally. Fluff cooked rice with a fork. Add mushrooms, onion, and parsley. Spoon into a greased 1-quart ring mold and set in a pan of hot water. Bake in a preheated 350°F. oven for 30 minutes. Turn out onto a platter. Makes 6 servings.

	PROTEIN (grams)	FAT UNSATURATED (grams)	FAT SATURATED (grams)	CARBOHYDRATES (grams)	CALORIES
TOTAL RECIPE	20	0	0	155	740
EACH SERVING	3.3	0	0	16	123

CURRIED RICE

What a lovely way to enhance the flavor of rice! Choose the unhulled brown variety for extra nutrition and crunchy texture.

1 cup rice
3 cups chicken broth
1½ teaspoons curry powder
1 teaspoon grated onion

1 tablespoon chopped fresh parsley
⅛ teaspoon paprika

Combine all ingredients in a heavy saucepan. Cover and simmer for 25 minutes, or until all liquid is absorbed and rice is tender. Serves 6.

	PROTEIN (grams)	FAT UNSATURATED (grams)	FAT SATURATED (grams)	CARBOHYDRATES (grams)	CALORIES
TOTAL RECIPE	13	0	0	157	711
EACH SERVING	2	0	0	26	118

DIRTY RICE

This is a unappealing name for a wonderful dish. Use up leftover chicken, turkey, or meat, and serve with a simple salad.

1 green pepper, diced
1 onion, diced
2 tablespoons water
2 cups cooked brown rice

½ cup diced cooked chicken
1 teaspoon dried thyme
¼ teaspoon pepper

Simmer pepper and onion in water for several minutes. Combine with rest of ingredients in a 1½-quart casserole. Bake in a 325°F. oven for 45 minutes. Makes 4 servings.

	PROTEIN (grams)	FAT UNSATURATED (grams)	FAT SATURATED (grams)	CARBOHYDRATES (grams)	CALORIES
TOTAL RECIPE	35	1.9	1	110	639
EACH SERVING	8.6	.47	.26	28	160

ORANGE RAISIN RICE

Did you know that orange juice can be used in place of water to give rice an extra punch of flavor and nutrition? Produces an interesting color too.

1 cup brown rice
2 cups orange juice
½ cup chicken broth or water
½ cup seedless white raisins

3 scallions, sliced fine, including tops
½ teaspoon dried dillweed

Combine rice, orange juice, broth or water, raisins, scallions, and dillweed in a heavy saucepan. Bring to a boil, then reduce heat to a simmer and cover tightly. Cook for 25 minutes, adding additional water if necessary. Fluff once during cooking time. Makes 6 servings.

	PROTEIN (grams)	FAT UNSATURATED (grams)	FAT SATURATED (grams)	CARBOHYDRATES (grams)	CALORIES
TOTAL RECIPE	20	0	0	262	1149
EACH SERVING	3	0	0	44	192

HERB RICE CASSEROLE

The carrots give a hint of sweetness and the herbs a final kick to this rice casserole of unique flavor and finesse.

¾ cup brown rice
1½ cups chicken broth
¾ cup dry white wine
2 onions, diced fine

2 carrots, shredded
¼ teaspoon dried oregano
¼ teaspoon dried marjoram
⅛ teaspoon pepper

Place all ingredients in a casserole. Mix well. Cover tightly with lid or aluminum foil. Bake in a 350°F. oven for 1 hour. Fluff rice and serve. Makes 4 servings.

	PROTEIN (grams)	FAT UNSATURATED (grams)	FAT SATURATED (grams)	CARBOHYDRATES (grams)	CALORIES
TOTAL RECIPE	15	0	0	145	665
EACH SERVING	3.8	0	0	36	166

SALADS

Fresh and crisp raw vegetables are almost bursting with vitamins and minerals. That's why it's most important to brighten your menu with a variety of uncooked combinations of these easy-to-prepare food. Salads, a natural way to serve vegetables, should be an important part of your daily diet.

Raw vegetables also contribute a good deal of cellulose bulk to your digestive system. They are nature's present to you to prevent colon problems. Pare vegetables as thin as possible and only if you must. Sometimes a brisk scrubbing with a vegetable brush is all that is needed.

Salads can be a kind of free-for-all dish, developing textures and flavors with available ingredients in the refrigerator. Do you have half a cup of rice left over from last night's dinner? Toss it with the salad for economy, health, and a different taste. Do the same with cold macaroni, or peel and dice a leftover chilled baked potato into the crisp greens. Small amounts of leftover chicken, turkey, fish, or meat can also be used to stretch a simple vegetable salad into a complete meal.

It's the dressing that pulls a salad together. But Aerobic Nutrition means that you will avoid all high-saturated-fat dressings and limit your intake of the unsaturated fats. When the amount of oil is not specified in recipes, it is not computed in the fat breakdown. *Be sure to use as little as possible.*

This chapter will show you how to make your own mayonnaise in the blender and then how to turn it into a rémoulade sauce. You will find recipes that use low-fat yogurt as the basis of the dressing, enabling you to limit your saturated fat intake mostly to the animal fat in your meat dishes.

Remember that herbs liven up a simple vinegar and unsaturated oil dressing. Add oregano, thyme, tarragon, a bit of dry mustard, and you're off to a good start. Discover the interesting flavors of greens such as arugula, dandelion leaves, and chopped chives. Perk up your salads with chopped fresh parsley and chopped fresh dill. And always think of lemon—just a squeeze of lemon juice will enhance the simplest of salads.

Here is a wide assortment of salad recipes to get you interested in the wonderful possibilities that await your palate.

SUPER SALAD

When you want a quick highly nutritious lunch, try this version of the French niçoise salad. We've left out the high-sodium anchovies, but the rest is quite authentic.

1 small head lettuce, torn up
1 carrot, scraped and sliced
½ small red onion, sliced thin
    7½-ounce can water-packed
    tuna
2 tomatoes, quartered

1 cup cooked corn
1 green or red pepper, cut in
    strips
    Wine vinegar
    Salad oil

Combine lettuce, carrots, onion, tuna (broken up), tomatoes, corn, and pepper. Toss well. Pass cruets of wine vinegar and oil. Makes 4 servings.

	PROTEIN (grams)	FAT UNSATURATED (grams)	FAT SATURATED (grams)	CARBOHYDRATES (grams)	CALORIES
TOTAL RECIPE	71	0	0	80	602
EACH SERVING	18	0	0	20	150

VITAMIN C SALAD

You can get lots of vitamin C from the foods you eat. Prepare a salad this way and see how much C you can include.

1 quart fresh torn spinach leaves
1 red pepper, cut in strips and seeded
2 tomatoes, cut in wedges
2 tablespoons salad oil
¼ cup orange juice
2 tablespoons lemon juice
½ teaspoon garlic powder
¼ teaspoon celery seed

Combine spinach, red pepper, and tomatoes in a salad bowl. In a jar, combine salad oil, orange and lemon juices, garlic powder, and celery seed; shake well. Pour over salad and toss. Makes 4 servings.

	PROTEIN (grams)	FAT UNSATURATED (grams)	FAT SATURATED (grams)	CARBOHYDRATES (grams)	CALORIES
TOTAL RECIPE	20	22	3	49	488
EACH SERVING	5	5.5	.75	12	122

COTTAGE CHEESE VEGETABLE SALAD

What a wonderful diet lunch this can be. Herbs turn the yogurt into a zesty topping.

1 large tomato, diced
1 large cucumber, peeled and diced
1 green pepper, seeded and diced
2 stalks celery, sliced
1 carrot, scraped and sliced thin
2 cups low-fat cottage cheese
1 cup plain low-fat yogurt
2 tablespoons chopped chives
½ teaspoon dried tarragon

Combine tomato, cucumber, pepper, celery, and carrot. Add cottage cheese and stir lightly until mixed through. Stir yogurt, chives, and tarragon together; use as a topping for the cottage cheese vegetable salad. Makes 4 servings.

	PROTEIN (grams)	FAT UNSATURATED (grams)	FAT SATURATED (grams)	CARBOHYDRATES (grams)	CALORIES
TOTAL RECIPE	55	Trace	Trace	35	372
EACH SERVING	13	Trace	Trace	9	93

YOGURT SLAW

When you are yearning for slaw and don't want a mayonnaise dressing, consider using this low-fat yogurt dressing instead. It defies you to complain.

1 small head cabbage, shredded	1 teaspoon dried dillweed
¼ cup chopped scallions, including tops	1 cup plain low-fat yogurt
	¼ teaspoon dry mustard
⅓ cup chopped fresh parsley	1 tablespoon lemon juice

Combine cabbage, scallions, parsley, and dillweed. Stir together yogurt, dry mustard, and lemon juice; pour over cabbage mixture and toss lightly until well coated. Cover bowl and chill for several hours. Makes 6 servings.

	PROTEIN (grams)	FAT UNSATURATED (grams)	FAT SATURATED (grams)	CARBOHYDRATES (grams)	CALORIES
TOTAL RECIPE	13	Trace	Trace	55	246
EACH SERVING	2	Trace	Trace	9	41

CELERY-CARROT SLAW

All slaw is not made from cabbage. Here is one that is made from celery and carrots. Add green pepper if you wish, and make your own low-fat yogurt.

4 cups thinly sliced celery	2 tablespoons cider vinegar
½ cup coarsely shredded carrots	½ teaspoon white pepper
½ cup raisins	⅔ cup plain low-fat yogurt

In a large bowl combine celery with carrots and raisins. In a separate bowl, blend together vinegar and pepper. Stir in yogurt, mixing until smooth. Pour dressing over celery mixture and toss until well combined. Chill. Makes 8 servings.

	PROTEIN (grams)	FAT UNSATURATED (grams)	FAT SATURATED (grams)	CARBOHYDRATES (grams)	CALORIES
TOTAL RECIPE	13	1	1.5	90	401
EACH SERVING	1.6	.11	.19	11.3	50

AVOCADO GARDEN SALAD

Yes, avocado has a higher fat content than most vegetables, but it's an unsaturated fat, thank goodness. So enjoy a small portion in your salad and be glad that the flavor of avocado can be yours.

½ fresh lime or lemon
1 avocado, peeled and sliced
1 head romaine lettuce
½ head iceberg lettuce

½ cup tiny raw cauliflower pieces
⅓ cup thinly sliced carrots
2 tomatoes, cut in wedges

Squeeze lime or lemon juice over avocado slices; set aside. Line a salad bowl with romaine lettuce. Tear remaining romaine and iceberg lettuce into bite-size pieces; add to salad bowl. Add avocado slices, cauliflower, carrots, and tomatoes. Cover and chill until serving time. Makes 6 servings.

	PROTEIN (grams)	FAT UNSATURATED (grams)	FAT SATURATED (grams)	CARBOHYDRATES (grams)	CALORIES
TOTAL RECIPE	19	17	7	66	621
EACH SERVING	3	3	1	11	103

PICKLED CUCUMBER SALAD

Most of the calories are in the marinade. If you don't ingest it, don't count these calories as indicated below.

2 cucumbers, peeled and sliced
   thin
1 large onion, sliced thin
2 tablespoons corn oil

¼ cup wine vinegar
2 tablespoons water
1 teaspoon dried dillweed
¼ teaspoon pepper

Combine all ingredients in a bowl. Marinate in the refrigerator for several hours before serving. Can be kept for about 1 week if refrigerated and covered. To serve, lift out of the marinade with a slotted spoon. Discard marinade when cucumbers are consumed. Makes 8 servings.

	PROTEIN (grams)	FAT UNSATURATED (grams)	FAT SATURATED (grams)	CARBOHYDRATES (grams)	CALORIES
TOTAL RECIPE	3	22	2.7	18	316
EACH SERVING	.38	2.7	.34	2.2	39

SPINACH-ORANGE SALAD BOWL

Fresh spinach leaves are brimming with calcium and other nutrients. What better way to eat them than in a bath of high vitamin C dressing?

¼ cup lemon juice
½ cup orange juice
2 tablespoons corn oil
½ teaspoon paprika
1 teaspoon garlic powder
⅛ teaspoon pepper

1 quart torn fresh spinach leaves
1 quart torn lettuce leaves
½ cup sliced radishes
2 oranges, peeled and cut into
  bite-size pieces

In a jar or blender, combine lemon juice, orange juice, corn oil, paprika, garlic powder, and pepper. Cover and refrigerate until ready to use; shake again just before serving. Arrange spinach leaves, lettuce, radishes, and oranges in a salad bowl. Pour dressing over salad and toss lightly. Makes 8 servings.

	PROTEIN (grams)	FAT UNSATURATED (grams)	FAT SATURATED (grams)	CARBOHYDRATES (grams)	CALORIES
TOTAL RECIPE	23	22	3	80	607
EACH SERVING	2.8	2.7	.4	10	76

SPINACH SALAD

Here's a simple salad that will get rave notices every time you serve it. Don't forget the thinly sliced red onion—it gives just the needed tang.

1 pound fresh spinach, trimmed
  and washed
1 clove garlic, halved
1 small red onion, sliced thin
6 large fresh mushrooms, sliced
  thin

¼ cup tomato juice
2 tablespoons olive oil
3 tablespoons wine vinegar
½ teaspoon dry mustard
⅛ teaspoon dried tarragon

Place torn-up pieces of spinach in a salad bowl that has been rubbed well with cut clove of garlic. Discard remaining garlic. Add onion and mushroom slices. Combine tomato juice, olive oil, vinegar, mustard, and tarragon in a cruet bottle; shake well and pour over spinach. Toss well and serve. Makes 8 servings.

	PROTEIN (grams)	FAT UNSATURATED (grams)	FAT SATURATED (grams)	CARBOHYDRATES (grams)	CALORIES
TOTAL RECIPE	20	22	3	41	460
EACH SERVING	2.5	2.75	.38	5	57

YOGURT WALDORF SALAD

Here's a way to keep the calories low and the fat content down while you relax and enjoy a famous apple concoction.

3 apples, pared and diced
2 tablespoons lemon juice
1 cup thinly sliced celery
½ cup coarsely chopped walnuts

½ cup plain low-fat yogurt
½ teaspoon celery seed
½ teaspoon grated lemon rind
Lettuce leaves

Combine apples and lemon juice, tossing well to coat. Add celery and walnuts. Combine yogurt, celery seed, and grated lemon rind; toss with apple mixture. Serve on lettuce leaves. Makes 6 servings.

	PROTEIN (grams)	FAT UNSATURATED (grams)	FAT SATURATED (grams)	CARBOHYDRATES (grams)	CALORIES
TOTAL RECIPE	14.6	30	3.8	47	576
EACH SERVING	2.4	5	.6	7.8	96

YOGURT SPINACH RING MOLD

A good hostess always needs another new gelatin mold to spring on buffet guests. This one will please you so much, and your dieting friends will be grateful. If you like, garnish the serving platter with sliced tomatoes, or fill the ring with cherry tomatoes.

2 envelopes (2 tablespoons) unflavored gelatin
2 cups water
1 tablespoon lemon juice
2 cups chopped raw spinach

1 cup low-fat cottage cheese
½ cup plain low-fat yogurt
½ cup finely diced celery
1 tablespoon grated onion
¼ teaspoon ground nutmeg

Dissolve gelatin in 1 cup water, then bring to a boil. Add 1 cup cold water and lemon juice. Add rest of ingredients. Pour into 6-cup ring mold. Chill until firm. Unmold on large round plate. Serves 8.

	PROTEIN (grams)	FAT UNSATURATED (grams)	FAT SATURATED (grams)	CARBOHYDRATES (grams)	CALORIES
TOTAL RECIPE	38	0	0	14	218
EACH SERVING	5	0	0	2	27

CRANBERRY VEGETABLE ASPIC MOLD

Here's a way to use no-calorie unflavored gelatin to hold some vegetables and fruit juice together. Pretty party fare, or special food for a family occasion.

2 envelopes (2 tablespoons) unflavored gelatin
2 cups cranberry juice
1½ cups apple juice
2 tablespoons lemon juice
½ cup chopped scallions
1 cup cooked peas
1 cup sliced cooked carrots
1 cup sliced celery
Salad greens

In a small saucepan, sprinkle gelatin over ½ cup cranberry juice. Let stand 5 minutes to soften, then heat and stir until gelatin is completely dissolved. Pour into remaining cranberry juice; add apple juice and lemon juice. Mix well. Chill until mixture is the consistency of unbeaten egg whites. Fold in scallions, peas, carrots, and celery. Pour mixture into a 2-quart ring mold. Chill until firm. Unmold on salad greens. Makes 8 servings.

	PROTEIN (grams)	FAT UNSATURATED (grams)	FAT SATURATED (grams)	CARBOHYDRATES (grams)	CALORIES
TOTAL RECIPE	13	0	0	173	728
EACH SERVING	1.6	0	0	21	91

ORANGE SESAME DRESSING

Those who diet can't afford to overlook a low-calorie, great-tasting dressing. Here's one that has an especially fine flavor.

1 cup plain low-fat yogurt
2 teaspoons grated orange peel
2 teaspoons frozen orange juice
   concentrate

2 tablespoons toasted sesame
   seeds

Open container of yogurt. Stir in grated orange peel, juice, and sesame seeds. Use as a dressing for salad. Makes 1 cup.

	PROTEIN (grams)	FAT UNSATURATED (grams)	FAT SATURATED (grams)	CARBOHYDRATES (grams)	CALORIES
TOTAL RECIPE	11	8	3.5	18	229
EACH TBS.	.7	.5	.2	1	14

BLUE CHEESE YOGURT DRESSING

No need for blue cheese to be part of a high-calorie dressing when you can shake it up in yogurt as below. At a mere 14 calories a tablespoon it's a dieter's dream. It would make a great dip too.

1 cup plain low-fat yogurt
¼ cup crumbled blue cheese
1 clove garlic, crushed

½ teaspoon dried crushed
   tarragon

Open container of yogurt. Stir in blue cheese, crushed garlic, and tarragon. Use as a salad dressing. Makes 1¼ cups.

	PROTEIN (grams)	FAT UNSATURATED (grams)	FAT SATURATED (grams)	CARBOHYDRATES (grams)	CALORIES
TOTAL RECIPE	18	6	8	18	280
EACH TBS.	.9	.3	.4	.9	14

FRENCH DRESSING

If you are tired of the high price and high caloric content of the salad dressings you use, make your own and know just what goes into the cruet. If dressing separates, shake well before using.

⅔ cup corn oil

⅓ cup vinegar

¼ teaspoon dry mustard

¼ teaspoon paprika

⅛ teaspoon pepper

Combine all ingredients in a cruet and shake well. Store, covered, in refrigerator until ready to use. Shake well before using. Makes 1 cup dressing.

	PROTEIN (grams)	FAT UNSATURATED (grams)	FAT SATURATED (grams)	CARBOHYDRATES (grams)	CALORIES
TOTAL RECIPE	0	118	14	0	1291
EACH TBS.	0	7	.87	0	80

HERB DRESSING

Measure the amount of dressing you use to keep careful count of the calories on your salad. Be sure to use tarragon vinegar for its spectacular flavor punch.

⅔ cup salad oil

⅓ cup tarragon vinegar

1 clove garlic, minced fine

¼ teaspoon dried oregano

¼ teaspoon dried thyme

⅛ teaspoon pepper

Combine all ingredients in a cruet and shake well. Store, covered, in the refrigerator until ready to use. Shake well before using. Makes 1 cup dressing.

	PROTEIN (grams)	FAT UNSATURATED (grams)	FAT SATURATED (grams)	CARBOHYDRATES (grams)	CALORIES
TOTAL RECIPE	.2	118	15	.9	1295
EACH TBS.	.01	7	1	.05	81

ITALIAN DRESSING

It's hard to explain how a little bit of dry mustard lifts the oil and vinegar dressing into another dimension of flavor. But it does, so don't skip it.

⅔ cup corn oil
¼ cup vinegar
¼ cup water
 1 clove garlic, minced fine

¼ teaspoon cayenne pepper
¼ teaspoon dry mustard
¼ teaspoon dried oregano

Combine all ingredients in a cruet. Shake well. Store in the refrigerator until ready to serve. Shake before serving. Makes about 1¼ cups dressing.

	PROTEIN (grams)	FAT UNSATURATED (grams)	FAT SATURATED (grams)	CARBOHYDRATES (grams)	CALORIES
TOTAL RECIPE	.2	118	15	.9	1295
EACH TBS.	.01	6	.75	.04	65

BLENDER MAYONNAISE

When you make this mayonnaise at home, you may never buy it at the store again. The trick is to drizzle the oil slowly into the egg so the mixture doesn't separate.

 1 egg
½ teaspoon dry mustard
½ teaspoon paprika

1 tablespoon vinegar
1 tablespoon lemon juice
1 cup corn oil

Put the egg, mustard, paprika, vinegar, lemon juice, and ¼ cup of the corn oil into an electric blender or food processor. Cover and process. Remove cover and pour remaining oil in a slow steady stream while blender is on. Turn off blender as soon as all is absorbed. Refrigerate until time to use. Makes 1¼ cups of mayonnaise.

	PROTEIN (grams)	FAT UNSATURATED (grams)	FAT SATURATED (grams)	CARBOHYDRATES (grams)	CALORIES
TOTAL RECIPE	6	179	24	1.7	1680
EACH TBS.	.3	9	1	.08	84

BLENDER RÉMOULADE SAUCE

Here's a quick way to turn your homemade mayonnaise into a remarkable fish sauce. Measure it by the tablespoon serving so your calorie and fat count is controlled.

1 cup Mayonnaise *(see preceding recipe)*
2 tablespoons skim milk
2 tablespoons chopped fresh parsley

1 teaspoon dried tarragon
1 teaspoon dried chervil
½ fresh cucumber, peeled and cut up

Place all ingredients in an electric blender or food processor. Blend together. Makes 1½ cups sauce.

	PROTEIN (grams)	FAT UNSATURATED (grams)	FAT SATURATED (grams)	CARBOHYDRATES (grams)	CALORIES
TOTAL RECIPE	2.8	84	21	6	1369
EACH TBS.	.12	3.5	.88	.25	57

BREAKFASTS

We have declared war on buttered, syrup-dripping pancakes, waffles, and French toast. This chapter has many pancake formulas, some without any wheat for those who are sensitive to gluten, and all taste quite good alone. Where did the idea for unhealthful goppy coverings begin? Let them end with this book, please. If you feel the need for a sauce for pancakes and the like, toss some berries into the electric blender and whirl them into an instant fruit topping. If you want a sweeter taste (do try to wean yourself of sweets) add a spoonful or two of concentrated apple juice or honey.

Learn to read cereal labels with an eye to finding sugar-free products. Make your own minimally sweetened granola. Start the day off with a serving of bran to bulk up the bowels and to fight the colon diseases that are thought to be caused by our overrefined diet. Bake muffins with bran and place them in the freezer to be reheated for breakfast as needed. Get in the habit of cooking old-fashioned oatmeal and other whole-grain cereals. Pop in some raisins for a punch of protein and potassium. Use only skim milk in your cereal and your coffee. To keep your nerves unjangled, drink decaffeinated coffee, herb tea, or weak tea for breakfast and through all the "coffee breaks" of the day.

An excellent choice for breakfast would be fresh fruit and low-fat cottage cheese with a slice of whole-wheat toast. Find a really good-tasting bread, or bake your own. If the quality is great, you won't need to mask your bread with gobs of butter or jelly. You can start to strip sugar and fat out of your food right at the breakfast table.

The Aerobic Nutrition concept includes several servings of eggs a week. But learn how to cook them without a lot of butter or grease. Get a skillet with a premium nonstick surface that won't scratch easily and will permit you to cook without fat. Also, learn how to poach eggs, how to make perfect soft-cooked and hard-cooked eggs, and how to make a great omelet. A large egg contains a mere 75 calories and offers many desirable trace minerals and a perfect offering of protein. If you have been told to restrict your use of egg yolks, don't overlook the possibility of making an omelet with one yolk and many whites, or with the whites alone. Whip the whites a little until bubbles appear and then cook them in a nonstick skillet.

Always cook eggs over low heat so they don't get tough. Remember that eggs separate better when they are cold, but the whites beat higher when they are at room temperature.

Here are a few pointers on cooking eggs—the Aerobic Nutrition way:

TO BOIL EGGS.   Choose a saucepan that won't darken (aluminum always darkens) and that is deep enough so that water will cover the eggs completely but not splash over during cooking. Bring the water to a boil first, and then reduce the heat to a low simmer. Place eggs in the water with a slotted spoon. Cook soft-cooked eggs for 2 to 4 minutes, depending on how solid you prefer them. Cook hard-cooked eggs for 12 to 15 minutes. Rinse immediately under cold water and the shells will slip off with no trouble after you crack the surface in several places.

TO POACH EGGS.   Use a skillet full of boiling water. Add a teaspoon of vinegar to the water and reduce the heat. Stir a circle in the water with a spoon, break an egg into the circle, and push the spreading white back over the yolk with a spoon until it solidifies. Cook for about 4 minutes. Remove egg with a slotted spoon and serve on whole-wheat toast.

TO "FRY" EGGS.   Heat a nonstick-surface skillet. Break each egg carefully into the skillet and cook until done to your liking. Turn over with a spatula if you prefer your egg "once over lightly," or just spoon a bit of white over the yolk and cover the skillet for a moment until a thin film forms. Remove eggs with a spatula.

TO SCRAMBLE EGGS.   Heat a nonstick skillet and pour in beaten eggs. Let egg mixture solidify around the edges and then gently push the cooked egg toward the center to permit the uncooked mixture to flow around the edges and set. Avoid any vigorous stirring or the mixture will crumble into tiny particles. Remove from heat when the mixture is still moist, or it will be overcooked by the time you serve it.

SUPER SHAKE

If you're the kind of person who needs a breakfast drink on the run, here's a fantastic combination for fast nutrition that will last you through the morning. Lecithin granules, torula yeast and brewers' yeast can be found in a health food store.

1 cup orange juice
1 banana
1 apple, peeled and cored, cut up
¼ cup low-fat dry milk
½ cup skim milk

1 tablespoon lecithin granules
1 tablespoon torula yeast or
   brewers' yeast
1 teaspoon honey

Place all ingredients in an electric blender. Blend at high speed until completely combined and frothy. Serve at once. Makes 2 servings.

	PROTEIN (grams)	FAT UNSATURATED (grams)	FAT SATURATED (grams)	CARBOHYDRATES (grams)	CALORIES
TOTAL RECIPE	18	Trace	Trace	102	477
EACH SERVING	9	Trace	Trace	51	239

SLIM SKIMNOG

You can make this the night before and have it ready to pour for the morning in a hurry. Gives you a low-fat punch of protein with a pleasant vanilla flavor.

2 cups low-fat dry milk
3¼ cups skim milk
1 tablespoon frozen apple juice
   concentrate

1 teaspoon vanilla extract
1 egg white

Combine all ingredients in a large bowl; mix with an electric or hand beater until frothy. Refrigerate. Makes 1½ quarts.

	PROTEIN (grams)	FAT UNSATURATED (grams)	FAT SATURATED (grams)	CARBOHYDRATES (grams)	CALORIES
TOTAL RECIPE	118	Trace	Trace	174	1204
EACH SERVING	20	Trace	Trace	29	201

POACHED EGGS ON WHOLE-WHEAT TOAST

This is just about the perfect breakfast to order when traveling. Everything else will be high in fat and swimming in grease. When you make poached eggs at home, garnish the plate with orange slices, melon slices, or berries.

2 cups water	2 eggs
1 teaspoon vinegar	2 slices whole-wheat toast

Bring water to a boil in a large skillet; add vinegar and reduce heat. Stir a circle in the water and break an egg into the circle; push spreading white back over the yolk with a spoon until it solidifies. Repeat for second egg. Cook for about 4 minutes. Remove eggs with a slotted spoon and serve each on a slice of whole-wheat toast. Makes 2 servings.

	PROTEIN (grams)	FAT UNSATURATED (grams)	FAT SATURATED (grams)	CARBOHYDRATES (grams)	CALORIES
TOTAL RECIPE	18	4	7	23	276
EACH SERVING	9	2	3.5	11.5	138

SCRAMBLED COTTAGE CHEESE

If you are eating fewer eggs but want to have a good portion once in a while, try this way of stretching an egg with cottage cheese.

4 eggs	½ cup cottage cheese
⅛ teaspoon pepper	1 tablespoon chopped chives
1 tablespoon corn oil margarine	Dash of paprika

Beat eggs and pepper together. Melt margarine in a skillet; pour in egg mixture. Push cooked egg to the center as uncooked egg flows to the edges to solidify. Stir cottage cheese quickly through the egg mixture the last moment of cooking. Remove from heat. Sprinkle with chives and a colorful dash of paprika. Makes 4 servings.

	PROTEIN (grams)	FAT UNSATURATED (grams)	FAT SATURATED (grams)	CARBOHYDRATES (grams)	CALORIES
TOTAL RECIPE	43	23	8.7	4	534
EACH SERVING	11	6	2	1	133

HERB WHEAT-GERM OMELET

Add some vitamin B to your egg and some yogurt protein too. Combine with herbs to make this a real breakfast treat.

3 eggs, separated
1 cup plain low-fat yogurt
⅓ cup wheat germ
2 tablespoons chopped fresh parsley

½ teaspoon dried rosemary
⅛ teaspoon pepper

Beat egg yolks lightly; add yogurt, wheat germ, parsley, rosemary, and pepper. Beat well. In a separate bowl, beat egg whites until very stiff peaks form; fold into egg yolk mixture. Pour into an ovenproof nonstick skillet. Bake in the oven at 350°F. for 15 to 18 minutes, or until set. Loosen edges of omelet with a spatula, tip pan, and fold omelet in half. Invert onto a warm serving plate. Makes 4 servings.

	PROTEIN (grams)	FAT UNSATURATED (grams)	FAT SATURATED (grams)	CARBOHYDRATES (grams)	CALORIES
TOTAL RECIPE	30	11	6	20	388
EACH SERVING	7	3	1.5	5	97

OATMEAL PANCAKES

If you are sensitive to wheat or just wish another grain for a change, try this oatmeal pancake. Forget the syrup and butter of days behind—this time just see how fine the pancakes taste alone.

1 egg
¾ cup skim milk
1 teaspoon frozen apple juice concentrate

1 cup quick rolled oats
1½ teaspoons baking powder

Beat egg. Add milk and apple juice. Add oats (or if a finer pancake is desired, pour oats into an electric blender to make a fine flour and then add). Add baking powder. If batter is too thick, add a little more milk; if too thin, add a little more oats. Drop by spoonfuls onto a hot nonstick

skillet and cook until lightly browned; turn to brown the other side.
Makes 4 pancakes.

	PROTEIN (grams)	FAT UNSATURATED (grams)	FAT SATURATED (grams)	CARBOHYDRATES (grams)	CALORIES
TOTAL RECIPE	24	7	3	68	477
EACH SERVING	6	2	.75	17	119

BANANA PANCAKES

*Here's a trick with a banana and a pancake mix. If you have fresh blueberries on
hand, just stir some in and drop on the griddle as directed.*

1 cup unbleached flour
2 teaspoons baking powder
1 cup skim milk

1 egg, slightly beaten
1 teaspoon corn oil
1 ripe banana, mashed

Combine flour and baking powder. Add milk. Stir in egg and oil. Then stir in
mashed banana. Pour batter by heaping tablespoonfuls onto a hot nonstick
griddle. When brown on one side, turn and brown the other. Serve at once.
Makes 4 servings.

	PROTEIN (grams)	FAT UNSATURATED (grams)	FAT SATURATED (grams)	CARBOHYDRATES (grams)	CALORIES
TOTAL RECIPE	28	6	2.3	141	792
EACH SERVING	7	1.5	.6	35	198

BLUEBERRY-RICE PANCAKES

*Rice flour has a slightly gritty texture, but is a marvelous treat for those who can't
eat wheat. The rice flour varies with the short- and long-grain varieties, so add a
little more liquid, if needed.*

2 eggs
1 cup skim milk
¾ cup rice flour
1½ teaspoons baking powder

1 teaspoon frozen apple juice
   concentrate
½ cup fresh blueberries, washed
   and dried

Beat eggs and half of the milk together. Combine rice flour and baking powder; add to egg mixture. Stir in remaining milk and apple juice. If batter is too stiff, add a few more tablespoons of milk; if too thin, add a little more rice flour. Add blueberries. Spoon batter onto a hot nonstick skillet. Cook on one side until lightly browned, then flip to brown on other side. Makes 4 pancakes.

	PROTEIN (grams)	FAT UNSATURATED (grams)	FAT SATURATED (grams)	CARBOHYDRATES (grams)	CALORIES
TOTAL RECIPE	32	6	3.7	146	846
EACH SERVING	8	1.5	.93	36	211

CORN MEAL COTTAGE CHEESE PANCAKES

Use a yellow meal if you want color, and be sure to include the vanilla extract. This is a great way to start the day. Blend some fresh berries into a sauce and skip the sweet and sticky stuff.

1 egg
¼ cup skim milk
¼ cup low-fat cottage cheese

½ cup ground corn meal
1 teaspoon vanilla extract

Beat egg lightly with a fork. Add milk and beat together. Stir in cottage cheese. Stir in corn meal and vanilla. If batter is too thin, add a little more corn meal; if too thick, add a little more milk. Mix well. Spoon batter onto a hot nonstick skillet, forming 4-inch diameter pancakes. Brown on one side, then turn and brown other side. Makes 4 pancakes.

	PROTEIN (grams)	FAT UNSATURATED (grams)	FAT SATURATED (grams)	CARBOHYDRATES (grams)	CALORIES
TOTAL RECIPE	23	4.80	2.11	50	364
EACH SERVING	5.75	1.20	.53	12.5	91

YOGURT PANCAKES

See how yogurt joins the pancake act, making light and fluffy treats every time.

1 cup flour
1 tablespoon sugar
1 teaspoon baking powder
½ teaspoon baking soda

1 egg
1 cup skim milk
½ cup plain low-fat yogurt

Combine flour, sugar, baking powder, and baking soda together. Beat egg slightly and add milk; stir into dry ingredients. Stir in yogurt. Pour ¼ cupfuls onto a hot nonstick skillet. When browned, turn over to brown other side. Makes 6 pancakes.

	PROTEIN (grams)	FAT UNSATURATED (grams)	FAT SATURATED (grams)	CARBOHYDRATES (grams)	CALORIES
TOTAL RECIPE	29	0	0	130	719
EACH SERVING	5	0	0	22	120

CINNAMON FRENCH TOAST

Here's a way to stretch one egg to serve four with flair. Vanilla gives just the taste kick that's needed, and cinnamon makes it simply divine.

1 egg
½ cup skim milk
½ teaspoon vanilla extract

4 slices whole-grain bread
Ground cinnamon

Beat egg lightly; add milk and mix through. Add vanilla. Dip bread slices into the batter, one at a time, coating each side well. Place on a hot nonstick griddle or skillet surface; cook until browned on one side, then turn and brown other side. Lift to serving plates and sprinkle lightly with cinnamon. Makes 4 servings.

	PROTEIN (grams)	FAT UNSATURATED (grams)	FAT SATURATED (grams)	CARBOHYDRATES (grams)	CALORIES
TOTAL RECIPE	21	5	2.41	62	398
EACH SERVING	5	1.25	.60	15	100

ORANGE–WHOLE-WHEAT FRENCH TOAST

If you are allergic to milk or just want a change of pace, use orange juice with the egg to make a significant difference.

2 eggs
⅓ cup orange juice
½ teaspoon vanilla extract

4 slices whole-wheat bread
½ cup strawberries, puréed

Beat eggs lightly; add orange juice and vanilla. Dip bread slices into batter, covering both sides well. Cook on one side in a skillet with a premium nonstick surface; turn and brown other side. Serve hot with puréed strawberries as sauce. Makes 4 servings.

	PROTEIN (grams)	FAT UNSATURATED (grams)	FAT SATURATED (grams)	CARBOHYDRATES (grams)	CALORIES
TOTAL RECIPE	24	8	4	60.	450
EACH SERVING	6	2	1	15	125

APRICOT OATMEAL

We're always looking for a new taste or a new trick, and here are both in one. Add finely chopped dried apricots to plain old oatmeal and watch those smiles all around the table.

4 cups water
2 cups quick-cooking oatmeal
½ cup finely chopped dried
  apricots

1 teaspoon ground cinnamon
½ cup wheat germ
  Skim milk

Pour water into a large saucepan; bring to a boil. Gradually stir in oatmeal, apricots, and cinnamon. Simmer, stirring occasionally, until oatmeal is thick. Remove from heat; stir in wheat germ. Spoon into serving bowls; serve hot with skim milk. Makes 6 servings.

	PROTEIN (grams)	FAT UNSATURATED (grams)	FAT SATURATED (grams)	CARBOHYDRATES (grams)	CALORIES
TOTAL RECIPE	58	12	3.4	201	1153
EACH SERVING	10	2	.6	34	192

COOKED WHOLE-GRAIN CEREAL AND RAISINS

Apple juice and raisins are such a wonderful natural sweetening team. No need for sugar. Serve with skim milk if desired.

2 cups whole-grain cereal, such as oatmeal

2 teaspoons frozen apple juice concentrate, thawed

½ cup seedless raisins

Skim milk

Cook whole-grain cereal as directed on package. Spoon into bowls. Stir 1 teaspoon apple juice concentrate into each bowl. Add ¼ cup raisins to each bowl. Makes 6 servings.

	PROTEIN (grams)	FAT UNSATURATED (grams)	FAT SATURATED (grams)	CARBOHYDRATES (grams)	CALORIES
TOTAL RECIPE	23	2.82	.86	160	750
EACH SERVING	4	.47	.14	27	125

FRUIT AND NUT GRANOLA

If you are concerned about the high sugar count of store-bought granola, here's the way to make your own controlled version. Store in a tightly closed jar.

4 cups uncooked old-fashioned oat cereal

½ cup wheat germ

¼ cup sesame seeds

1 tablespoon brown sugar

½ cup unsalted chopped cashew nuts

½ cup unsalted slivered almonds

3 tablespoons corn oil

1 cup raisins

½ cup dried apricots, cut into bits

Combine oats, wheat germ, sesame seeds, brown sugar, cashew nuts, and slivered almonds; toss with corn oil until well coated. Spread mixture in a thin layer on two baking pans. Bake at 350°F. for 30 minutes, stirring the mixture occasionally. Remove from oven; cool and add raisins and apricots. Use as a cereal with skim milk, or as a munching snack. Makes 14 (½ cup) servings.

	PROTEIN (grams)	FAT UNSATURATED (grams)	FAT SATURATED (grams)	CARBOHYDRATES (grams)	CALORIES
TOTAL RECIPE	98	103	18.4	446	3172
EACH SERVING	7	7.3	1.3	31.8	226

PLAIN LOW-FAT YOGURT

Yes, those new electric yogurt makers do work just fine. It's so easy to do, and you'll know that the yogurt you eat is pure and as low in fat as you can make it. Jelly may be added to bottom of glasses before adding yogurt mixture. Flavorings and fruit may be added after yogurt is made.

2 cups nonfat dry milk
5 cups water

¼ cup commercial plain low-fat yogurt

In a saucepan, combine dry milk and water; stir well. Heat to 120°F. (use a candy thermometer or thermometer that is included in an electric yogurt maker). Pour ½ cup of the mixture into ¼ cup commercial plain low-fat yogurt; stir well until smooth. Return this mixture to the warm milk. Heat again to 120°F., only a moment. Pour into individual glass jars of the electric yogurt maker. Cover jars with lids and place in electric yogurt maker. Process according to directions, from 3 to 12 hours depending on the degree of firmness desired. Refrigerate at least 3 hours before using. This yogurt may be used as a starter, as may several subsequent batches before a commercial starter will again have to be used. Makes 6 cups.

	PROTEIN (grams)	FAT UNSATURATED (grams)	FAT SATURATED (grams)	CARBOHYDRATES (grams)	CALORIES
TOTAL RECIPE	88	.37	.57	129	902
EACH SERVING	15	.06	.09	21	150

BREADS AND MUFFINS

Just when dieters were convinced that it was a good idea to skip all bread in their diets, along came the nutritionists and medical doctors to explain that bread is indeed the staff of life. Why? Because it is an easy and satisfactory way to eat grains that represent the complex carbohydrates that are good for you. Preferably they will be the unrefined grains and unrefined flours.

Many people think that the only flour for baking is refined white wheat flour. Others have discovered that unbleached wheat flour, whole-wheat flour, rye flour, oatmeal flour, potato flour, cornstarch, corn meal (both fine and coarse), millet flour, and other grains may be used to bake tasty muffins and breads. Some of these are available in your local supermarket, some in your health food store, and some can be whirled fine in your electric food processor.

When you choose to bake your own breads and muffins, you have total control of the ingredients, use no preservatives or artificial additives, and always have wholesome products to eat. Get in the habit of freezing extras and you will soon have a nice assortment of baked breads and muffins on hand.

This chapter offers a wide assortment of recipes, from the easy-to-bake muffins to the more time-consuming yeast breads. In between are batter breads, a recipe for making your own crackers, and a crêpe that is made with wheat germ.

When baking with yeast, be sure that the yeast is active and fresh. Keep yeast in the refrigerator for best results. Try to use dry yeast before the expiration date stamped on the package.

When mixing the yeast dough, follow directions carefully for the kneading step. Then place the dough in a warm place out of a draft, cover it, and let it rise. It's fun to make yeast bread—it is really easy and the aroma when baking is a sheer delight.

It is not wise to change the basic formula of bread recipes, but do think of adding a handful of raisins, perhaps some crushed herbs, or a bit of grated onion, to get a change of pace and flavor. You will be limited only by your kitchen supplies and your imagination.

OATMEAL MUFFINS

These would make a good breakfast for those mornings when you haven't got a minute to spare. Keep them in the freezer, defrost in the refrigerator the night before, and pop them in the toaster oven at the last minute.

1 cup raw oatmeal	1 cup sifted unbleached flour
½ cup brown sugar	2 teaspoons baking powder
1 cup buttermilk	½ teaspoon baking soda
1 egg, beaten	½ teaspoon salt
¼ cup salad oil	¼ teaspoon ground cinnamon

Preheat oven to 375°F. Combine oatmeal and brown sugar; add buttermilk and stir well. Stir together egg and salad oil; add to oatmeal mixture. Sift together flour, baking powder, baking soda, salt, and cinnamon; stir into oatmeal mixture, just until all ingredients are moistened. Spoon mixture into a greased and floured muffin tin, filling each cup two-thirds full. Bake for 25 minutes, or until lightly browned. Makes 1 dozen.

	PROTEIN (grams)	FAT UNSATURATED (grams)	FAT SATURATED (grams)	CARBOHYDRATES (grams)	CALORIES
TOTAL RECIPE	41	52	8	244	1743
EACH MUFFIN	3	4	.7	20	145

OATMEAL BRAN RAISIN MUFFINS

Here's another fast oatmeal muffin, this time with whole bran and raisins added. What a wonderful way to start or end the day.

1 cup raw oatmeal
2 tablespoons whole-bran cereal
½ cup brown sugar
1 cup buttermilk
1 egg, beaten
¼ cup corn oil

1 cup sifted unbleached flour
2 teaspoons baking powder
½ teaspoon baking soda
¼ teaspoon ground cinnamon
½ cup raisins

Preheat oven to 375°F. Combine oatmeal, bran, and brown sugar; add buttermilk and stir well. Stir together egg and corn oil; add to oatmeal mixture. Sift together flour, baking powder, baking soda, and cinnamon; stir most of it into the oatmeal mixture. Toss the remaining flour mixture with the raisins to coat them well; then add all to the oatmeal mixture. Mix thoroughly. Spoon mixture into a greased and floured muffin tin, filling each cup two-thirds full. Bake for 25 minutes, or until lightly browned. Makes 1 dozen muffins.

	PROTEIN (grams)	FAT UNSATURATED (grams)	FAT SATURATED (grams)	CARBOHYDRATES (grams)	CALORIES
TOTAL RECIPE	41	28	8	288	1888
EACH MUFFIN	3	2.3	.7	24	157

APPLE MUFFINS

If you are cutting calories but want a toothful treat, bake these muffins in tiny tins and get three times as many for your batter.

1 egg
1 cup skim milk
¼ cup corn oil
2 cups unbleached flour
3 tablespoons sugar
1 tablespoon baking powder

½ teaspoon ground cinnamon
⅛ teaspoon ground nutmeg
½ teaspoon salt
1 cup finely chopped peeled apples

In a small bowl, beat egg lightly. Add milk and corn oil; beat until well mixed. In a large bowl, stir together flour, sugar, baking powder, cinnamon, nutmeg, and salt. Add chopped apples, mixing well. Make a well in the center of the flour mixture and add the milk mixture. Stir lightly, just until the flour mixture is moistened. Batter will be lumpy. Spoon into paper-lined muffin pans, filling cups two-thirds full. Bake in a 400°F. oven for 25 to 30 minutes, or until lightly browned. Makes 1 dozen muffins.

	PROTEIN (grams)	FAT UNSATURATED (grams)	FAT SATURATED (grams)	CARBOHYDRATES (grams)	CALORIES
TOTAL RECIPE	44	47	7	291	1925
EACH MUFFIN	4	4	.5	24	160

BLUEBERRY MUFFINS

Why buy the store offerings when you can stir up a muffin in minutes? These are good even if you omit the blueberries.

1 egg
1 cup skim milk
¼ cup corn oil
2 cups unbleached flour
¼ cup sugar

1 tablespoon baking powder
½ teaspoon salt
1 cup fresh or frozen
    unsweetened whole blueberries

In a small bowl, beat egg lightly. Add milk and corn oil; beat until well mixed. In a large bowl, stir together flour, sugar, baking powder, and salt. Add blueberries, coating well to distribute through the mixture. Make a well in the center of the flour mixture and add the milk mixture. Stir lightly, just until the flour mixture is moistened. Batter will be lumpy. Spoon into paper-lined muffin pans, filling cups two-thirds full. Bake in a 400°F. oven for 25 to 30 minutes, or until lightly browned. Makes 1 dozen muffins.

	PROTEIN (grams)	FAT UNSATURATED (grams)	FAT SATURATED (grams)	CARBOHYDRATES (grams)	CALORIES
TOTAL RECIPE	45	47	7	297	1947
EACH MUFFIN	4	4	.6	25	162

DATE AND NUT MUFFINS

Here's a very low-sugar product that can double as a dessert. Make them tinier or cut in half if you are counting calories for weight loss.

8-ounce package pitted dates,
  chopped
¾ teaspoon baking soda
¾ cup boiling water
1 egg

¼ cup corn oil
1½ cups unbleached flour
⅓ cup sugar
¼ cup chopped nuts
½ teaspoon vanilla extract

Combine dates and baking soda in a large bowl. Add boiling water, stir and set aside. Beat together the egg and corn oil; gradually stir it into the date mixture. Combine flour, sugar, and nuts; add to batter. Add vanilla and stir just until dry ingredients are moistened. Pour into paper-lined muffin pans, filling cups two-thirds full. Bake in a 375°F. oven for 25 minutes, or until golden brown. Makes 1 dozen muffins.

	PROTEIN (grams)	FAT UNSATURATED (grams)	FAT SATURATED (grams)	CARBOHYDRATES (grams)	CALORIES
TOTAL RECIPE	37	62	9	393	2383
EACH MUFFIN	3	5	.7	33	198

BUTTERMILK BRAN BREAD

Want to bake a bread without the bother of proofing yeast? Here's a quick and nutritious bran bread that is sweetened with apple juice concentrate—it gives you four times the sweetening power of its reconstituted counterpart.

1⅔ cups crushed whole-bran
  cereal
4⅓ cups sifted unbleached flour
1 tablespoon baking soda

1 teaspoon salt
2½ cups buttermilk
2 teaspoons frozen apple juice
  concentrate, thawed

Preheat oven to 350°F. Mix together bran, flour, baking soda, and salt. Make a well in the center and pour in buttermilk and apple juice concentrate. Work quickly and knead dough lightly. Shape dough into a loaf and press into a greased 9-by-5-inch loaf pan. Bake 1 hour, or until firm and lightly browned. Makes 1 loaf, 16 slices.

	PROTEIN (grams)	FAT UNSATURATED (grams)	FAT SATURATED (grams)	CARBOHYDRATES (grams)	CALORIES
TOTAL RECIPE	98	3	1	566	2652
EACH SERVING	6	.2	.06	35	166

PUMPKIN MUFFINS

If you can stew your own pumpkin at home in season, go to it. Otherwise, the canned variety is the only way to get good cheap pumpkin for baking breads and muffins. The flavor is stunning.

1½ cups sifted unbleached flour
2½ teaspoons baking powder
1 teaspoon salt
1 teaspoon ground cinnamon
½ teaspoon ground nutmeg
1¼ cups whole-bran cereal

⅔ cup skim milk
¾ cup seedless raisins
1 cup canned pumpkin
½ cup soft brown sugar
1 egg
⅓ cup corn oil

Preheat oven to 400°F. Sift together flour, baking powder, salt, cinnamon, and nutmeg; set aside. Combine bran cereal, milk, raisins, pumpkin, and brown sugar in a mixing bowl. Let stand 2 minutes to soften bran. Add egg and oil; beat well. Add sifted ingredients, stirring only until all ingredients are moistened. Fill greased muffin-pan cups three-fourths full. Bake 35 minutes, or until muffins are golden brown. Serve hot. Makes 1 dozen.

	PROTEIN (grams)	FAT UNSATURATED (grams)	FAT SATURATED (grams)	CARBOHYDRATES (grams)	CALORIES
TOTAL RECIPE	49	66	13	409	2481
EACH MUFFIN	4	5.5	1	34	206

RAISIN RICE MUFFINS

For those who can't eat wheat, and those who'd like to try rice flour. It doesn't have the wonderful gluten quality that produces a fine texture, but it does taste mighty good.

1½ cups rice flour
⅔ cup hot water
2 tablespoons butter
¼ cup sugar
3 tablespoons baking powder

¼ teaspoon salt
1 teaspoon vanilla extract
1 teaspoon grated lemon rind
½ cup seedless raisins

Preheat oven to 375°F. Combine half the rice flour with hot water; set aside. Beat together butter and sugar until light and fluffy. Add flour mixture and beat well. Stir together the remaining rice flour, sugar, baking powder, and salt. Add dry mixture to batter. Add vanilla and grated lemon rind. Stir in raisins.

Spoon into 8 cups of a greased muffin tin and bake 20 minutes, or until lightly browned. Makes 8 muffins.

	PROTEIN (grams)	FAT UNSATURATED (grams)	FAT SATURATED (grams)	CARBOHYDRATES (grams)	CALORIES
TOTAL RECIPE	21	12	3	352	1646
EACH MUFFIN	2.7	1.5	.37	44	206

PEANUT BUTTER CARROT BREAD

There's a tablespoon of sugar in every slice, so serve this on a day when you've otherwise been sugar-free.

1 cup packed brown sugar
½ cup chunk-style peanut butter
½ cup corn oil
2 eggs
2 cups shredded scraped carrots
1¾ cups unbleached flour
1 teaspoon baking powder

1 teaspoon baking soda
½ teaspoon ground cinnamon
¼ teaspoon ground allspice
¼ teaspoon ground nutmeg
½ cup skim milk
1 teaspoon vanilla extract

Mix brown sugar, peanut butter, corn oil, and eggs in a large bowl until creamy. Stir in carrots. In another bowl, stir together flour, baking powder, baking soda, cinnamon, allspice, and nutmeg. In yet another bowl, combine milk and vanilla. Then alternately stir the dry ingredients and the milk mixture into the carrot mixture. Turn into a greased 9-by-5-by-3-inch loaf pan. Bake in a preheated 350°F. oven for 70 minutes, or until a wooden toothpick inserted in the center of loaf comes out clean. Cool in the pan 10 minutes; then remove from pan and cool completely on a wire rack. Cut into thin slices to serve. Makes 16 servings.

	PROTEIN (grams)	FAT UNSATURATED (grams)	FAT SATURATED (grams)	CARBOHYDRATES (grams)	CALORIES
TOTAL RECIPE	46	94	14	358	2710
EACH SERVING	3	6	.8	22	169

IRISH SODA BREAD

This is such an easy and fast bread to make, it's a wonder the whole world doesn't know how to do it by now.

2 cups unbleached flour	½ teaspoon salt
1½ teaspoons baking powder	1 tablespoon sugar
¼ teaspoon baking soda	1 cup buttermilk

Sift flour, baking powder, baking soda, salt, and sugar together; mix well. Add buttermilk, stirring to make a soft dough. Knead dough on a lightly floured board for a minute. Then shape dough into a round loaf and put it into an 8-inch greased round pan. Pat flour lightly over the top surface, then cut crosswise into the top. Bake in a preheated 350°F. oven for 40 minutes, or until lightly browned. Bread should have a hollow sound when you tap it. Makes 8 servings.

	PROTEIN (grams)	FAT UNSATURATED (grams)	FAT SATURATED (grams)	CARBOHYDRATES (grams)	CALORIES
TOTAL RECIPE	37	0	0	234	1139
EACH SERVING	4	0	0	29	142

MOLASSES BROWN BREAD

Save those heavy tin-lined cans for baking brown bread. Be sure to brush them well with oil, or you'll have quite a time sliding the goodies out.

1 cup whole-bran cereal	1 egg
½ cup seedless raisins	1 cup sifted unbleached flour
2 tablespoons butter	1 teaspoon baking soda
⅓ cup molasses	½ teaspoon salt
¾ cup boiling water	½ teaspoon ground cinnamon

Preheat oven to 350°F. Combine bran cereal, raisins, butter, and molasses. Add boiling water, stirring until butter is melted. Add egg and beat well. Sift together flour, baking soda, salt, and cinnamon; add to bran mixture, stirring only until all ingredients are moistened. Pour batter into 2 well-greased cans, 4¼ inches deep and 3 inches in diameter, or a well-greased 9-by-5-inch loaf pan. Bake 35 to 45 minutes, or until browned. Remove from baking cans or pan and slice. Serve hot. Makes 2 round small loaves, or 1 large loaf, 16 slices.

	PROTEIN (grams)	FAT UNSATURATED (grams)	FAT SATURATED (grams)	CARBOHYDRATES (grams)	CALORIES
TOTAL RECIPE	30	17	5	276	1343
EACH SERVING	1.8	1	.31	17	84

YOGURT CORN BREAD

This bread will complement a poultry or fish dish with grace. Stirs up easy and bakes just fine.

1 cup flour
1 cup yellow corn meal
2 tablespoons sugar
2 teaspoons baking powder
½ teaspoon baking soda
½ teaspoon salt

1 egg
⅓ cup skim milk
2 tablespoons corn oil
2 tablespoons chopped pimiento
1 teaspoon minced onion flakes
1 cup plain low-fat yogurt

Combine flour, corn meal, sugar, baking powder, baking soda, and salt in a large bowl. In a small bowl, beat together egg and milk; add corn oil, pimiento, and onion. Add to the dry ingredients along with the yogurt; stir just until blended. Turn into a buttered 8-inch-square baking pan. Bake in a preheated 400°F. oven for 20 to 25 minutes. Cut into squares; serve warm. Makes 9 servings.

	PROTEIN (grams)	FAT UNSATURATED (grams)	FAT SATURATED (grams)	CARBOHYDRATES (grams)	CALORIES
TOTAL RECIPE	33	27	5	226	1390
EACH SERVING	4	3	.5	25	154

RHUBARB WALNUT BREAD

This recipe is for adventurous cooks, when rhubarb is in season. It freezes well, so plan to double everything and make some for another season too.

3 eggs	1 cup whole-wheat flour
1 cup salad oil	1 teaspoon baking powder
1¾ cups brown sugar	2 teaspoons baking soda
2 teaspoons vanilla extract	2 teaspoons ground cinnamon
2½ cups finely diced rhubarb	½ teaspoon salt
½ cup chopped walnuts	½ teaspoon ground nutmeg
2 cups unbleached flour	½ teaspoon ground allspice

Combine eggs, oil, sugar, and vanilla in a large mixing bowl; beat until thick and foamy. Using a spoon, stir in rhubarb and walnuts. In a separate bowl, combine two kinds of flour, baking powder, baking soda, cinnamon, salt, nutmeg, and allspice. Add to the rhubarb mixture and stir gently just until blended. Divide the batter equally between two greased 9-by-5-inch loaf pans. Bake at 350°F. for 1 hour, or until an inserted wooden pick comes out clean. Cool in pans 10 minutes, then turn out on a wire rack to cool thoroughly. Makes 2 loaves, 16 slices each.

	PROTEIN (grams)	FAT UNSATURATED (grams)	FAT SATURATED (grams)	CARBOHYDRATES (grams)	CALORIES
TOTAL RECIPE	75	217	30	562	4963
EACH SERVING	2	7	1	18	155

WHOLE-WHEAT BRAIDED HERB BREAD

Braiding yeast dough is fun. Just when you think you have the dough where you want it, the yeast action seems to make it move right out of your hands. Hang on and braid it all into shape.

1 cup wheat germ
2 envelopes (½ ounce) active
dry yeast
2–2½ cups all-purpose flour
2 tablespoons sugar
¾ teaspoon salt
½ teaspoon dried oregano
½ teaspoon dried marjoram

½ cup skim milk
½ cup water
¼ cup softened margarine
2 eggs
½ cup whole-wheat flour
Egg wash (1 egg beaten
with 1 tablespoon water)

Combine wheat germ, undissolved yeast, 1 cup all-purpose flour, sugar, salt, and herbs. Warm milk, water, and margarine to 120° to 130°F. Combine with wheat germ mixture. Add eggs. Beat at low speed 2 minutes. Mix in whole-wheat flour and enough of remaining all-purpose flour to form dough. Turn onto floured surface. Knead 1 minute. Place in greased bowl, turning dough to coat. Cover. Let rise in warm draft-free place about 1½ hours or until doubled. Cut off a quarter of the dough. Divide into 3 equal parts and shape each into 10-inch rope. Braid ropes. Form remaining dough into oblong and place in greased 8½-by-4½-by-2½-inch loaf pan. Top with braid. Brush with egg wash. Sprinkle with additional wheat germ as desired. Cover. Let rise in warm place about 45 minutes or until doubled. Bake in 375°F. oven 30 minutes or until golden brown. Cover with foil last 10 minutes if crust browns too quickly. Makes 1 loaf, 16 slices.

	PROTEIN (grams)	FAT UNSATURATED (grams)	FAT SATURATED (grams)	CARBOHYDRATES (grams)	CALORIES
TOTAL RECIPE	95	51	13	336	2260
EACH SERVING	6	3	.8	21	141

WHOLE-WHEAT BUNS

What a wonderful way to get whole-wheat nutritious bread. Freeze the extra buns for another time.

2 envelopes (½ ounce) active
dry yeast
3 tablespoons sugar
1 teaspoon salt
3½ cups all-purpose flour
¼ cup softened margarine

2 cups skim milk
3 eggs
1 cup wheat germ
2–2½ cups stone-ground
whole-wheat flour
Vegetable oil

Combine yeast, sugar, salt, and 2 cups all-purpose flour in large mixer bowl. Add margarine. Heat milk until warm to the touch (not scalding). Add to flour mixture and beat with electric mixer at medium speed 2 minutes, scraping bowl occasionally. Add remaining 1½ cups all-purpose flour and 2 eggs. Beat at high speed 1 minute or until thick and elastic. Stir in wheat germ. Gradually add just enough whole-wheat flour, about 2 cups, to make a soft dough which leaves sides of bowl. Turn onto floured surface. Knead 5 to 8 minutes or until dough is smooth and elastic. Cover with plastic wrap, then a towel. Let rest 20 minutes. Punch down. Divide dough in half. Shape each half into 10 equal portions. Form into smooth balls. Place 10 balls into each of two greased 9-inch round pans. Brush lightly with oil. Cover loosely with plastic wrap. Refrigerate overnight. When ready to bake, remove from refrigerator, uncover, and let stand 30 minutes. Brush with remaining egg, beaten. Sprinkle with additional wheat germ. Bake in 400°F. oven 25 to 30 minutes or until done. Remove from pans. Makes 20 buns.

	PROTEIN (grams)	FAT UNSATURATED (grams)	FAT SATURATED (grams)	CARBOHYDRATES (grams)	CALORIES
TOTAL RECIPE	154	49	13	651	3826
EACH SERVING	8	2	.6	32	191

EGG-FREE BANANA BREAD

There are those who cannot eat eggs at all due to an allergy. For them, and for anyone else who is eating eggs sparingly, try serving this delicious egg-free bread.

2 cups whole-wheat flour
1 cup yellow corn meal
¾ teaspoon salt
1 teaspoon baking soda

1 cup mashed bananas
1 cup buttermilk
¾ cup unsulfured molasses
¾ cup raisins

In a large bowl, mix together flour, corn meal, salt, and baking soda. Stir in mashed bananas, buttermilk, molasses, and raisins. Turn into 3 greased and floured 1-pound cans (from canned fruit or vegetables). Bake in a preheated

350°F. oven for 45 minutes. Cool 10 minutes, turn out of cans, and serve warm. Loaves may be frozen. Thaw, wrap in foil, and reheat in a 350°F. oven for about 20 minutes. Makes 3 loaves, 8 slices each.

	PROTEIN (grams)	FAT UNSATURATED (grams)	FAT SATURATED (grams)	CARBOHYDRATES (grams)	CALORIES
TOTAL RECIPE	56	8	.5	547	2372
EACH SERVING	2.3	.33	.02	23	99

EGG-FREE WHOLE-WHEAT BREAD

Making a yeast bread is easy, especially if you have a dough hook on an electric mixing machine. Otherwise, get the heels of your hands into good action of kneading until dough is smooth and elastic.

1 envelope (¼ ounce) active
  dry yeast
2¼ cups warm water
1 teaspoon sugar
3½ cups wheat flour

3 tablespoons soft margarine,
  melted
2 tablespoons molasses
1½ teaspoons salt
2 cups whole-wheat flour

Dissolve yeast in water; add sugar and 2½ cups wheat flour. Mix well and let rise until bubbly, about 20 minutes. Add margarine, molasses, salt, and 2 cups whole-wheat flour; beat well. Knead in just enough of the remaining 1 cup wheat flour to make a soft dough. Knead dough until it is smooth and elastic. Let rise in a lightly greased bowl until dough doubles. Punch down; divide in two and roll out each piece to fit into two lightly greased 8½-by-4½-inch loaf pans. Allow to rise again. Bake in a 375°F. oven for 40 minutes, or until bread sounds hollow when tapped. Turn breads out to cool on a wire rack. Makes 2 loaves, 16 slices each.

	PROTEIN (grams)	FAT UNSATURATED (grams)	FAT SATURATED (grams)	CARBOHYDRATES (grams)	CALORIES
TOTAL RECIPE	85	23	4	568	2885
EACH SERVING	2.6	.72	.12	18	90

WHEAT-GERM CRÊPES

The nice thing about crêpes is that you can make them at your leisure, freeze them in stacks, and then use them at will. This recipe adds wheat germ for extra nutrition. Crêpes may be filled with stewed fruit, then lightly dusted with confectioners' sugar. Or fill with cooked chicken, fish, or vegetables, and dust with chopped fresh parsley.

2 eggs	3 tablespoons wheat germ
⅔ cup skim milk	1 tablespoon corn oil
⅓ cup unbleached flour	

Combine all ingredients in an electric blender. Blend until smooth. Pour about ¼ cup of the mixture into a hot nonstick skillet; quickly tilt skillet to coat bottom and then cook over medium heat until top is dry, about 30 seconds. Turn and cook other side until lightly browned. Repeat until all the batter is used. Stack crêpes between layers of wax paper until ready to fill. Makes about 8 crêpes.

	PROTEIN (grams)	FAT UNSATURATED (grams)	FAT SATURATED (grams)	CARBOHYDRATES (grams)	CALORIES
TOTAL RECIPE	29	18	5	53	576
EACH CRÊPE	3.6	2	.6	6.6	72

CRISSCROSS WHEAT-GERM CRACKERS

This recipe is included so you can have fun making your own mighty tasty crackers. Store in a tightly closed canister to keep crisp.

1½ cups grated Parmesan cheese	1¼ cups unbleached flour
¾ cup soft shortening	¾ cup wheat germ
1 tablespoon water	½ teaspoon baking powder
2 drops red pepper liquid seasoning	

Beat cheese, shortening, water, and red pepper liquid together, using an electric mixer or food processor. Cut in flour, wheat germ, and baking powder, until mixture forms a dough. Divide dough and shape into 36 small balls. Place on an ungreased baking sheet. Flatten to ¼-inch thickness, pressing with the bottom of a glass. Press with the tines of a fork to make a crisscross design. Bake in a 350°F. oven about 10 minutes, or until lightly browned. Remove from baking sheet and cool on a rack. Makes 3 dozen.

	PROTEIN (grams)	FAT UNSATURATED (grams)	FAT SATURATED (grams)	CARBOHYDRATES (grams)	CALORIES
TOTAL RECIPE	94	128	60	171	2818
EACH SERVING	2.6	3.5	1.6	5	78

DESSERTS

The dessert course is the downfall of most American diets. Generally high in fat and sugar content, made of refined white grains, desserts are astronomically high in calories. Aerobic Nutrition concepts aim at a change to healthier dessert choices.

Picture an archer's target as representing your aims for conforming to a lower-fat, lower-sugar dessert intake. Place fresh fruit right on the bull's eye. In the next two circles, place cooked fruit and frozen fruits that are sugar-free, then desserts made with unrefined grains, small amounts of sugar, and unsaturated fat; in the last circle baked goods that have natural ingredients, refined grains, unsaturated fat, and limited amounts of sugar, to be used for special occasions. Off target completely are all high-fat, high-sugar bakery concoctions, with sweet toppings and enough calories to support a normal person for an entire day. If you can't pass them up completely because of pressure from peers or family, then take a congenial taste and spread the rest of the portion around your plate or dump it in the garbage when no one's looking. It's just not worth sending your triglycerides into a jam-up over nonnutritious party food.

You'll find a gamut of recipes in this chapter to help you to prepare sensible desserts. But the most recommended dessert is a bowl of fresh fruit on the table or a simple dish of berries in season.

The nutritional data at the end of each recipe will help you to restrict portions and yet to enjoy some baked cookies and cakes as desired.

Pay particular attention to the innovative Frozen Fruit Frappé made from frozen bananas or berries; prepared just before serving, it looks like sherbet, and without a drop of added sugar manages to taste quite rich.

All of these dessert recipes are on target. It's up to you to pace them throughout your menus, selecting a cake dessert for a day when you have an otherwise low intake of fat and sugar, so that your total intake will fall within the Aerobic Nutrition guidelines.

ABOUT FRUIT

APPLES.   Select firm, well-colored fruit; avoid those that lack good color, those that are bruised or decayed, and those that have a shriveled appearance. Over-ripe apples yield to slight pressure on the skin, and will have soft, mealy flesh. Store unripe or hard apples at cool room temperature (69° to 70°F.) until ready to eat. Store mellow apples, uncovered, in the refrigerator, and use within a week.

APRICOTS.   Select plump, uniform-colored golden-orange, juicy-looking fruit; avoid those that are bruised or decayed, dull-looking, pale yellow or greenish yellow in appearance. Store ripe fruit, uncovered, in the refrigerator. Use within three to five days.

AVOCADOS.   Select slightly soft fruit that yields to gentle pressure on the skin; avoid those with dark sunken spots, or those with cracked or broken surfaces. When unripe, allow to ripen at room temperature, not in direct sunlight. Store ripe fruit, uncovered, in the refrigerator, and use within three to five days.

BANANAS.   Select yellow, firm fruit; avoid those with decay marks. Bananas with green tips have not developed their fullest flavor; those with brown flecks have. Store at room temperature.

BLUEBERRIES.   Select plump, firm, uniform-size berries; avoid those that are soft, bruised, or discolored. Keep in the refrigerator for use within one to two days. Wash just before using.

CHERRIES.   Select well-colored fruit with bright, glossy, plump-looking surfaces; avoid those with shriveled appearance, dried stems, and soft, leaking flesh with brown discolorations. Wash just before using. Use within one or two days.

CRANBERRIES.   Select plump, firm berries, with good red color; avoid soft, spongy, or leaky berries that may be of poor flavor. Store in refrigerator for one or two days, and wash just before using.

GRAPEFRUIT.   Select firm, well-shaped fruit that seems heavy for its size; avoid those with soft discolored areas on the peel near the stem end, and peel that breaks easily under finger pressure—they are signs of internal decay. Grapefruit is picked "tree-ripe," so store in the refrigerator and use within five to seven days.

GRAPES.   Select well-colored, plump grapes that are firmly attached to the stem, which itself should be green and pliable. Avoid soft or wrinkled grapes with whitened areas around the stem end, and leaking grapes, which are a sign of decay. Refrigerate and use within one or two days.

LEMONS.   Select those that have a rich yellow color, a smooth-textured skin, and feel firm and heavy for their size. Avoid lemons that are off-color, dull in appearance, and those with hard or shriveling skin or soft spots. Refrigerate and use within one week.

LIMES.   Select limes with glossy skin; they should feel firm and heavy for their size. Avoid those with dull, dry skin, and those with soft spots, mold, and skin breaks. Store in the refrigerator and use within one week.

MELONS.   For *cantaloupes* (muskmelons), select those with well-defined netting marks and a background color that is yellowish. The melon should yield slightly to thumb pressure on the blossom end; avoid overripeness that is indicated by a soft rind, and avoid those that are bruised or have mold near the stem scar. Full maturity is indicated by a pleasant melon odor noticeable when fruit is held to the nose.

For *casaba* melons; select those with a golden-yellow rind and a slight softening at the blossom end; avoid those with dark, sunken, or water-soaked spots, as this indicates internal decay.

For *honey ball* and *honeydew,* select melons of yellowish white to creamy rind color, with slight softening at the blossom end, and a pleasant aroma. Avoid those with dead-white or greenish white color, smooth rather than velvety feel, and bruised or punctured appearance.

For *Persian* melons, follow selection procedure used with cantaloupes.

For *watermelons,* look for smooth surface with a slight dullness of color and a cream-colored underbelly. If cut, select those with good red color, firm flesh, free from white streaks, and with seeds that are dark brown or black. Avoid pale-colored flesh, whitish seeds (which indicate immaturity), and mealy or watery flesh.

All melons should be kept at room temperature until ripened and should be refrigerated until used. Use within one or two days.

NECTARINES.   Select plump, rich-colored fruit with a slight softening along the seam; avoid hard, dull-colored fruit, shriveled and soft fruit, or overripe fruit with signs of decay. Store at room temperature until ripe, then store in the refrigerator until ready to use. Use within three to five days.

ORANGES.   Select firm fruit with fresh and bright-looking skin. Avoid those that are lightweight for their size, have dull, dry skin, or pitted skin and discolored appearance. Refrigerate and use within five to seven days.

PEARS.   Select those that have begun to soften but have a firm appearance. Avoid wilted fruit with dull-looking skin and weakness of skin near the stem. Ripen at room temperature and refrigerate until wanted. Use within three to five days.

PINEAPPLES.   Select fruit that is heavy for its size, those of good color for the variety, and those whose leaves can easily be pulled out. Avoid those with dried appearance, bruises or discolorations, an unpleasant odor, or traces of mold. Pineapples will ripen at room temperature, and should then be refrigerated until wanted. Use within one to two days.

PLUMS AND PRUNES.   Select fruit of a good color for the variety, and those that feel slightly soft to the touch. Avoid fruit with discolorations or breaks in the skin, and those that are leaking or decaying. Store in refrigerator until wanted. Use within three to five days.

STRAWBERRIES.   Select those with full, red color and firm flesh, with stem intact and a dry, clean appearance. Avoid berries that are soft, bruised, or discolored. Keep whole in the refrigerator until ready to use. Wash just before using. Use within one to two days.

TANGERINES.   Select those of deep orange color and good luster. Avoid those that are off-color or greenish, and those with any signs of decay. Refrigerate until wanted, and use within five to seven days.

FRESH STRAWBERRY DELIGHT

This is the kind of dessert we wish you would eat. It's low-calorie and very delicious.

1 pint fresh strawberries, hulled
½ cup plain low-fat yogurt

½ teaspoon vanilla extract
1 tablespoon slivered almonds

Wash strawberries and drain well. Spoon berries into 4 stemmed wineglasses. Combine yogurt and vanilla; mix only until well blended. Spoon over berries. Sprinkle with slivered almonds. Makes 4 servings.

	PROTEIN (grams)	FAT UNSATURATED (grams)	FAT SATURATED (grams)	CARBOHYDRATES (grams)	CALORIES
TOTAL RECIPE	3.5	4	.35	26	158
EACH SERVING	.87	1	.09	6.5	40

FRUIT DELIGHT

Substitute whatever fruit you wish for those listed below. The yogurt topping makes it taste very special.

1 banana, sliced
½ cantaloupe, cut into 1-inch chunks
1 kiwi fruit, peeled and sliced thin

1 cup plain low-fat yogurt
¼ teaspoon ground nutmeg
1 teaspoon grated orange rind
½ teaspoon vanilla extract

Combine fruit and spoon into 6 stemmed wineglasses. Combine yogurt, nutmeg, orange rind, and vanilla extract; spoon over fruit. Top with a dash of nutmeg. Makes 6 servings.

	PROTEIN (grams)	FAT UNSATURATED (grams)	FAT SATURATED (grams)	CARBOHYDRATES (grams)	CALORIES
TOTAL RECIPE	3	0	0	47	185
EACH SERVING	.5	0	0	8	31

HIGH-POTASSIUM FRUIT SALAD

This is the perfect fruit salad to serve the carbohydrate-loading athlete the day before the marathon. For all others, it's a high vitamin C treat too.

1 orange, cut into segments
1 grapefruit, cut into segments
½ cantaloupe, cut into chunks or balls

1 cup strawberries, cut in half
1 cup pineapple juice

Combine fruits in a large bowl. Pour pineapple juice over fruits and toss lightly to coat well. Chill until ready to serve. Makes about 6 servings, containing 440 mg potassium each.

	PROTEIN (grams)	FAT UNSATURATED (grams)	FAT SATURATED (grams)	CARBOHYDRATES (grams)	CALORIES
TOTAL RECIPE	6	0	0	103	418
EACH SERVING	1	0	0	17	70

MELON SALAD BOWL

When you are concerned about potassium intake, here's a high and mighty way to fulfill the need. All ingredients have a natural high potassium count in this super melon salad.

½ cantaloupe
1 banana
½ cup pitted dates

4 large pitted prunes
¼ cup pineapple juice

Remove seeds of melon and scoop out fruit into balls; place in a bowl. Add sliced banana, dates, and prunes. Toss with pineapple juice. Fill dessert dishes with this mixture and serve. Makes 4 servings.

	PROTEIN (grams)	FAT UNSATURATED (grams)	FAT SATURATED (grams)	CARBOHYDRATES (grams)	CALORIES
TOTAL RECIPE	7	0	0	169	647
EACH SERVING	1.8	0	0	42	162

BAKED AMBROSIA

What a lovely little taste treat! If you get really ambitious, cut a slit into the top of each orange half almost to the middle, then pull up each side and tie into a basket handle.

3 oranges
¼ cup pitted dates
2 tablespoons coconut

½ cup chopped walnuts
½ cup plain low-fat yogurt
½ teaspoon vanilla extract

Cut oranges in half and scoop out the fruit, leaving the half-shells intact. Chop dates and mix with cut-up orange segments. Add coconut and chopped walnuts. Spoon into the orange shells and place in a baking dish. Bake for 25 minutes in a 350°F. oven. Remove from oven. Stir yogurt and vanilla together; spoon mixture on top of each baked orange. Sprinkle with additional grated coconut. Serve at once. Makes 6 servings.

	PROTEIN (grams)	FAT UNSATURATED (grams)	FAT SATURATED (grams)	CARBOHYDRATES (grams)	CALORIES
TOTAL RECIPE	18	0	0	90	741
EACH SERVING	3	0	0	15	123

BAKED APPLES

*Make these in the microwave oven in just a few minutes if you are in a hurry. No
need for sugar when the apples are filled with natural sweet stuff.*

6 large baking apples	½ teaspoon ground cinnamon
⅓ cup golden raisins	⅛ teaspoon ground nutmeg
⅓ cup frozen apple juice concentrate	1 cup boiling water

Wash and core apples. Place in a flat baking dish. Combine raisins, apple juice
concentrate, cinnamon, and nutmeg in a bowl; mix well. Stuff cores of apples
with raisin mixture. Pour boiling water around apples. Bake, uncovered, in
a 350°F. oven for 35 minutes, or until tender. Baste apples occasionally with
pan liquid. Makes 6 servings.

	PROTEIN (grams)	FAT UNSATURATED (grams)	FAT SATURATED (grams)	CARBOHYDRATES (grams)	CALORIES
TOTAL RECIPE	4	0	0	260	1031
EACH SERVING	.6	0	0	43	172

BAKED RHUBARB

*If you have a rhubarb patch in the garden, or if you just plain love rhubarb, here's
a way to bake it up tasty and terrific.*

3 cups fresh rhubarb, cut into ½-inch chunks	¼ cup grated orange rind
1½ cups unflavored bread crumbs	¼ cup frozen apple juice concentrate

Trim rhubarb and peel only if stalks are old. Sprinkle ½ cup bread crumbs
on a well-buttered 1-quart baking dish. Cover with a layer of rhubarb. Sprinkle
with 2 tablespoons grated orange rind and 2 tablespoons apple juice. Top

with another layer of bread crumbs. Cover with remaining rhubarb. Sprinkle with remaining orange rind and apple juice. Top with a layer of bread crumbs. Cover loosely with foil. Bake in a 350°F. oven for 45 minutes. Remove cover to brown during the last 10 minutes of baking. Makes 6 servings.

	PROTEIN (grams)	FAT UNSATURATED (grams)	FAT SATURATED (grams)	CARBOHYDRATES (grams)	CALORIES
TOTAL RECIPE	9	2	.5	83	387
EACH SERVING	1.5	.33	.08	14	64

STEWED FIGS

Figs have a natural high-sugar content, but it's the healthful kind. Add some apricots and other dried fruit if desired.

1 pound dried figs	1 tablespoon lemon juice
1½ cups water	1 tablespoon honey

Soak figs in water for several hours. Then pour into a saucepan and add lemon juice and honey. Cover and simmer over low heat for 30 minutes. Cool and refrigerate until well chilled. Makes 6 servings.

	PROTEIN (grams)	FAT UNSATURATED (grams)	FAT SATURATED (grams)	CARBOHYDRATES (grams)	CALORIES
TOTAL RECIPE	5	0	0	109	428
EACH SERVING	.9	0	0	18	71

APRICOT FLUFF

Here is a dessert to please the sweet tooth and the waistline too.

5-ounce jar strained apricots for babies	1 teaspoon grated lemon rind
1 tablespoon sugar	1 teaspoon unflavored gelatin
1 teaspoon vanilla extract	1 tablespoon cold water
1 teaspoon lemon juice	2 egg whites

Stir together strained apricots, sugar, vanilla, and lemon juice and rind. Soften gelatin in cold water, then dissolve over hot water in a double boiler. Beat egg whites until frothy; add gelatin and beat until very stiff. Fold into apricot mixture and spoon into sherbet glasses. Chill. Makes 4 servings.

	PROTEIN (grams)	FAT UNSATURATED (grams)	FAT SATURATED (grams)	CARBOHYDRATES (grams)	CALORIES
TOTAL RECIPE	8	0	0	41	191
EACH SERVING	2	0	0	10	48

PRUNE FLUFF

This makes good use of baby's strained prunes in a grown-up dessert. It's a wonderful mouthful of fluff that will seem richer than it is. If you wish, garnish with walnut halves.

5-ounce jar strained prunes, no sugar added	1 teaspoon lemon juice
1½ teaspoons frozen apple juice concentrate	1 teaspoon grated lemon rind
	1 teaspoon unflavored gelatin
1 teaspoon vanilla extract	1 tablespoon cold water
	2 egg whites

Blend prunes, apple juice, vanilla, lemon juice, and lemon rind together. Soften gelatin in the cold water, then dissolve over hot water in a double boiler. Beat egg whites until frothy, add gelatin, and beat very stiff. Fold into prune mixture and pile lightly into dessert glasses. Chill. Makes 4 servings.

	PROTEIN (grams)	FAT UNSATURATED (grams)	FAT SATURATED (grams)	CARBOHYDRATES (grams)	CALORIES
TOTAL RECIPE	8	0	0	45	202
EACH SERVING	2	0	0	11	50

FROZEN FRUIT FRAPPÉ

This idea is from Vicky Mannerberg's kitchen to yours. No need to add sugar or anything else. Just freeze the fruit and process it into a sherbetlike consistency.

4 bananas   1 pint fresh strawberries

Place bananas in their skins into the freezer for several hours until frozen through. Rinse strawberries, remove hulls, and freeze in a single layer, using a flat pan that is uncovered, just until berries are solid. Remove bananas and set aside for a few minutes until the skins slip off with ease. Remove berries. Process with a food processor or an electric homogenizer until frozen fruit is puréed together. Mixture will resemble the texture of soft ice cream. Serve at once. Makes 4 servings.

	PROTEIN (grams)	FAT UNSATURATED (grams)	FAT SATURATED (grams)	CARBOHYDRATES (grams)	CALORIES
TOTAL RECIPE	7	0	0	131	514
EACH SERVING	1.8	0	0	33	128

ORANGE-PINEAPPLE SHERBET

This sherbet is so easy to make it's almost sinful to write about. Keeps awhile in the freezer, so you might want to double everything.

6-ounce can frozen
unsweetened orange juice
concentrate
6-ounce can frozen
unsweetened pineapple juice
concentrate

3½ cups cold water
1 cup nonfat dry milk
1 teaspoon vanilla extract

Put all ingredients into a large mixing bowl and beat just enough to blend thoroughly. Pour into ice cube trays. Freeze 1 to 2 hours, until half frozen. Remove to large chilled mixer bowl; beat on low speed until mixture is softened, then beat on high speed 3 to 5 minutes until creamy but not liquid. Pour into freezer containers or ice cube trays. Freeze until ready to serve. Makes about 16 (½ cup) servings.

	PROTEIN (grams)	FAT UNSATURATED (grams)	FAT SATURATED (grams)	CARBOHYDRATES (grams)	CALORIES
TOTAL RECIPE	51	0	0	245	1185
EACH SERVING	3	0	0	15	74

PINEAPPLE WHIP

The calorie count is low and the flavor is very up when you make this gelatin-based sherbet. No need to freeze—the refrigerator does this job just fine.

2 tablespoons unflavored gelatin
3½ cups unsweetened pineapple
juice
1 tablespoon frozen apple juice
concentrate

¼ teaspoon ground nutmeg
2 teaspoons grated lemon rind

In a small mixer bowl, soften gelatin in ½ cup of the pineapple juice. Heat remaining juice and add to gelatin, stirring to dissolve completely. Add apple juice concentrate, nutmeg, and lemon rind. Chill until mixture begins to thicken. Beat on high speed of an electric mixer until fluffy and double in volume. Chill a few minutes until mixture mounds from spoon. Spoon into 6 sherbet glasses. Chill until set. Makes 6 servings.

	PROTEIN (grams)	FAT UNSATURATED (grams)	FAT SATURATED (grams)	CARBOHYDRATES (grams)	CALORIES
TOTAL RECIPE	3.5	0	0	126	510
EACH SERVING	.5	0	0	21	85

BERRY YOGURT EGG CUSTARD

Serve this as a berry topping only on a day when you have not had eggs for breakfast. For an elegant touch, serve in long-stemmed wineglasses.

4 egg yolks
2 tablespoons sugar
¼ cup orange juice

½ cup plain low-fat yogurt
1 pint fresh strawberries or
  blueberries, washed

Place egg yolks in the top of a double boiler; beat at medium speed of hand mixer until thick and lemon-colored. Gradually add sugar, beating until soft peaks form. Place over simmering water; beat in orange juice. Continue cooking and beating until mixture is fluffy. Remove from heat and beat until cool. Fold in yogurt. Divide berries equally among 6 dessert dishes. Spoon sauce over top. Makes 6 servings.

	PROTEIN (grams)	FAT UNSATURATED (grams)	FAT SATURATED (grams)	CARBOHYDRATES (grams)	CALORIES
TOTAL RECIPE	12	3	.9	111	535
EACH SERVING	2	.4	.15	18	89

LEMON-RICE RING

This is for times when you feel compelled to serve a fancy-looking dessert. Fill the ring with fresh berries, if desired.

½ cup rice
½ cup boiling water
2½ cups skim milk
1 envelope (1 tablespoon) unflavored gelatin
¼ cup cold water

4 eggs, separated
2 tablespoons frozen apple juice concentrate
1 tablespoon lemon rind
2 tablespoons lemon juice
1 teaspoon vanilla extract

Combine rice and boiling water in the top of a double boiler; bring to a boil and cook about 2 minutes. Add milk and cook 10 minutes more. Soften gelatin in cold water and set aside. Combine egg yolks, apple juice concentrate, lemon rind, lemon juice, and vanilla. Add some of the hot rice mixture to the egg yolk mixture, then pour the egg yolk mixture back into the rice and cook 5 minutes more, stirring constantly. Remove from heat, stir in softened gelatin, mix thoroughly, then chill slightly. Beat egg whites until stiff; fold into rice mixture. Spoon into a 2-quart lightly oiled ring mold and chill until set. Makes 8 servings.

	PROTEIN (grams)	FAT UNSATURATED (grams)	FAT SATURATED (grams)	CARBOHYDRATES (grams)	CALORIES
TOTAL RECIPE	55	11	7	130	972
EACH SERVING	7	1.4	.9	16	121

MANDARIN RICE MOLD

Here's a low-calorie gelatin mold that looks rich with calories. But it's the kind of sleight-of-hand dessertmaking that makes great sense. Serve cut into wedges with fresh berries or other fruit.

1 envelope (1 tablespoon) unflavored gelatin
4-ounce can water-packed mandarin oranges
1¼ cups skim milk

3-ounce package low-fat cream cheese, softened
2 eggs, separated
1 cup cooked rice
1 teaspoon vanilla extract

Soften gelatin in ¼ cup drained juice of mandarin oranges; set aside. Blend milk and cream cheese together; stir in lightly beaten egg yolks. Add gelatin mixture. Cook over low heat, stirring constantly, until mixture coats the spoon. Add rice and vanilla; cool slightly. Add drained orange segments. Beat egg whites until stiff peaks form; fold into rice mixture. Turn into a 1-quart mold. Chill until firm. Makes 8 servings.

	PROTEIN (grams)	FAT UNSATURATED (grams)	FAT SATURATED (grams)	CARBOHYDRATES (grams)	CALORIES
TOTAL RECIPE	41	6	3.7	54	504
EACH SERVING	5	.7	.4	7	63

SHORTBREAD COOKIES

Not an egg in sight, and still the cookies are pleasantly textured and delicious. Keep covered in a tight container for best results.

2 cups sifted flour
1 cup cornstarch
Dash of salt

1 cup soft shortening
½ cup sugar

Sift flour, cornstarch, and salt together. Beat shortening with sugar until light and fluffy. Add dry ingredients gradually until dough is stiff enough to work with hands. Knead on a lightly floured board until well blended and smooth. Press into an 8-by-12-inch rectangle on a greased baking sheet. Smooth the top with a spatula. Score almost through with a knife, making 1-by-2-inch rectangles. Prick with a fork. Bake in a 325°F. oven for 30 to 40 minutes, or until golden brown. Recut where previously scored. Sprinkle with additional sugar while still hot, if desired. Cool completely. Remove from baking sheet. Store in an airtight container. Makes 4 dozen cookies.

	PROTEIN (grams)	FAT UNSATURATED (grams)	FAT SATURATED (grams)	CARBOHYDRATES (grams)	CALORIES
TOTAL RECIPE	29	144	50	420	3614
EACH COOKIE	.6	3	1	8.7	75

BRAN COCONUT COOKIES

You get a lot of cookies for a little effort. It's not every day that you can munch on bran and coconut together.

2 cups unbleached flour	2 eggs
½ teaspoon baking soda	1 teaspoon vanilla extract
1 cup butter, softened	1 cup whole-bran cereal
1½ cups sugar	½ cup shredded coconut

Preheat oven to 375°F. Sift together flour and baking soda; set aside. Cream butter and sugar until fluffy. Add eggs and vanilla. Stir in bran cereal and coconut. Stir in sifted dry ingredients and mix well. Drop by level tablespoonfuls onto an ungreased baking sheet. Bake for 12 minutes, or until lightly browned. Makes about 5 dozen cookies.

	PROTEIN (grams)	FAT UNSATURATED (grams)	FAT SATURATED (grams)	CARBOHYDRATES (grams)	CALORIES
TOTAL RECIPE	50	153	66	556	4367
EACH COOKIE	.8	2	1	9	73

CRISP PEANUT BUTTER COOKIES

If you have a very tiny ice cream scoop, now's the time to use it. Otherwise, follow directions and roll with lightly floured hands.

1 cup creamy peanut butter	1 teaspoon vanilla extract
1 cup soft shortening	2½ cups sifted flour
½ cup sugar	1 teaspoon baking powder
1 cup brown sugar	1 teaspoon baking soda
2 eggs, beaten	½ teaspoon salt

Stir together peanut butter, shortening, and sugars until blended. Beat in eggs and vanilla. Sift together flour, baking powder, baking soda, and salt; add to sugar mixture and mix well. Chill dough until it can be easily handled. Shape into 1-inch balls. Place about 2 inches apart on a greased cookie sheet. Flatten with the floured bottom of a glass or with a floured fork, making crosswise pattern. Bake in a 350°F. oven 12 to 15 minutes, or until lightly browned. Makes 6 dozen cookies.

	PROTEIN (grams)	FAT UNSATURATED (grams)	FAT SATURATED (grams)	CARBOHYDRATES (grams)	CALORIES
TOTAL RECIPE	49	150	53	502	4110
EACH COOKIE	.6	2	.7	7	57

COCOA BROWNIES

This is for those chocoholics who should cut down on sugar but can't resist a chocolate flavor. Cocoa is unsweetened and sugar is controlled to a mere 1½ teaspoons per piece.

½ cup unbleached flour
6 tablespoons unsweetened cocoa
1 cup sugar
¼ teaspoon salt

¼ cup corn oil
2 eggs
1 cup coarsely chopped walnuts
1 teaspoon vanilla extract

Combine flour, cocoa, sugar, and salt in a large bowl. Stir in corn oil. Add eggs, one at a time, beating well after each addition. Stir in nuts and vanilla. Pour into an 8-inch-square nonstick baking pan or a regular greased and floured pan. Bake in a 350°F. oven for 25 minutes, or until cake tester inserted in center comes out clean. Cut into 1-by-2-inch pieces while still warm. Makes 32 pieces.

	PROTEIN (grams)	FAT UNSATURATED (grams)	FAT SATURATED (grams)	CARBOHYDRATES (grams)	CALORIES
TOTAL RECIPE	686	182	118	271	6148
EACH PIECE	21	6	4	8	192

APPLE CRISP

This is sort of an upside-down cake. Apples on the bottom, crumbs on the top, and none will be left over.

4 large apples, pared and sliced
½ cup brown sugar
½ cup sifted unbleached flour
½ cup rolled-oat cereal

¼ cup soft margarine
1 teaspoon ground cinnamon
½ teaspoon ground nutmeg

Arrange sliced apples evenly over the bottom of an 8-inch-square nonstick baking pan or greased regular pan. Combine sugar, flour, oats, margarine, cinnamon, and nutmeg; mix until crumbly. Spread over the apples. Bake at 375°F. for 30 minutes, or until lightly browned. Cut into squares. Makes 9 servings.

	PROTEIN (grams)	FAT UNSATURATED (grams)	FAT SATURATED (grams)	CARBOHYDRATES (grams)	CALORIES
TOTAL RECIPE	15	26	6	272	1440
EACH SERVING	1.6	3	.6	30	160

APPLESAUCE CAKE

Make your own applesauce or use a can of sugar-free sauce. Either way, this is a wonderful-tasting treat.

2⅓ cups sifted flour
1 teaspoon ground cinnamon
½ teaspoon salt
½ teaspoon ground cloves
½ teaspoon ground nutmeg
⅔ cup corn oil margarine

1 cup sugar
1⅓ cups warm unsweetened applesauce
1¼ teaspoons baking soda
⅓ cup raisins
⅓ cup chopped nuts

Grease a 9-inch-square baking pan; line bottom with waxed paper and grease again. Sift together flour, cinnamon, salt, cloves, and nutmeg. Mix margarine and sugar until blended. Stir in 2 tablespoons of the applesauce. Add baking soda to remaining applesauce in small bowl, stirring until mixture foams and looks bubbly. Stir into margarine mixture alternately with sifted dry ingredients, mixing until smooth after each addition. Pour into prepared pan. Bake in 350°F. oven 45 to 50 minutes or until cake springs back when touched. Cool in pan. Cut into 1½-by-3-inch bars. Makes 18 servings.

	PROTEIN (grams)	FAT UNSATURATED (grams)	FAT SATURATED (grams)	CARBOHYDRATES (grams)	CALORIES
TOTAL RECIPE	41	138	16	520	3752
EACH SERVING	2.2	8	9	29	208

APPLESAUCE OATMEAL CAKE

If you prefer to serve cake bars, cut these into 1-by-3-inch size. Either way, it's a good mouthful.

2 cups unsweetened applesauce	1 teaspoon vanilla extract
½ cup soft shortening	1½ cups flour
1 cup quick rolled oats	1 teaspoon baking soda
1 cup sugar	1 teaspoon ground cinnamon
1 cup brown sugar	⅛ teaspoon salt
2 eggs, beaten	

Combine applesauce and shortening in a saucepan. Heat until shortening is melted, stirring constantly. Remove from heat and stir in oats; set aside. Beat together sugar, brown sugar, eggs, and vanilla. Stir in oat mixture. Add flour, baking soda, cinnamon, and salt. Pour into a greased 8-by-12-inch baking dish. Bake in a 350°F. oven for 35 to 40 minutes, or until lightly browned. Makes 24 servings, 2 by 2 inches each.

	PROTEIN (grams)	FAT UNSATURATED (grams)	FAT SATURATED (grams)	CARBOHYDRATES (grams)	CALORIES
TOTAL RECIPE	47	82	30	603	3619
EACH SERVING	2	3	1.25	25	150

NO-YOLK CHIFFON CAKE

Designed for those who are avoiding egg yolks because of conviction or cholesterol, this makes a lovely low-calorie offering and a wonderful base for sliced berries.

1 cup unsifted flour	¼ cup corn oil
¼ cup sugar	¼ teaspoon almond extract
1 teaspoon baking powder	4 egg whites
½ teaspoon salt	¼ teaspoon cream of tartar
½ cup water	2 tablespoons sugar

In a large bowl, stir together flour, ¼ cup sugar, baking powder, and salt. Add water, corn oil, and almond extract. With mixer at medium speed, beat until smooth. In a small bowl, beat the egg whites and cream of tartar at high speed until foamy. Gradually add 2 tablespoons sugar, beating until stiff peaks form. Gently fold egg whites into flour mixture. Pour into a greased 8-inch-square pan. Bake in a 325°F. oven for 45 minutes, or until cake springs back when lightly touched. Immediately upon taking cake out of the oven, invert the pan over a rack. Let cake cool in the pan. Remove by loosening sides with a spatula. Makes 12 servings.

	PROTEIN (grams)	FAT UNSATURATED (grams)	FAT SATURATED (grams)	CARBOHYDRATES (grams)	CALORIES
TOTAL RECIPE	29	44	5	179	1333
EACH SERVING	2.4	4	.4	15	111

NO-YOLK ORANGE CAKE

The subtle orange flavor makes this a grand and easy cake. Be sure to beat the egg whites long enough to make stiff peaks when you raise the beaters, but not so long that the peaks look dry.

1½ cups sifted flour	½ cup corn oil
1 cup sugar	2 teaspoons grated orange rind
2 teaspoons baking powder	½ cup orange juice
¼ teaspoon salt	4 egg whites

In a large bowl, stir together flour, sugar, baking powder, and salt. Add corn oil, orange rind, and orange juice; beat until smooth. In a separate bowl, beat egg whites until stiff peaks form. Fold egg whites into flour mixture. Pour into a 9-by-5-inch loaf pan that has been greased and floured, or one with a nonstick surface. Bake in a 350°F. oven for 50 minutes, or until cake springs back when lightly touched. Cool 10 minutes in the pan. Then remove from pan and cool completely on a wire rack. Makes 12 servings.

	PROTEIN (grams)	FAT UNSATURATED (grams)	FAT SATURATED (grams)	CARBOHYDRATES (grams)	CALORIES
TOTAL RECIPE	15	88	11	213	1858
EACH SERVING	1.2	7.3	.9	18	155

ORANGE SPONGE CAKE

So low in calories and so easy to do. The most important thing to remember is to turn the sponge cake upside down on a rack or suspend it from an empty soda bottle if you've used an angel-food cake pan.

4 eggs, separated
1 cup sugar
½ cup orange juice

2 tablespoons grated orange rind
1 cup unbleached flour, sifted
1 teaspoon baking powder

Beat egg yolks until lemon-colored. Add sugar and beat well. Add orange juice and orange rind; beat well. Add sifted flour and baking powder. Beat egg whites until stiff peaks form; fold gently through the batter until well mixed. (Be careful not to break down the air bubbles of the beaten egg whites.) Pour into an ungreased angel-food cake pan and bake for 30 to 40 minutes in a 325°F. oven, or until lightly browned. Immediately upon removing from oven, invert pan on a wire rack to cool upside down. Cool completely. Then turn right side up and slice. Makes 16 slices.

	PROTEIN (grams)	FAT UNSATURATED (grams)	FAT SATURATED (grams)	CARBOHYDRATES (grams)	CALORIES
TOTAL RECIPE	41	12	7.4	322	1667
EACH SERVING	2.5	.7	.5	20	104

EGGLESS CAKE

Some readers with egg allergy pray for a recipe like this. All others won't even know the difference, it's so very good.

1¾ cups unsifted flour	1 teaspoon ground cinnamon
1 teaspoon baking powder	1 teaspoon ground cloves
½ teaspoon baking soda	½ teaspoon salt
1 cup water	¼ teaspoon ground nutmeg
½ cup sugar	¼ teaspoon ground allspice
½ cup raisins	½ cup corn oil

In a small bowl, stir together flour, baking powder, and baking soda. In a medium saucepan, bring water, sugar, raisins, cinnamon, cloves, salt, nutmeg, and allspice to a boil over medium heat. Reduce heat and simmer 3 minutes. Cool. Pour into a large mixing bowl; add oil and beat. Add flour mixture. Beat until blended. Pour into a greased 8-inch-square baking pan. Bake in a 350°F. oven for 40 minutes, or until cake springs back when lightly touched. Serve warm. Makes 12 servings.

	PROTEIN (grams)	FAT UNSATURATED (grams)	FAT SATURATED (grams)	CARBOHYDRATES (grams)	CALORIES
TOTAL RECIPE	27	88	11	339	2436
EACH SERVING	2	7	1	28	203

OIL PASTRY SHELL

Pie crust is a high-fat offering no matter how you slice it. A one-crust pie (use half the following ingredients) is sensibly better than two crusts, but at least this crust is unsaturated fat. Think of keeping the pie fat-free when you fill it with your own recipe of fruit.

2 cups sifted unbleached flour	3 tablespoons cold water
½ cup corn oil	

Mix flour and corn oil in a bowl, using a fork. Add water a little at a time and mix well. Press firmly into a ball with your hands. If slightly dry, mix in a small amount of additional water. Divide dough almost in half. Flatten larger portion between 2 pieces of waxed paper. Roll out to a 12-inch circle. Peel off top paper; place dough in a 9-inch pie pan, paper side up. Peel off paper and fit pastry loosely into pan. Fill as desired. Trim dough ½ inch beyond rim of pan. Roll out remaining dough for top crust. Peel off paper after placing over pan. Trim ½ inch beyond rim of pan. Fold edges of both crusts under; seal and flute. Cut slits into top crust to let steam escape. Bake pie according to recipe directions for filling used. Makes 2 crusts for an 8-serving pie.

	PROTEIN (grams)	FAT UNSATURATED (grams)	FAT SATURATED (grams)	CARBOHYDRATES (grams)	CALORIES
TOTAL RECIPE	28	88	11	208	1961
EACH SERVING	3.5	11	1.3	26	245

BIBLIOGRAPHY

1. THE SECRET TO GOOD HEALTH

Brewster, Letitia, and Jacobson, Michael F., Ph.D. "The Changing American Diet." Center for Science in the Public Interest, 1978.

Cheraskin, E., M.D., D.M.D., and Ringsdorf, W. M., Jr., D.M.D. *Predictive Medicine.* Keats Publishing Co., 1973.

Enos, W. F.; Homes, R. H.; and Beyer, J. C. "Coronary Disease among United States Soldiers Killed in Action in Korea." *JAMA* 152 (1953): 1090.

Sebag, Jerry. "Diagnosis of Health." *Preventive Medicine* 8 (1979): 76.

Stomer, Jeremiah, M.D. "Lifestyles, Major Risk Factors, Proof, and Public Policy." *Circulation* 58 (1978): 3.

2. TRIGLYCERIDES

Albrink, Margaret J., M.D., and Man, Evelyn R., Ph.D. "Serum Triglycerides in Coronary Artery Disease." *Arch. Int. Med.* 103 (1959): 4.

Brown, David R., M.B.; Kinch, Sandra H., M.S.; and Doyle, Joseph T., M.D. "Serum Triglycerides in Health and in Ischemic Heart Disease." *NEJM* 273 (1963): 947.

Brunner, D. S.; Altman, K.; Loebl, K.; Schwartz, S.; and Leven, S. "Serum Cholesterol and Triglycerides in Patients Suffering from Ischemic Heart Disease and in Healthy Subjects." *Atherosclerosis* 28 (1977): 197.

Cheraskin, E., M.D., D.M.D., and Ringsdorf, W. M., Jr., D.M.D., M.S. " 'Normal' vs. 'Normal' Criteria." *Internat. Acad. Prevent. Med.* 4 (1977): 5.

Crombie, J. B., M.D.; Thomason, K. J., M.D.; Cullimore, O. S., M.S.; and Beach, E. F., Ph.D. "Studies in Serum Lipids." *Circulation* 27 (1963): 360.

Denborough, M. A. "Alimentary Lipaemia in Ischaemic Heart Disease. *Clin. Sci.* 25 (1963): 115.

Fredrickson, Donald S. "The Regulation of Plasma Lipoprotein Concentrations as Affected in Human Mutants." *Annals N.Y. Acad. Sci.* 64 (1969): 1138.

Friedman, Meyer, M.D.; Rosenman, Ray H., M.D.; and Byers, Sanford, Ph.D. "Serum Lipids and Conjunctival Circulation after Fat Ingestion in Man Exhibiting Type A Behavior Pattern." *Circulation* 24 (1964): 874.

Friedman, Meyer, et al. "Serum Lipids and Conjunctival Circulation after Fat Ingestion." *Circulation* 29 (1964): 874.

Gibson, Thomas C., and Whorton, Elbert B. "The Prevalence of Hyperlipidemia in a Natural Community." *J. Chron. Dis.* 26 (1973): 227.

Hatch, Fredrick T., M.D., Ph.D. "Interactions between Nutrition and Heredity in Coronary Heart Disease." *Amer. J. Clin. Nutr.* 27 (1974): 80.

Hollister, Leo F., M.D.; Beckman, Wallace G., M.D.; and Baker, Martha, M.S. "Comparative Variability of Serum Cholesterol and Serum Triglycerides." *Am. J. Med. Sc.* 34 (1964): 329.

Holister, T. E., and Wright, A. "Diurnal Variation of Serum Lipids." *J. Atherosclerosis Research* 5 (1956): 445.

Kuo, Peter T., and Carson, John C. "Dietary Fats and the Diurnal Serum Triglycerides Levels in Man." *J. Clin. Invest.* 38 (1959): 1384.

Nestel, P. J. "Relationship between Plasma Triglycerides and Removal of Chylomicrons." *J. Clin. Invest.* 43 (1964): 943.

Schlierf, G., and Raetyer, H. "Diurnal Patterns of Blood Sugar, Plasma, Insulin, Free Fatty Acid and Triglyceride Levels in Normal Subjects and in Patients with Type IV Hyperlipoproteinemia and the Effect of Meal Frequency." *Nutr. Metabol.* 14 (1972): 113.

Tyagournis, Emanuel. "Triglycerides in Clinical Medicine." *Amer. J. Clin. Nutr.* 31 (1978): 360.

Wood, Peter D. S., Ph.D.; Stern, Michael P., M.D.; Silvers, Abraham, Ph.D.; Reaven, Gerald M., M.D.; and van der Groeben, Jobst, M.D. "Prevalence of Plasma Lipoprotein Abnormalities in a Free-Living Population of the Central Valley, California." *Circulation* 45 (1972): 114.

Zwears, A.; Yaron, E.; and Groen, J. J. "A Study of Fasting and Postprandial Serum Triglycerides in Connection with Epidemiological Surveys." *Clin. Chem. Acta.* 19 (1968): 267.

EFFECT OF TRIGLYCERIDES

Aarli, Johan A., M.D. "Neurological Manifestations in Hyperlipidemia." *Neurology* 18 (1968): 883.

Bagdads, John D., and Ways, Peter O. "Erythrocyte Membrane Lipid Composition in Exogenous and Endogenous Hypertriglyceridemia." *J. Lab. Clin. Med.* 75 (1970): 53.

Cullen, Chester F., and Swank, Roy L., M.D., Ph.D. "Intravascular Aggregation and Adhesiveness of the Blood Elements Associated with Alimentary Lipemia and Injections of Large Molecular Substances. Effect on Blood-Brain Barrier." *Circulation* 9 (1954): 335.

de Dechere, E. A. M., and Hoor, F. ten. "Effects of Dietary Fats on the Coronary Flow Rate and the Left Ventricular Function of the Isolated Rat Heart." *Nutr. Metab.* 23 (1979): 88.

Fahraeus, Robin. "The Influence of the Rouleau Formation of the Erythrocytes on the Rheology of the Blood." *Acta Medica Scandinavica,* CLXI (1958): 151.

Friedman, Meyer, M.D. "Type A Behavior Pattern: Some of Its Pathophysiological Components." *Bull. of New York Acad. of Med.* 53 (1977): 593.

Friedman, Meyer, M.D; Byers, Sanford O., Ph.D.; and Rosenman, Roy H., M.D. "Effect of Unsaturated Fats upon Lipemia and Conjunctival Circulation." *JAMA* 193 (1965): 110.

Fukuzake, Hisashi; Okamoto, Ryozo; and Matsuo, Takefumi. "Studies on Pathophysiological Effects of Postalimentary Lipemia in Patients with Ischemic Heart Disease." *Japanese Circulation Journal* 39 (1975): 317.

Green, Harry T., M.D.; Hoylett, David, M.D.; and Demacee, Richard, Ph.D. "Relationship between Intralipid-Induced Hyperlimpemia and Pulmonary Function." *Amer. J. Clin. Nutr.* 29 (1976); 127.

Hazlett, David R., M.D. "Dietary Fats Appear to Reduce Lung Functions." *JAMA* 223 (1973): 15.

Knisely, Marvin H; Bloch, Edward H.; Eliot, Thoedore S.; and Warmer, Louis. "Sludged Blood." *Science* 106 (1947): 431.

Knisely, Marvin H. "Intravascular Erythrocyte Aggregation (Blood Sludge)." *Handbook of Physiology: Circulation III,* Ch. 63.

Joyner, Claude R., Jr., M.D.; Horwitz, Orville, M.D.; and Williams, Phyllis G., B.S. "The Effect of Lipemia upon Tissue Oxygen Tension in Man." *Circulation* 22 (1960): 901.

Kuo, Peter T., M.D., and Joyner, Claude R., Jr., M.D. "Angina Pectoris Induced by Fat Ingestion in Patients with Coronary Artery Disease." *JAMA* 158 (1955): 1008.

Nestel, C. J. "Relationship between Plasma Triglycerides and Removal of Chylomicrons." *J. Clin. Invest.* 5 (1964): 943.

Reagan, Timothy G., M.D.; Binak, Kenan, M.D.; Gordon, Seymour, M.D.; Defazio, Valentino, M.D.; and Hellems, Harper K., M.D. "Myocardial Blood Flow and Oxygen Consumption During Postprandial Lipemia and Heparin-Induced Lipolysis." *Circulation* 23 (1961): 55.

Swank, R. A. Biochemical Basis of Multiple Sclerosis. Springfield: C. C. Thomas, 1961.

Swank, Roy. L. "Changes in Blood Produced by a Fat Meal and by Intravenous Heparin." *Amer. J. Physiology* 164 (1951): 798.

Swank, Roy L. "Changes in Blood of Dogs and Rabbits by High Fat Intake." *Am. J. Physiol.* 196 (1959) (3): 473.

Swank, Roy L., and Nakamura, Haruomi, M.D. "Oxygen Availability in Brain Tissue after Lipid Meals." *Amer. J. Physiol.* 198 (1960): 217.

Well, Roe E., Jr., M.D. "Rheology of Blood in the Microvasculature." *NEJM* 270 (1964): 832.

Williams, Arthur V., M.D.; Higginbotham, A. Curtis, M.D.; and Knisely, Marvin H. "Increased Blood Cell Agglutination Following Ingestion of Fat: A Factor Contributing to Cardiac Ischemia, Coronary Insufficiency and Angina Pain." *Angiology* 8 (1957): 29.

Zauner, Christian W., and Swenson, Edward W. "Effects of Hyperlipemia on Oxygen Uptake, Oxygen Extraction and Ventilation." *J. Sports Med.* 12 (1972): 157.

WHAT AFFECTS TRIGLYCERIDES?

Antonis, A., Ph.D., and Bersohn, I., M.B., B.SC. "The Influence of Diet on Serum Triglycerides." *Lancet,* 7 Jan. 1961.

Albrink, Margaret J., M.D., and Man, Evelyn B., Ph.D. "Serum Triglycerides in Health and Diabetes." *Diabetes* 7 (1958): 194.

Barter, Philip J.; Carroll, Kevin F.; and Nestel, Paul J. "Diurnal Fluctuations in Triglyceride Free Fatty Acids and Insulin During Sucrose Consumption and Insulin Infusion in Man." *J. of Clin. Invest.* 50 (1971): 583.

Becker, H.; Meyer, Jacob; and Necheles, H. "Fat Absorption and Atherosclerosis." *Science* 110 (1949): 529.

Cromie, J. B., M.D. "Studies in Serum Lipids: Effect of Short-term Dietary Changes." *Circulation* 27 (1963): 360.

Day, J. T.; Simpson, N.; Metcalfe, J. et al. "Metabolic Consequences of Atenolol and Propranolol in Treatment of Essential Hypertensions." *Br. Med. J.* 1 (1979): 77.

Ford, Starr, Jr., M.D.; Bozian, Richard C., M.D.; and Knowles, Harvey C., M.D. "Interactions of Obesity and Glucose and Insulin Levels in Hypertriglyceridemia." *Amer. J. Clin. Nutr.* 21 (1968): 904.

Garn, S. M.; Block, W. D.; and Clark, D. C. "Level of Fatness and Lipid Levels." *Ecol. Food Nutr.* 4 (1976): 235.

Ginsberg, Harry, M.D.; Olefsky, Jerrold, M.D.; Farquhar, John, M.D.; and Reaven, Gerald M., M.D. "Moderate Ethanol Ingestion and Plasma Triglyceride Levels." *Annals of Int. Med.* 80 (1974): 143.

Hennekens, Charles H., M.D.; Evans, Denis A., M.D.; Castelli, William P., M.D.; Taylor, James O., M.D.; Rosner, Bernard, Ph.D.; and Kass, Edward H., M.D., Ph.D. "Oral Contraceptive Use and Fasting Triglyceride, Plasma Cholesterol, and HDL Cholesterol." *Circulation* 60 (1979): 486.

Johnson, R. H., and Walton, J. L. "Metabolic Fuels During and After Severe Exercise in Athletes and Non-Athletes." *Lancet,* 30 Aug. 1969, 452.

Kaufmann, Nathan A., M.D.; Poznanski, M. S.; Blondheim, S. H., M.D.; and Stein, Yechizkiel, M.D. "Changes in Serum Lipid Levels of Hyperlipemic Patients Following the Feeding of Starch, Sucrose and Glucose." *Amer. J. Clin. Nutr.* 18 (1966): 261.

Kershbaum, Alfred, M.D., and Bellet, Samuel, M.D. "Cigarette Smoking and Blood Lipids." *JAMA* 187 (1964): 32.

Kudzma, D. J., and Schonfeld, G. "Alcoholic Hyperlipidemia: Induction by Alcohol But Not by Carbohydrates." *J. Lab. Clin. Med.* 77 (1971): 384.

Kuo, Peter T. "Dietary Sugar in the Production of Hyperglyceridemia." *Annals of Int. Med.* 62 (1965): 1199.

Kuo, Peter T., M.D., and Bassett, David R., M.D. "Dietary Sugar in the Production of Hyperglyceridemia." *Annals of Int. Med.* 62 (1965): 1199.

Lifton, Lester, M.D., and Scheig, Robert, M.D. "Ethanol-Induced Hypertriglyceridemia, Prevalence and Contributing Factors." *Amer. J. Clin. Nutr.* 31 (1978): 614.

Lopez, A.; Vial, S. R.; Balart, T.; and Arroyove, G. "Effect of Exercise and Physical Fitness on Serum Lipids and Lipoproteins." *Atherosclerosis* 20 (1974): 1.

Mann, J. I.; Truswell, A. S.; Hendricks, D. A.; and Manning, E. "Effects on Serum Lipids in Normal Men of Reducing Dietary Sucrose or Starch for Five Months." *Lancet,* 25 April 1970.

Nestel, Paul F.; Carroll, Kevin F.; and Havenstein, Nathalie. "Plasma Triglyceride Response to Carbohydrates, Fats and Caloric Intake." *Metabolism* 19 (1970): 1.

Olefsky, M. M., M.D.; Crapo, Phyllis, R.D.; and Reaven, Gerald M., M.D. "Postprandial Plasma Triglyceride and Cholesterol Response to a Low Fat Meal." *J. Clin. Nutr.* 29 (1976): 535.

Oscai, Lawrence B. et al. "Normalization of Serum Triglycerides and Lipoprotein Electrophoretic Patterns by Exercise." *Amer. J. Card.* 30 (1972): 775.

Ringsdorf, W. M., Jr., D.M.D., M.S.; Cheraskin, E., M.D., D.M.D.; and Medford, F. H., B.S. "Smoking and Serum Triglycerides." *J. Med. Assoc. of the State of Alabama,* Oct. 1975.

Simonelli, Christine, and Eaton, R. Philip. "Reduced Triglyceride Secretion: A Metabolic Consequence of Chronic Exercise." *Amer. J. Physiol.* 234 (3) (1978): E221.

Stone, Daniel B., M.B., and Connor, William E. "The Prolonged Effects of a Low Cholesterol, High Carbohydrate Diet upon the Serum Lipids in Diabetic Patients." *Diabetes* 12 (1963): 127.

"Sucrose, Starch, and Hyperlipidemia." *Nutrition Reviews* 33 (1975): 44.

Taggert, Peter, and Carruthers, Malcolm. "Endogenous Hyperlipidemia Induced by Emotional Stress of Race Driving." *Lancet,* 20 Feb. 1971.

Tosowsky, M. S., M.D., M.R.C.P.; Jones, D. P., M.D.; Davidson, C. S., M.D.; and Lieber, C. S., M.D. "Studies of Alcoholic Hyperlipemia and Its Mechanisms." *Amer. J. Med.* 35 (1963): 794.

Turner, John L., M.D.; Bierman, Edwin T., M.D.; Brunzell, John D., M.D.; and Chait, Alan, M.D., "Effect of Dietary Fructose on Triglyceride Transport and Glucoregulatory Hormones in Hypertriglyceridemic Men." *Amer. J. Clin. Nutr.* 32 (1979): 1043.

Wilson, Dana, E.; Schreibman, Paul H.; Brewster, Alan C.; and Arky, Ronald A. "The Enhancement of Alimentary Lipemia by Ethanol in Man." *J. Lab Clin. Med.* 75 (1970): 264.

Wood, Peter D.; Haskell, William; Klein, Herbert; Lewis, Steven; Stern, Michael P.; and Farquhar, John W. "The Distribution of Plasma in Middle-Aged Male Runners." *Metabolism* 25 (1976): 1249.

Zorrilla, Eduardo; Hulse, Mildred; Hernandez, Alfredo; and Gershberg, Herbert. "Severe Endogenous Hypertriglyceridemia During Treatment with Estrogen and Oral Contraceptives." *J. Clin. Endocr.* 28 (1968): 1783.

SLUDGING

Biecher, H. I.; Bruley, D.; Knisely, M. H.; and Reneau, D. D. "Effect of Microcirculation Changes on Brain Tissue Oxygenation." *J. Physiology* 217 (1971): 689.

Fajers, C. M., and Gelin, L. E. "Kidney, Liver and Heart Damages from Trauma and from Induced Intravascular Aggregation of Blood Cells." *Acta PathMicro-Biol., Scand.* 46 (1959): 97.

"Intravascular Erythrocyte Aggregation (Blood Sludge)," *Handbook of Physiology: Circulation,* chap. 63, p. 2249.

Richer, H. I., and Beemer, A. M. "Induction of Ischemic Myocardial Damage by Red Cell Aggregation (Sludge) in the Rabbit." *Atherosclerosis Res.* 7 (1967): 409.

Zederfeldt, Bengt. "Studies on Wound Healing and Trauma." *Acta Chirurgica Scandinavica Suppl.* 224 (1957).

3. YOUR OXYGEN DELIVERY SYSTEM

Andersen, Per. "Capillary Density in Skeletal Muscle of Man." *Acta Physiol. Scand.* 95 (1975): 203.

Edwards, Miles J.; Novy, Miles J.; Walters, Carrie-Lou; and Metcalfe, James. "Improved Oxygen Release: An Adaptation of Mature Red Cells to Hypoxia." *J. Clin. Invest.* 47 (1968): 1851.

Hansen, Dr. A. Tybjaery. "Osmotic Pressure Effect of the Red Blood Cells—Possible Physiological Significance." *Nature* 190 (1961): 504.

Hechtmen, Herbert B., M.D.; Grindlinger, Gene A., M.D.; Vegos, Armando M., M.D.; Manny, Jonah, M.D.; and Valeri, C. Robert, M.D. "Importance of Oxygen Transport in Clinical Medicine." *Critical Care Medicine* 7 (1979): 419.

Holmgren, A. "Cardiorespiratory Determinates of Cardiovascular Fitness." *Canad. Med. Assoc. J.* 96 (1967): 697.

Kessler, M., ed. *Oxygen Supply, Theoretical and Practical Aspect of Oxygen Supply and Microvasculature of Tissue.* Baltimore: University Park Press, 1971.

Lauer, N. V., ed. "The Oxygen Regime of the Organism and Its Regulation (Symposium)." 1969.

Lubber, D. W., ed. *Oxygen Transport in Blood and Tissue.* New York: Intercontinental Medical Book Corp., 1968.

Mueggler, Paul A.; Peterson, James S.; Koler, Robert D.; Metcalfe, James; and Black, John A. "Postnatal Regulation of Oxygen Delivery: Hematologic Parameters of Postnatal Dogs." *Amer. J. Physiol.* 237 (1) (1979): H71.

Pietra, Giuseppe G., and Magno, Michael. "Pharmacological Factors Influencing Permeability of the Bronchial Microcirculation." *Federation Proceedings* 37 (1978): 2466.

Rosen, Arthur L., Ph.D.; Gould, Steven, M.D.; Sehgal, Lakshman R., Ph.D.; Noud, Geroge, M.D.; Sehgal, Hansa T., B.S.; Rice, Charles, L., M.D.; Moss, Gerald S., M.D. "Cardiac Output Response to Extreme Hemodilution with Hemoglobin Solutions of Various P_{50} Values." *Critical Care Medicine* 7 (1979): 380.

Salhany, J. M., and Swanson, J. C. "Kinetics of Passive Anion Transport Across the Human Erythrocyte Membrane." *Biochemistry* 17 (1978): 3354.

Woodson, Robert D., M.D. "Physiological Significance of Oxygen Dissociation Curve Shifts." *Critical Care Medicine* 7 (1979): 368.

OXYGEN DELIVERY AND SMOKING, ALCOHOL, AND STRESS

Aronow, Wilbert S., M.D., F.A.C.P., and Cassidy, John, M.D. "Effect of Carbon Monoxide on Maximal Treadmill Exercise: A Study in Normal Persons." *Annals of Internal Med.* 83 (1975): 496.

Aronow, Wilbert S. M.D.; Stemmer, Edward A., M.D.; and Isbell, Michael W. "Effect of Carbon Monoxide Exposures on Intermittent Claudication." *CPT Circulation* 49 (1974): 415.

Beary, John F., B.S., and Benson, Herbert, M.D. "A Simple Psychophysiologic Technique Which Elicits the Hypometabolic Changes of the Relaxation Response." *Psychosomatic Medicine* 36 (1974): 115.

Benson, Herbert; Beary, John F.; and Carol, Mark P. "The Relaxation Response." *Psychiatry* 37 (1974): 37.

Burch, G. E., and DePasquale, N. P. "Alcoholic Cardiomyopathy." *Amer. J. Card.* 23 (1969): 723.

Carlson, Lars A.; Levi, Lennard; and Oro, Lars. "Plasma Lipids and Urinary Excretion of Catecholamines in Man During Experimentally Induced Emotional Stress and Their Modification by Nicotinic Acid." *J. Clin. Invest.* 47 (1968): 1795.

Cooper, Michael J., M.D., and Aygen, Maurice M., M.D. "A Relaxation Technique in the Management of Hypercholesterolemia." *J. Human Stress,* Dec. 1979, p. 24.

Dales, Loring G.; Friedman, Gary D.; Siegelaub, A. B.; and Seltzer, Carl C. "Cigarette Smoking and Serum Chemistry Tests." *J. Chron. Dis.* 27 (1974): 293.

Da Silva, Angelo M. T., and Hamosh, Paul. "Effect of Smoking a Single Cigarette on the Small Airways." *J. Applied Physiology* 34 (1973): 361.

Dreyfuss, F., M.D., and Cyaczkes, J. W., M.Sc. "Blood Cholesterol and Uric Acid of Healthy Medical Students Under Stress of an Examination." *Arch. Int. Med.* 103 (1959): 708.

Ebblom, Bjorn, and Huot, Roger. "Response to Submaximal and Maximal Exercise at Different Levels of Carboxyhemoglobin." *Acta. Physiol. Scand.* 86 (1972): 474.

Forsander, O., and Suomainen, H. "Alcoholic Intake and Erythrocyte Aggregation." *Quart. J. Studies Alc.* 16 (1955): 614.

Ginsberg, Harry, M.D.; Olefsky, Jerrold, M.D.; Farquhar, John, M.D.; and Reaven, Gerald M., M.D. "Moderate Ethanol Ingestion and Plasma Triglyceride Levels." *Annals of Internal Med.* 80 (1974): 143.

Hlastala, M. P.; McKenna, H. P.; Franada, R. T.; and Detter, J. C. "Influence of Carbon Monoxide on Hemoglobin-Oxygen Binding." *J. Applied Physiol.* 44 (1976): 893.

Jones, Maxwell, and Melhersh, Veronica. "A Comparison of the Exercise Response in Anxiety States and Normal Controls." *Psychosomatic Med.* 8 (1946): 180.

Kershbaum, Alfred, M.D., and Bellet, Samuel, M.D. "Cigarette Smoking and Blood Lipids." *JAMA* 187 (1964): 32.

Kershbaum, Alfred, M.D.; Bellet, Samuel, M.D., F.A.C.C.; Caplan, Raymond F., M.D.; and Feinberg, Leonard J., Ph.D. "Effect of Cigarette Smoking on Free Fatty Acids in Patients with Healed Myocardial Infarction." *Amer. J. Card.* 6 (1962): 204.

Kershbaum, Alfred, M.D.; Bellet, Samuel, M.D.; Dickstein, Edward R., M.D.; and Finelberg, Leonard J., Ph.D. "Effect of Cigarette Smoking and Nicotine on Serum Free Fatty Acids." *Circulation Res.* 9 (1961): 631.

Loskowsky, M. S., M.D., M.R.C.P.; Jones, I. P., M.D.; Davidson, C. S., M.D.; and Lieber, C. S., M.D. "Studies of Alcholic Hyperlipemia and Its Mechanism." *Amer. J. Med.* 35 (1963): 794.

Moskow, Herbert A.; Pennington, Raymond C.; and Knisely, Marvin H. "Alcohol, Sludge and Hypoxic Areas of Nervous System, Liver and Heart." *Microvascular Research* 1 (1968): 174.

Nizami, Riaz M., and Khan, Rahmeth S. "Smoking: Evidence of Its Adverse Effects Increases." *Modern Medicine,* Sept. 15–Sept. 30, 1979, p. 25.

Regan, T. J.; Khan, M. I.; and Ettinger, P. O. "Myocardial Function and Lipid Metabolism in the Chronic Alcoholic Animal." *J. Clin. Invest.* 54 (1974): 740.

Toggard, Peter. "Endogenous Hyperlipidemia Induced by Emotional Stress of Race Driving." *Lancet,* 20 Feb. 1971.

Tevander, V. T.; Benson, H.; Wheeler, R. C.; and Wallace, R. K. "Increased Forearm Blood Flow During a Wakeful Hypometabolic State." *Federation Proceedings* 31 (1972): 405.

Wallace, Robert Keith. "Physiological Effects of Transcendental Meditation." *Science* 167 (1970): 1751.

Wallace, Robert Keith; Benson, Herbert; and Wilson, Archie F. "Wakeful Hypometabolic Physiologic State." *Amer. J. Physiol.* 221 (1971): 795.

Whitehorn, J. C., M.D.; Lundholm, Helge, Ph.D.; Fox, E. T.; and Benedict, Francis G., Ph.D. "The Metabolic Rate in 'Hypnotic Sleep.' " *NEJM* 206 (1932): 777.

Wolf, Steward, M.D.; McCabe, William R., M.D.; Yamamoto, Joe, M.D.; Adsett, C. A., M.D.; and Schottstaedt, W. W., M.D. "Changes in Serum Lipids in Relation to Emotional Stress During Rigid Control of Diet and Exercise." *Circulation* 26 (1962): 379.

4. BIOCONTAMINATION

OBESITY

Chirico, Anna-Marie, M.D., and Sternbard, Albert J., M.D. "Physical Activity and Human Obesity." *NEJM* 263 (1960): 935.

Cohn, Clarence, M.D., and Joseph, Dorothy. "Effects on Metabolism Produced by the Rate of Ingestion of the Diet." *J. Clin. Nutr.* 8 (1960): 682.

Darn, S. M.; Block, W. D.; and Clard, D. C. "Level of Fatness and Lipid Levels." *Ecol. Food Nutr.* 4 (1976): 235.

Durnin, J. V. G., M.A., M.D., Ch.B., D.Sc., M.R.C.P. "The Influence of Nutrition." *Canadian Med. Assoc. J.* 96 (1967): 715.

Essen, Birgitta. "Intramuscular Substrate Utilization During Prolonged Exercise." *Annals N.Y. Acad. Sc.* 301 (1977): 30.

Fabry, Pavel, M.D., D.Sc., and Tepperman, Joy, M.D. "Meal Frequency—A Possible Factor in Human Pathology." *Amer. J. Clin. Nutr.* 8 (1970): 1059.

Garby, Lars, and Tansmert, Ole. "Effect of the Preceding Day's Energy Intake on the Total Energy Cost of Light Exercise." *Acta. Physiol. Scand.* 101 (1977) 411.

Gollnick, Phillip D. "Free Fatty Acid Turnover and the Availability of Substrates as a Limiting Factor in Prolonged Exercise." *Annals N.Y. Acad. Sc.* 301 (1977).

Katch, Victor T.; Martin, Robert; and Margin, John. "Effects of Exercise Intensity on Food Consumption in the Male Rat." *Amer. J. Clin. Nutr.* 32 (1979): 1401.

Krogh, Auguest, and Lindhard, Johannes. "Relative Value of Fat and Carbohydrate as Sources of Muscular Energy." *Biochemical J.* 14 (1920): 290.

March, M. Elizabeth, and Murlin, John R. "Muscular Efficiency on High Carbohydrate and High Fat Diets." *J. Nutr.* 1 (1928): 105.

Martin, Bruce. "Influence on Diet Uptake of Glucose During Heavy Exercise." *Am. J. Clin. Nutr.* 31 (1978): 62.

Mayer, Jean, and Thomas, Donald W. "Regulation of Food Intake and Obesity." *Science* 156 (1967): 328.

Naughton, John P., M.D., and Hellerstein, Herman K., M.D., eds. *Exercise Testing and Exercise Training in Coronary Heart Disease.* New York: Academic Press, 1973.

Newsholme, E. A. "The Regulation of Intracellular and Extracellular Fuel Supply During Sustained Exercise." *Annals N.Y. Acad. Sc.* 301 (1977): 81.

Tuttle, W. W.; Wilson, Marjorie; and Daum, Kate. "Effect of Altered Breakfast on Physiological Response." *J. of Applied Physiol.* 1 (1949): 545.

Tuttle, W. W.; Daum, Kate; Myers, Loraine; and Martin, Constance. "Effect of Omitting Breakfast on the Physiologic Response of Men." *J. Amer. Dietetic Assoc.* 26 (1950): 332.

CHOLESTEROL

Beaglehole, Robert; LaRosa, John C.; Heiss, Geraldo; Davis, C. E.; Williams, O. Dale; Tyroder, H. A.; and Rifkind, B. M. "Serum Cholesterol, Diet and the Decline in Coronary Heart Disease Mortality." *Preventive Medicine* 8 (1979): 538.

Bersohn, J., and Oelofse, P. J. "Correlation of Serum, Magnesium and Serum Cholesterol Levels in South African Bantu and European Subjects." *Lancet,* 18 May 1957, p. 1020.

Bronsgeest-Schoute, Driek C.; Hautvast, Joseph G. A. J.; and Hermus, Rudd J. J. "Dependence of the Effects of Dietary Cholesterol and Experimental Conditions on Serum Lipids in Man." *Amer. J. Clin. Nutr.* 33 (1979): 2188.

Bronsgeest-Schoute, Driek C.; Hautvast, Joseph G. A. J.; and Hermus, Rudd J. J. "Dependence of the Effects of Dietary Cholesterol and Experimental Conditions of Serum Lipids in Man. Effects of Dietary Cholesterol in a Linoleic Acid Rich Diet." *Amer. J. Clin. Nutr.* 32 (1973): 2183.

Bronto-Steward, B., M.D.; Antonio, A., Ph.D.; Eales, L., M.D.; and Brock, J. F., M.D. "Effects of Feeding Different Fats on Serum Cholesterol." *Lancet,* 28 April 1956.

Carroll, K. K., Ph.D. "Dietary Protein in Relation to Plasma Cholesterol Levels and Atherosclerosis." *Nutrition Reviews* 36 (1978): 1.

Cheraskin, E., M.D.; Ringsdorf, W. M., Jr., M.D.; and Brecker, Arline. *Psycho-Dietetics.* New York: Bantam Books, 1972.

Cohn, Clarence. "Feeding Patterns and Some Aspects of Cholesterol Metabolism." *Federation Proceedings* 23 (1964): 76.

Conner, William E.; Hodges, Robert E.; and Bleiler, Roberts E. "The Serum Lipids in Men Receiving High Cholesterol and Cholesterol Free Diets." *Circulation* 22 (1960): 735.

de Groot, A. P.; Tayben, R.; and Pibaar, N. A. "Cholesterol-Lowering Effect of Rolled Oats." *Lancet,* 10 August 1963.

Flynn, Margaret A., Ph.D; Nolph, Georgia B., M.D.; Flynn, Timothy C., B.A.; Kahrs, Ruth, M.S.; and Krause, Gary, Ph.D. "Effect of Dietary Egg on Cholesterol and Triglycerides." *Amer. J. Clin. Nutr.* 32 (1979): 1051.

Friedman, Meyer; Sanford, Byers, O.; Michaelis, Fred. "Production and Excretion of Cholesterol in Mammals." *Journal of Biol. Chem.* 164 (1951): 789.

Grundy, Scott M., B.S., and Griffin, Clark A., Ph.D. "Effects of Periodic Mental Stress on Serum Cholesterol Levels." *Circulation* 19 (1959): 496.

Gwineys, Gront, M.D.; Bryon, Richard C., M.D.; Roush, William H., M.D.; Kruger, Fred A., M.D.; and Hamavi, George J., M.D. "Effect of Nibbling Versus Gorging on Serum Lipids in Man." *Amer. J. Clin. Nutr.* 13 (1963): 209.

Hanson, Dale T.; Lorentzen, James A.; Morris, Alfred E.; Ahrens, Richard A.; and Wilson, James E., Jr. "Effects of Fat Intake and Exercise on Serum Cholesterol and Body Composition in Rats." *Amer. J. Physiol.* 213 (1967): 347.

Hepner, Gershon, M.D.; Fried, Richard, M.D.; Jeor, Sachika St., Ph.D.; Fusetti, Lydia, M.D.; and Morin, Robert, M.D. "Hypocholesterolemic Effect of Yogurt and Milk." *Amer. J. Clin. Nutr.* 32 (1979): 19.

Hodges, Robert E., M.D., and Krehl, W. A., M.D., Ph.D. "The Role of Carbohydrates in Lipid Metabolism." *Amer. J. Clin. Nutr.* 17 (1965): 334.

"Hypocholesterolemic Effect of Substituting Soybean Protein for Animal Protein in the Diet of Healthy Young Women." *Amer. J. Clin. Nutr.* 31 (1978): 1312.

Kannel, William B., M.D., M.P.H.; Castelli, William P. M.D.; and Gordon, Tavia. "Cholesterol in the Prediction of Atherosclerotic Disease." *Annals Int. Med.* 90 (1979): 50.

Kannel, William B., M.D., M.P.H.; Castelli, William P., M.D.; and Gordon, Tavia. "Cholesterol in the Prediction of Atherosclerotic Disease." *Annals of Internal Med.* 90 (1979): 50.

Kay, M., Ph.D., and Truswell, A. Stewart, M.D. "Effect of Citrus Pectin on Blood Lipids and Fecal Steroid Excretion in Man." *Amer. J. Clin. Nutr.* 30 (1977): 171.

Kay, R. M., and Truswell, A. S. "The Effect of Wheat Fiber on Plasma Lipids and Fecal Steroid Excretion in Man." *B. J. Nutr.* 37 (1977): 227.

Keys, Ancel; Anderson, Joseph T.; and Grande, Francisco. "Diet-Type (Fats Constant) and Blood Lipids in Man." *J. Nutr.* 70 (1960): 257.

Keys, Ancel, Ph.D. "Human Atherosclerosis and Diet." *Circulation* 5 (1952): 115.

Keys, Ancel; Grande, Francisco; and Anderson, Joseph T. "Fiber and Pectin in the Diet and Serum Cholesterol Concentrations in Man." *Amer. S. Clin. Nutr.* 30 (1974): 171.

Kritchevsky, David. "Food Products and Hyperlipidemia." *Arch. of Surgery* 113 (1978): 52.

Kritchevsky, David; Teppor, Shirley A.; Morrissey, Robert B.; Czarnoske, Susanne K.; and Klurfield, David. "Influence of Whole or Skim Milk on Cholesterol Metabolism in Rats." *Amer. J. Clin. Nutr.* 32 (1979): 597.

Mann, George V.; Spoerry, Ann; Gray, Margarete; and Jarashaw, Debra. "Atherosclerosis in the Masai." *Amer. J. of Epidemiology* 26 (1972): 95.

Mann, G. V.; Shaffer, R. D.; Anderson, R. S.; and Handstead, H. H. "Cardiovascular Disease in the Masai." *J. of Atherosclerosis Res.* 4 (1964): 289.

Mann, George V. "A Factor in Yogurt Which Lowers Cholesterolemia in Man." *Atherosclerosis* 26 (1977): 335.

Mann, George V., Sc.D., M.D., and Spoerry, Anne, DT.H., M.B. "Studies of a Surfactant and Cholesteremia in the Masai." *Am. J. Clin. Nutr.* 27 (1974): 464.

Mann, J. I.; Watermeyear, G. S.; Manning, E. B.; Randles, J.; and Truswell, A. S. "Effects of Serum Lipids of Different Dietary Fats Associated with a High Sucrose Diet." *Clinical Sci.* 44 (1973): 610.

"New Confusion on Linking Cholesterol, Heart Disease Caused by European Test." *Wall Street Journal,* 14 December 1978, p. 14.

Olson, Robert E., Ph.D., M.D.; Vestes, John W., M.D.; Gurshey, Deha, M.D.; Davis,

Norman, M.D.; and Longman, Doris, M.D. "The Effect of Low Protein Diets upon Serum Cholesterol in Man." *Amer. J. Clin. Nutr.* 6 (1958): 310.

Peterson, John E., M.D.; Keith, Robert A., Ph.D.; Wilcox, Alan A., Ph.D. "Hourly Changes in Serum Cholesterol Concentrations: Effects of Anticipation of Stress." *Circulation* 25 (1962): 798.

Pinchney, Edward R., M.D., and Pinchney, Cathey. *The Cholesterol Controversy.* Los Angeles: Sherbourne Press, 1973.

Reiser, Robert. "Oversimplification of Diet: Coronary Heart Disease Relationship and Exaggerated Diet Recommendation." *Amer. J. Clin. Nutr.* 31 (1978): 865.

Robertson, J., B.Sc.; Brydon, W. G., B.Sc.; Tadesse, M. C. B. K., M.D.; Wendam, P., M.Sc.; Walls, A., F.R.C.S.; Eastwood, M. A., M.Sc., F.R.C.P. "The Effect of Raw Carrot on Serum Lipids and Colon Function." *Amer. J. Clin. Nutr.* 32 (1979): 1889.

Simmons, L. A.; Gibson, J. Corey; Paino, C.; Hosking, M.; Bullock, J.; and Trim, J. "The Influence of a Wide Range of Absorbed Cholesterol on Plasma Cholesterol Levels in Man." *Amer. J. Clin. Nutr.* 31 (1978): 1334.

Socks, Frank M., Sc.B.; Cosetelli, William P., M.D.; Donner, Allen, Ph.D.; and Kass, Edward H., M.D., Ph.D. "Plasma Lipids and Lipoproteins in Vegetarians and Controls." *NEJM* 292 (1975): 1148.

Stamler, Jeremiah. "Dietary and Serum Lipids in the Multi-Factorial Etiology of Atherosclerosis." *Archives of Surgery* 113 (1978): 21.

Stasse-Walthius, Marianne, M.Sc., et. al. "The Effect of a Natural High Fiber Diet on Serum Lipids, Fecal Lipids and Colonic Function." *Amer. J. Clin. Nutr.* 32 (1979): 1881.

"Thiazides Increase Cholesterol." *Primary Cardiology,* Sept. 1979, p. 96.

Truswell, A. S., and Kay, Ruth M. "Bran and Blood Lipids." *Lancet,* 14 Feb. 1976.

Truswell, A. S., and Mann, J. I. "Epidemiology of Serum Lipids in Southern Africa." *Atherosclerosis* 16 (1972): 15.

Walden, Richard T., M.D.; Schoefer, Louis E., M.D.; Lemon, Frank R., M.D.; and Wynder, Ernest T., M.D. "Effect of Environment or the Serum Cholesterol-Triglyceride Distribution Among Seventh-Day Adventists." *Amer. J. of Med.* 36 (1964): 269.

"Weight Loss, Not Exercise, Changes Levels of Cholesterol." *Internal Med. News,* 12 (1979).

Wells, V. M., and Bronte-Stewart, B., M.D. "Egg Yolk and Serum-Cholesterol Levels: Importance of Dietary Cholesterol Intake." *Brit. Med J.,* March 2, 1963, p. 577.

"Which Drugs May Elevate Serum Cholesterol?" *Modern Medicine,* Sept. 30–Oct. 15, 1979, p. 119.

Williams, Roger. *Nutrition Against Disease.* chap. 5, New York: Pitman Publishing Corp. 1971.

Wissler, Robert W., et al. "Conference on the Effects of Blood Lipids: Optimal Distribution for Populations." *Preventive Med.* 8 (1979): 715.

Wynder, Ernest L., and Hill, Peter. "Blood Lipids: How Normal Is Normal?" *Preventive Med.* 1 (1972): 161.

Zilversmit, D. B. "Mechanism of Cholesterol Accumulation in the Arterial Wall." *Amer. J. Cardiol.* 35 (1975): 559.

Zilversmit, D. B. "Role of Triglyceride-Rich Lipoproteins in Atherogenesis." *Annals N.Y. Acad. Sci.* 275 (1976): 138.

HIGH DENSITY LIPOPROTEINS

Brunner, D.; Weisbort, J.; Loebl, K.; Schwartz, S.; Altman, S.; Bearman, J. E.; and Levin, S. "Serum Cholesterol and High Density Lipoprotein-Cholesterol in Coronary Patients and Healthy Persons." *Atherosclerosis* 33 (1979): 9.

Glueck, C. J.; Fallat, R. W.; Millett, F.; Gortside, P.; Elston, R. C.; and Go, R. C. P. "Familial Hyper-alpha-lipoprotenemia: Studies in Eighteen Hundreds." *Metabolism* 24 (1975): 1243.

Glueck, C. J.; Gortside, P.; Gallat, R. W.; Sielski, J.; and Sleiner, P. M. "Longevity Syndromes: Familial Hypobeta, Familial Hyperalpha Lipoprotenemia."

"HDL Levels Clue to Heart Risk." *Internal Med. News,* 1 Feb. 1980, p. 26.

Hjermann, Ingvar, M.D.; Enger, Sven, M.D.; Helgeland, Anders, M.D.; Holme, Ingar; Teren, Paul, M.D.; and Trygg, Kerstin. "The Effect of Dietary Changes on High Density Lipoprotein Cholesterol." *Am. J. Medicine* 60 (1979): 105.

Hulley, Stephen B., M.D., M.P.H.; Cohen, Richard, M.A.; and Widdowson, Graham, Ph.D. "Plasma High-Density Lipoprotein Cholesterol Level." *JAMA* 238 (1977): 2269.

Kannel, W. B., M.D.; Castelli, W. P., M.D.; and Gordon, T. "Cholesterol in the Prediction of Atherosclerosis Disease: New Perspectives Based on the Framingham Study." *Annals Internal Med.* 90 (1979): 85.

Michele, Horace; Pometta, Daniel; Jornot, Constantin; and Scherrer, Jean-Roaul. "High Density Lipoprotein Cholesterol in Male Relatives of Patients with Coronary Heart Disease." *Atherosclerosis* 32 (1979): 269.

"Propranolol-Thiazide Combination Lowers HDL-Cholesterol," *Primary Cardiology.* Feb. 1979, p. 126.

Schaefer, E. J.; Anderson, D. W.; Brewster, H. B., Jr.,; Levey, R. I.; Danner, R. N.; and Blackwelder, W. C. "Plasma-Triglycerides in Regulation of HDL-Cholesterol Levels." *Lancet,* 19 August 1978, p. 391.

Schimell, C. J. "Cholesterol and Exercise: Is There a Connection?" *S. Afr. J. Sci.* 74 (1978): 407.

Sirtori, Cesare R.; Gianfranceschi, Gemme; Gritte, Ivana; Nappi, Giuseppe; Brambilla, Gianluigi; and Paoletti, Pietro. "Decreased High Density Lipoprotein-Cholesterol Levels in Male Patients with Transient Ischemic Attacks." *Atherosclerosis* 32 (1979): 205.

Wood, Peter D.; Haskell, William; Klein, Herbert; Lewis, Steven; Stern, Michael P.; and Farquhar, John W. "The Distribution of Plasma Lipoproteins in Middle Aged Runners." *Metabolism* 25 (1976): 1249.

Yano, Kaksuhiko, M.D.; Rhoads, George C., M.D., M.P.H.; and Kagan, Abraham, M.D. "Coffee, Alcohol, and Risk of Coronary Heart Disease Among Japanese Men Living in Hawaii." *NEJM* 297 (1977): 405.

FOOD ALLERGIES

Mandell, Marshall, M.D., and Scanlon, Lynne Waller. *Dr. Mandell's 5-Day Allergy Relief System.* New York: Thomas Y. Crowell, 1979.

Miller, Joseph B., M.D. *Food Allergy: Provocative Testing and Injection Therapy.* Springfield: C. C. Thomas, 1972.

Rinkel, Herbert J., M.D.; Randolph, Theron, G., M.D.; and Zeller, Michael, M.D. *Food Allergy.* Springfield: C. C. Thomas, 1951.

Roth, June. *Cooking for Your Hyperactive Child.* (Foreword by Kenneth Krischer, M.D.) Contemporary Books, Inc., 1977.

Roth, June. *The Food/Depression Connection.* (Foreword by David Hawkins, M.D.) Chicago: Contemporary Books, Inc., 1978.

Sheinkin, David, M.D.; Schachter, Michael, M.D.; and Hutton, Richard. *The Food Connection.* New York: Bobbs Merrill, 1979.

5. THE MANNERBERG METHOD OF MOVEMENT

EXERCISE

Astrand, P. O., M.D. "Measurement of Maximum Aerobic Activity." *Canadian Med. Assoc. J.* 96 (1967): 732.

Carson, Lars A., and Moafeldt, Folke. "Acute Effects of Prolonged Heavy Exercise on the Concentration of Plasma Lipids and Lipoproteins in Man." *Acta Physio. Scand.* 62 (1964): 51.

Cooper, Kenneth H., M.D.; Pollock, Michael L., Ph.D.; Martin, Randolph P., M.D.; White, Steve R.; Finnerud, Ardell C., Ph.D.; Jackson, Andrew, Ph.D. "Physical Fitness Levels vs. Selected Coronary Risk Factors." *JAMA* 236 (1976): 166.

deVries, Herbert A., Ph.D. "Physiological Effects of an Exercise Training Regimen upon Men Aged 52–88." *J. Gerontology* 25 (1970): 325.

Ducrouquet, Robert. *Walking and Limping.* Philadelphia: J.B. Lippincott Co., 1968.

Durning, J. V. G. A.; Brockway, J. M.; and Whitcher, H. W. "Effects of a Short Period of Training of Varying Severity on Some Measurements of Physical Fitness." *J. Applied Physiol.* 15 (1960): 161.

"Exercise Training Said Not to Foster Cardiovascular Fitness." *Internal Med. News,* 12 (1979).

Felig, Philip. "Amino Acid Metabolism in Exercise." *Annals N.Y. Acad. Science* 301 (1977): 56.

Fox, S. M.; Naughton, J. P.; and Gorman, P. A. "Physical Activity and Cardiovascular Health." *Modern Concepts Cardiovasc. Dis.* 41 (1972): 6.

Grimby, Gunnar, and Salten, Bengt. "Physiological Analysis of Physically Well Trained Middle Aged and Old Athletes." *Acta Medica Scandinavica* 179 (1966): 513.

Howath, S. M. "Review of Energetics and Blood Flow in Exercise." *Diabetes* 28 (1979): 33.

Howell, M. D., D.P.E., M.A., Ed.D., and Alderman, R. B., M.P.E., Ed.D. "Psychological Determinates of Fitness." *Canadian Med. Assoc. J.* 96 (1967): 721.

Kasch, F. W.; Philips, W. H.; Carter, J. E. F.; and Boyer, J. "Cardiovascular Changes in Middle Aged Men During Two Years of Training." *J. of Applied Physiol.* 54 (1973): 53.

Keys, Ancel. "Physical Performance in Relationship to Diet." *Federation Proceedings* 2 (1943): 164.

"Marathon Runners: Are They Immune to Fatal Atherosclerosis?" *Modern Medicine,* Nov. 30–Dec. 15, 1979.

Margaria, Rodolfo. *Biomechanics and Energetics of Muscular Exercise.* Oxford: Clarendon Press, 1976.

Mayer, Jean, and Bullen, Beverly. "Nutrition and Athletic Performance." *Physiological Reviews* 40 (1960): 369.

Noakes, Timothy D., M.D.; Opie, Lionel H., M.D.; Rose, Alan G., M.Med.; and Keynhans, Pieter H. T., M.Med. "Autopsy-Proved Coronary Atherosclerosis in Marathon Runners." *NEJM* 301 (1979): 86.

Passmore, R., and Durnin, J. N. G. "Human Energy Expenditure." *Physiological Reviews* 35 (1955): 801.

"A Monogram for Calculation of Aerobic Capacity (Physical Fitness) from Pulse Rate During Submaximal Work." *J. Applied Physiol.* 7 (1954): 218.

Pollock, Michael F.; Miller, Henry S., Jr.; Janeway, Richard; Finnerud, A. C.; Robertson, Bob; and Valentino, Richard. "Effects of Walking on Body Composition and Cardiovascular Function of Middle Aged Men." *J. Applied Physiol.* 30 (1971): 126.

"The Recommended Quantity and Quality of Exercise for Developing and Maintaining Fitness in Healthy Adults." *American College of Sports Medicine,* July 1977.

Rose, Charles L., and Cohen, Michael T. "Relative Importance of Physical Activity for Longevity." *Annals N.Y. Acad. Sci.* 301 (1977): 670.

Saltin, B.; Hartley, L. H.; Kilbom, Asa; and Astrand, Ira. "Physical Training in Sedentary Middle Aged and Older Men." *Scand. J. Clin. Lab. Invest.* 24 (1969): 323.

Thompson, Paul D., M.D.; Stern, Michael P., M.D.; Williams, Paul, M.S.; Duncan, Kirk, M.D.; Haskell, William T., Ph.D.; and Wood, Peter D., D.Sc. "Death During Jogging or Running, A Study of 18 Cases." *JAMA* 242 (1979): 1265.

"Update: Exercise and Some Coronary Risk Factors." *Physical Fitness Research Digest.* Series 9, No. 3, July 1979.

"Update: Physical Activity and Coronary Heart Disease." *Physical Fitness Research Digest,* Series 9, No. 2, April 1979.

6. VITAMINS AND MINERALS

Aizaua, Toyoyo, M.D., and Hamaya, Shoichi, M.D. "Cerebral Sclerosis Cerebral Circulation." *Japanese Heart J.* 2 (1961): 133.

Anderson, T. W.; Reid, D. B. W.; and Beaton G. H. "Vitamin C and Serum Cholesterol." *Lancet,* 21 Oct. 1972.

Barborka, Clifford J., M.D.; Foltz, Eliot E., M.D.; and Ivy, Andrew C., M.D. "Relationship between Vitamin B Complex Intake and Work Output in Trained Subjects." *JAMA* 122 (1943): 717.

Bayoumi, A., and Roselki, Sidney B. "Evaluation of Methods of Coenzyme Activation of Erythrocyte Enzymes for Detection of Deficiency of Vitamins B_1, B_2 and B_6." *Clinical Chemistry* 22 (1976): 333.

Bierenbaum, Marvin L.; Fleishman, Alan I.; and Raichelson, Robert I. "Long-term Human Studies on the Lipid Effects of Oral Calcium." *Lipids* 7 (1972): 202.

Bren, Myron; Shohet, Stephen S.; and Davidson, Charles S. "The Effect of Thiamine Deficiency on the Glucose Oxidative Pathway of Rat Erythrocytes." *J. Biol. Chem.* 230 (1958): 319.

Burch, G. E., M.D., and Geleio, T. D., M.D. "The Importance of Magnesium Deficiency in Cardiovascular Disease." *Amer. Heart J.* 94 (1977): 649.

Cheraskin, E., M.D., D.M.D.; Ringsdorf, W. M., Jr., D.M.D., M.S.; and Medord, F. H., B.S. "Daily Vitamin C Consumption and Fatigability." *J. Amer. Geriatric Soc.* 14 (1976): 136.

Cheraskin, E., M.D., D.M.D., and Ringsdorf, W. M., Jr., D.M.D., M.S. "Daily Vitamin E Consumption and Reported Cardiovascular Findings." *Nutrition Report International.*

Cheraskin, E.; Ringsdorf, W. M., Jr.; Medford, F. H.; and Hicks, B. S. "The 'Ideal' Daily B$_1$ Intake." *J. Oral Medicine 33* (1978).

Cheraskin, E.; Ringsdorf, W. M., Jr.; and Medford, F. H. "The 'Ideal' Daily Magnesium Intake," *IRCS Medical Science: Metabolism and Nutrition: Social and Occupational Medicine* 5 (1977): 588.

Cheraskin, E.; Ringsdorf, W. M., Jr.; and Medford, F. H. "The 'Ideal' Daily Vitamin A Intake." *International J. Vitamin Nutri. Res.* 46 (1976): 11.

Cheraskin, E.; Ringsdorf, W. M., Jr.; and Medford, F. H. "The 'Ideal' Daily Niacin Intake." *International J. Vitamin. Nutr. Res.* 46 (1976): 58.

Cheraskin, E., M.D., D.M.D.; Ringsdorf, W. M., Jr., D.M.D., M.S.; and Medford, F. H. B.S. "The 'Ideal' Daily Vitamin C Intake." *J. Medical Assoc. of the State of Alabama* 46 (1977): 12.

Cheraskin, E., M.D., D.M.D.; and Ringsdorf, W. M., Jr., D.M.D., M.S., A.T.S.H.; Setyaadmadja; and Barrett, R. A., D.D.S. "Thiamine Consumption and Cardiovascular Complaints." *J. Amer. Geriatrics Soc.* 15 (1967): 1074.

Cohen, Harold, M.D. "To the Editor." *NEMJ* 289 (1973): 980.

Cousins, Norman. "What I Learned from 3,000 Doctors." *Saturday Review,* 18 Feb. 1978.

Crondon, John H., M.D.; Tund, Charles C., M.D.; and Dill, David B., Ph.D. "Experimental Human Scurvy." *NEJM* 223 (1940): 366.

Dickerson, Dr. J. W. T. "There's More to Arterial Desease Than Just Fats." *Modern Medicine,* Aug. 15–Sept. 15, 1978.

Fleischman, A. I.; Yacowity, H.; Hayton, T.; and Bierenbaum, M. L. "Effects of Dietary Calcium upon Lipid Metabolism in Mature Male Rats Fed Beef Tallow." *J. Nutr.* 88 (1966): 255.

Genter, Emil, Ph.D. "What Is Truly the Maximum Body Pool Size of Ascorbic Acid in Man?" *Amer. J. Clin. Nutr.* 33 (1978): 538.

Genter, E.; Bobels, P.; and Vargova, D. "Tissue Levels and Optimum Dosage of Vitamin C in Guinea Pigs." *Nutr. Metabolism* 23 (1979): 217.

Herbert, Victor, M.D., J.D. "Pangamic Acid ('Vitamin B$_{15}$')." *Amer. J. Clin. Nutr.* 32 (1979): 1534.

Herting, David C., Ph.D. "Perspective on Vitamin E." *Amer. J. Clin. Nutr.* 19 (1967): 210.

Iacono, J. J., Ph.D., and Ammerman, C. B., Ph.D. "The Effect of Calcium in Maintaining Normal Levels of Cholesterol and Phospholipids in Rabbits During Acute Starvation." *Amer. J. Clin. Nutr.* 18 (1966): 197.

Jette, Maurice, Ph.D.; Pelletier, Omar, Ph.D.; Parker, Louise, M.Sc.; and Thoden, James, Ph.D. "The Nutritional and Metabolic Effects of a Carbohydrate Rich Diet in a Glycogen Supercompensation Training Regimen." *Amer. J. Clin. Nutr.* 31 (1978): 2140.

Johnson, Carl J., M.D.; Peterson, Donald R., M.D.; and Smith, Elizabeth K., Ph.D. "Myocardial Tissue Concentrations of Magnesium and Potassium in Men Dying

Suddenly from Ischemic Heart Disease." *Amer. J. Clin. Nutr.* 32 (1979): 967.

Kemp, George, D. O. "A Clinical Study and Evaluation on Pangamic Acid." *J. Amer. Osteropathic A.* 58 (1959): 714.

Keys, Ancel. "Physical Performance in Relationship to Diet." *Federation Proceedings* 2 (1943): 164.

Klevay, Leslie M., et al. "The Human Requirement for Copper." *Amer. J. Clin. Nutr.* 33 (1980.): 45.

Kohrs, Mary Bess, R.D. Ph.D., et al. "Nutritional Status of Elderly Residents in Missouri." *Amer. J. Clin. Nutr.* 31 (1978): 2186.

"Lecithin Helps Remove Tissue Cholesterol." *Geriatrics* 32 (1978): 15.

Leveille, G. A., and Sauberlich, H. E. "Mechanism of the Choesterol-depressing Effect of Pectin in the Cholesterol-fed Rat." *J. Nutr.* 88 (1966): 209.

Mayer, Jean, and Bullen, Beverly. "Nutrition and Athletic Performance." *Physiological Reviews* 40 (1960): 369.

Morrison, Lester M., M.D. "Serum Cholesterol Reduction with Lecithin." *Geriatrics* 31 (1958): 12.

Packer, J. E.; Slater, T. F.; and Wilson, R. L. "Direct Observation of a Free Radical Interaction between Vitamin E and Vitamin C. *Nature* 278 (1979): 737.

Pauling, Linus. "Are Recommended Daily Allowances for Vitamin C Adequate?" *Proc. Nat. Acad. Sci.* 71 (1974): 4442.

Ramp, W. K., and Thorton, P. A. "The Effect of Ascorbic Acid on the Glycolytic and Respiratory Metabolism of Embryonic Chick Tibias." *Calc. Tiss. Res.* 2 (1968): 77.

Seeling, Mitchel S., M.D., M.P.H., and Higgtvert, Alexander, M.D. "Magnesium Interrelationships in Ischemic Heart Disease." *Amer. J. Clin. Nutr.* 27 (1974): 59.

Solomon, Lawrence R., M.D., and Hillman, Robert S., M.D. "Regulation of Vitamin B_6 Metabolism in Human Red Cells." *Amer. J. Clin. Nutr.* 32 (1979): 1824.

Stah, S. A.; Johnson, Patricia, V.; and Kummerow, F. A. "The Effect of Pyridoxine on Cholesterol Metabolism." *J. Nutr.* 72 (1960): 81.

Sumes, Martti, A., M.D.; Refino, Canio, B.S.; and Dallman, Peter R., M.D. "Manifestation of Iron Deficiency at Various Levels of Dietary Iron Intake." *Amer. J. Clin. Nutr.* 33 (1980): 520.

Thompson, Christine D., Ph.D., M.H.Sc., and Robinson, Marion F., Ph.D., M.H.Sc. "Selenium in Human Health and Disease with Emphasis on Those Aspects Peculiar to New Zealand." *Amer. J. Clin. Nutr.* 33 (1980): 303.

Tsai, C.; Kelly, J. J.; Peng, Becky; and Cook, Nancy. "Study on the Effect of Megavitamin E Supplementation in Man." *Amer. J. Clin. Nutr.* 31 (1978): 831.

Van Dom, B. "Vitamins and Sport." *Brit. J. Sports Medcine* 12 (1978): 74.

"Vitamin, Amino Acid Supplements Improve Heavy Work Performance." *Modern Medicine,* April 30–May 15, 1979, p. 59.

Williams, M. A.; McIntosh, D. J.; and Hincenbergs, I. "Changes in Fatty Acid Composition in Liver Lipid Fractions of Pyridoxine-Deficient Rats Fed Cholesterol." *J. Nutr.* 88 (1966): 193.

Williams, Roger J., Ph.D., D.Sc. *Physicians Handbook of Nutritional Science.* chap. 9. Springfield: C. C. Thomas, 1975.

Wilson, Majorie; Tuttle, W. W.; Daum, Kate; Rhodes, Helen. "Influence of Various Levels of Thiamin Intake on Physiologic Response." *J. Amer. Diabetic Assoc.* 25 (1949): 221.

INDEX